MASTOLOGY

BREAST DISEASES

MASTOLOGY

BREAST DISEASES

Proceedings of the 8th International Congress on Senology (Breast Diseases), 8-12 May, 1994, Rio de Janeiro, Brazil

Editors:

Antonio S.S. Figueira Fo
President of the Senologic International Society
Professor of Mastology, Faculty of Medical Sciences
Recife, Brazil

Ezio Novais - Dias
Deputy Secretary of the Senologic International Society
Head of the Breast Unit, Department of Gynaecology
São Rafeal Hospital
Salvador, Brazil

Henrique M. Salvador - Silva
President of the Scientific Committee of the Brazilian Society of Mastology
Head of the Breast Unit, Materdei Hospital
Belo Horizonte, Brazil

Alfredo C.S.D. Barros
Assistent Professor of Gynaecology
University of São Paulo
Professor of Gynaecology and Obstetrics,
University of Santo Amaro
São Paulo, Brazil

1995

ELSEVIER
Amsterdam - Lausanne - New York - Oxford - Shannon - Tokyo

International Congress Series No. 1067
ISBN 0-444-82102-3

This book is printed on acid-free paper.

Published by:
Elsevier Science B.V.
P.O. Box 211
1000 AE Amsterdam
The Netherlands

Printed in the Netherlands

INTRODUCTION

It was a real pleasure for all of us to be informed that the proceedings of the 8th International Congress on Senology would be published soon.

We welcome this publication which will present not only the valuable scientific contributions of our colleagues, but it will also keep alive the memories of the excellent organization and warm hospitality of the organizers of this Congress in the beautiful city of Rio.

This important scientific event belongs now to history.

The valuable contribution of well known scientists from all over the world and huge participation from Latin America and especially from Brazil have ensured the success of the 8th International Congress on Senology.

The President of this congress, Professor Antonio Figueira Fo. and his colleagues have provided the participants with every opportunity to enjoy a very well organized congress of a high scientific level.

Welcoming the contribution of our colleagues as much for their research as for their clinical works and thanking the organizers for giving me this opportunity and the honor to introduce this book. I rest sure that this volume will serve as a valuable reference and an excellent review on the diagnosis and treatment of breast diseases.

Lydia Ioannidou-Mouzaka MD, PhD
President of the SIS
Athens, Greece

CONTENTS

I Benign Pathology

II Diagnosis

II.1 Mammography

II.2 Ultrasonography

II.3 Biopsy

II.4 Special Aspects

III Breast Cancer

III. 1. Epidemiology and risk factors

III. 2. Premalignant lesions

III. 3. In-situ carcinoma

III. 4. Surgical treatment

III. 5. Advanced diseases

III. 6. Recurrences

III. 7. Special forms

III. 8. Radiotherapy

III. 9. Prognosis

III. 10. Follow-up

III. 11. Special aspects

IV. Plastic surgery

V. General aspects

I Benign Pathology

Mastology - Breast Diseases
A.S.S. Figueira Fo et al., editors.

Histopathology of breast infections

Niki J. Agnantis, MD. PhD.

Department of Pathology, Ioannina University, Medical School, 5110 Ioannina, Greece

The anatomical structure of the breast comprises a ductal system which connects the glandular component with the skin surface of the nipple and creates possibilites for an invasion of different pathogenic microorganisms into the breast.

The term 'mastitis' has been widely used, in the past, for the definition of chronic cystic or fibrocystic or sclerosing mastopathies which represent the three forms of 'cystic disease' (C.D.) or 'fibrocystic changes' and in fact are not inflammatory. The use of this misleading term is due to the misinterpretation of the significance of interstitial lymphocytic infiltrates close to foci of pronounced epithelial hyperplasia or epitheliosis in C.D. Interestingly, polymorphonuclear leucocytes and plasma cells are never present within interstitial infiltrates of the stroma. Nowadays, we believe that this manifestation follows the parenchymatous changes of C.D. which are suggested to be the result of an unbalanced hormonal control.

Another inaccurate term concerns 'Chronic indurative mastitis' which was occasionally used as a synonym for the noninflammatory clinical entity 'fibrous disease'.

The only exception is the case of a ruptured tension apocrine cyst that has leaked the surrounding tissue and resulted to the production of a reactive inflammatory granuloma within C.D. lesions.

Needless to mention that an inflammation can coexist with C.D. in the same breast.

Classification of breast inflammatory lesions

- Acute or Chronic Lactational Mastitis
- Idiopathic granulomatous mastitis
- Duct Ectasia
- Subareolar Abscess
- Mammary duct fistula
- Eczema of the nipple
- Fat necrosis
- Foreign body granuloma
- Thrombophlebitis of the superficial veins

Conditions which might lead to inflammation
- Ruptured tension apocrine cyst*
- Ruptured galactocele*

- Infarct
- Massive necrosis

*Rare type of infections***
- Tuberculosis
- Sarcoidosis
- Syphilis
- Hydatidosis
- Filariasis
- Blastomycosis
- Sporotrichosis
- Leprosy
- Scleroderma
- Actinomycosis

Acute Mastitis (Lactational). This entity represents a common complication of nursing which occurs a few weeks after parturition. The most common pathogen is Staphylococcus aureus which gives rise to abscess formation, usually confined to one lobe. Beta haemolytic streptococcus may occasionally cause mastitis, which tends to produce more wide spread associated with regional lymphadenitis and general toxemia.

Idiopathic granulomatous mastitis. This entity is of unknown aetiology and it is characterized by the formation of noncaseating granulomas confined to the breast lobules. Since no microorganisms were detected, it is suggested that the disease may be immunologically mediated and therefore analogous to granulomatous thyroiditis or granulomatous orchitis.

Mammary Dust Ectasia (MDE). This common condition shows a long history in the literature under different names, such as 'varicocele tumor' (1923) Bloodgood, 'plasma cell mastitis' (1933) Adair, 'comedomastitis' (1948) Tice and Dockerty, 'mastitis obliterans' (1943) Payne et al, 'Galactoforitis', 'Mammary duct ectasia' (1951) Haagensen or 'periductal mastitis' etc. These two latter terms were widely accepted and still remain the most appropriate . Most of this misleading terminology reflects to the different stages of the same lesion. MDE differs from C.D. because it is an inflammatory disorder, usually of the major subareolar ducts, which spread in a segmental way through the ductal system and the lobules are affected by involution. Clinically, it presents a firm, solid, subareolar mass, which may mimic cancer. The perimenopausal period shows the higher incidence. Interestingly, one third of women over fifthies were found to have occult MDE in mastectomy specimens or in autopsy material. The aetiology remains obscure although it may be connected to breast feeding. Due to this uncertainty in the pathogenesis, there is a controversy to whether the inflammatory component preexists or follows the duct dilation. We agree with the believers of the concept, that the initial change is dilatation with retention of amorphous 'cheesy' secretions. Consequently, an acute inflammation occurs due to a rupture of the thin epithelial lining and leakage of the content to the fibrotic duct wall and the surrounding periductal stroma. This content is composed of neutral fat and some round to oval crystalline lipid bodies, which are characteristic of MDE. Furthermore, a chronic granulomatous reaction could be produced with foreign body giant cells and a pleomorphic inflammatory cell population. As MDE shows a long duration, sometimes the plasma cells predominates within the inflammatory infiltrates. This particular picture of MDE impressed some Pathologists who try to establish the misnomer 'plasma cell mastitis'. Other characteristics of MDE are the following. Serous or bloody nipple discharge in about 20% of the cases. Inversion of the nipple due to periductal fibrosis and ring or tubular calcifications at mammography, in the late stages of the disease. Apocrine metaplasia and/or epithelial hyperplasia do not exist. In fact, the epithelial lining is composed of flattened, atrophic cells. Finally, if MDE recurs often and the inflammation does not regress with antibiotics, the treatment of choise is surgical excision of the subareolar ducts.

Subareolar abscess. This lesion occurs in young women and shows a recurring low grade inflammation localized to the subareolar lactiferous sinuses without any connection with lactational disorders. Histologically, the lesion is characterized by squamous metaplasia of the epithelial layer of the sinuses, which become dilated and filled with keratin debris. Consequently, the infection through the nipple or by a blood spread shows the end results of this lesion, which is treated by broad spectrum antibiotics.

Mammary duct fistula. This condition is developed from a ruptured subareolar abscess into the areolar surface or in the vicinity skin area. This is a chronic non-healing lesion with a discontinuous discharge, which leads to a surgical excisional biopsy. The biopsy material should be as complete as possible, not fragmented, comprising the diseased duct from the skin surface towards an adequate depth of the mammary gland. By that way, the granulation tissue which lines the inner surface of the fistula track will be excised totally with healthy duct epithelium and recurrences are not developed.

Eczema of the nipple. It is an uncommon lesion, often bilateral and associated with atopic eczema elsewhere on the skin. The differential diagnosis (D.D.) from Paget's disease is clinically difficult, although it occurs in younger women and it shows a long duration. Histologically, there is a picture of a nonspecific chronic dermatitis. The dermis shows hyperkeratosis and hyperplasia (acanthosis) with intracellular oedema. There is a prominent lymphocytic infiltration of the papillary dermis. The whole lesion is devoted of atypia. Therefore the D.D. with Paget's disease is easy. Needless to say that the Pathologist should receive a full thickness skin biopsy in order to be able to identify the lesion.

Fat necrosis. It usually occurs in obese patients with large breasts. It is not bacterial. It is caused by a slow aseptic saponification of the nodular fat by the tissue or blood lipase. In most cases the aetiologic factor is a severe trauma and in rare cases a previous breast biopsy. Histologically, we observe a typical inflammatory granuloma of the fat tissue with areas of fibrosis and necrosis, fat vacuoles surrounded by histiocytes, multinucleated giant cells, blood pigments and lipid cristals.

Foreign Body Granulomas (Oleogranulomas). It consists of an inflammatory granulomatous reaction to substances such as polyvinyl plastic or silicone liquid used for mammoplasties. The main histological characteristic of the lesion is the presence of vacuolated histiocytes and giant cells around oily droplets.

Thrombophlebitis of the superficial veins (Mondor's Disease). This eponymic term was given to a peculiar thrombophlebitis involving the thoracoepigastric vein of the breast and the continuous thoracoabdominal wall. It similates carcinoma. It appears suddenly as a firm, slighty nodular cord beneath the skin with or without ecchymosis. Microscopically, it shows typical phlebitis and thrombosis.

Infarct. The microscopic changes which cause the greatest interpretive difficulty in this lesion present the margins . The compressed and distorted ducts associated with inflammation and organization of the infarct may cause difficulty in frozen section diagnosis. The recognition of two cell population helps towards to right diagnosis.

Massive necrosis. It occurs rarely and comprises the most dependent portion of the breast or usually both breasts. We observe this entity in patients under anticoagulent therapy.

Conclusion. Both Clinicians and Pathologists should have a deep knowledge of all these kind of infections, in order to avoid an overdiagnosis of breast cancer.

References***

1. Azzopardi JG. Problems in Breast Pathology. Philadelphia: WB Saunders Company Ltd, 1979.
2. Haagensen CD. Diseases of the Breast, 3rd edn. Philadelphia: WB Saunders Company Ltd, 1986.
3. Linell F. and Ljungberg O. Atlas of Breast Pathology. Copenhagen: Munksgaard, 1984.
4. Page DL. and Anderson TJ. Diagnostic Histopathology of the Breast. Edinburgh: Churchill Livingston, 1987.
5. Rogers K, Coup AJ. Surgical Pathology of the Breast. London: Wright Butterwarth & Co. Ltd, 1990.
6. Sloane JP. Biopsy Pathology of the Breast. London: Chapman and Hall Medical, 1985.
7. Summers WS. Systemic Pathology 2nd ed. London: Churchill Livingston, 1978; 1772-1773.

P.S. * No further description will be made, because they both present a nonspecific reactive inflammation.

** No description of these lesions will be made, because they don't present any particular features in the breast.

*** Alphabetical list of books used for the preparation of this manuscript, besides author's experience on the subject.

Mastology - Breast Diseases
A.S.S. Figueira Fo et al., editors.

Diagnosis of the Functional Disorders of the Breast

Dr. Román Torres Trujillo
Cirujano Oncologo Hospital de Mexico
Agrarismo 208 - 701 Mexico, D.F. 11800

During the early reproductive period, the maturity and involution of the breast present disorders which have different clinical manifestations: in the early reproductive period: fibroadenoma and juvenile hyperplasia; in the mature reproductive: cyclical mastalgia with or without discrete or generalized nodularity; and in the involution period: the macrocysts, sclerosing lesions, nipple discharge and epithelial hyperplasia. Clinic, ultrasonic and radiologic characteristics are mentioned, likewise, the transcendency of realizing a correct differential diagnosis from breast cancer is greatly emphasized.

The dynamic changes during the different stages of life (early reproductive, mature reproductive, and involution periods) originate the functional disorders of the breast.

The diagnosis of functional breast disorders must include the elaboration of clinical history with the evaluation of cancer risk factors and clinical characteristics as well as findings from image and histopathological studies.

Disorders in the Early Reproductive Period

The fibroadenoma is the most common disorder and develops during the childbearing years. Fifteen percent are multiple cases and eight percent are bilateral. Tumor size averages 2 to 3 centimeters in diameter, however large proportions are sometimes reached. Tumors can be pericanaliculars or intracanaliculars, but in any case they are solid mass, circumscribed, lobulated, moderately firm, mobile and occasionally cause pain. Pregnancy and lactation stimulate their growth which lead to clinical suspicion of carcinoma.

Ultrasonics show the presence of solid mass within well-defined limits. Mammographic patterns have smooth discrete edges and cannot be distinguished from cysts. The typical mammographic pattern in calcified fibroadenoma appears to be a 'popcorn'.

Juvenile hypertrophy of the breast may be present in either men or women, and is often unilateral. This is no cause for concern in girls.

Gynecomastia occurs between the ages of 13 to 17 years of age and is clinically a well-defined disc of 2 to 3 centimeters in diameter situated behind the areola. In most cases it disappears without treatment, however, exaggerated growth requires surgical removal.

Disorders in the Mature Reproductive Period

A frequent symptom in cyclical mastalgia is a slight breast pain which may o may not be accompanied with generalized or focal nodularity. Both pain and nodularity may be considered as normal cyclical changes, particularly if duration is less than seven days and disappears with menstruation. Focal nodularity, which is found in the superior external quadrant, may be confused with breast carcinoma. Cyclical mastalgia requires different diagnosis than the non-cyclical mastalgia (not related to menstrual cycle lasting more than seven days and present in older women) and the Tietze's Syndrome.

Ultrasonic and mammography are auxiliary means of diagnosis. When there is suspicion of carcinoma fine needle biopsy is required.

Disorders in the Involution Period

The aberrations of involution include macrocysts and sclerosing lesions during lobular involution. Duct dilatation fibrosis and epithelial hyperplasia appear during ductal involution.

Macrocysts are round, tender and limited lesions and are usually accompanied with pain (pain diminishes with menstruation). Tenderness and pain, have a relationship to the tension of the fluid within the cyst. Macrocysts can be multiple or bilateral.

The ultrasonic pattern is accurate and characteristic. In mammography, macrocysts may be confused with fibroadenoma. Obtainment of a liquid through fine needle aspiration clearly provides definite diagnosis of macrocysts.

Adenosis is the most common example of breast sclerosing lesions. Clinically, it is firm in consistence and poor delimited in the area of breast tissue in which it lies. These signs may be confused with breast cancer likely.

Mammographic patterns show round, regular-shaped macrocysts which are found isolated or in crops.

Nipple discharge is usually due to presence of one or more papillomas provoked by hyperplasia of cells of the internal layer of the ducts. Clinically papillomas are manifested by serous or bloody discharge, and occasionally skin dimpling. Nipple discharge with presence of a tumor demand a differential diagnosis from cancer.

Duct dilatation. Impaired drainage of duct secretions followed by dilatation are due to incomplete and prolonged involution of the terminal ducts of the breast. Dilatations and extravasation of retained secretions with high lipid content lead to plasma cell mastitis. Clinically duct ectasia is manifested by nipple retraction, skin thickening and inflammatory signs.

The development and involution aberrations of the breast are occasionally accompanied by hyperplasia with or without atipias. These findings correspond to the anatomopathological study interpretation and not to the clinical diagnosis.

References

Ashikari R, Farrow JH, O'Hara J. Fibroadenomas in the breast of juveniles, Surg Gynecol Obstet 1971;132:259-262.

Bauer BS, Jones KM, Talbot CW. Mammary masses in the adolescent female, Surg Gynecol Obstet 1987;165:63-65.

Cheatle GL. Hyperplasia of epithelial and connective tissues in the breast: Its relation to fibroadenoma and other pathological conditions, Br J Surg 1923;10:436-455.

Gold RH, Montgomery CK, Rambo ON. Significance of margination of benign and malignant infiltrative mammary lesions: Roentgenographic-pathological correlation, AJR 1973;119:881-894.

Goldman RL, Friedman NB. Carcinoma of the breast arising in fibroadenomas, with emphasis on lobular carcinoma, Cancer 1969;23: 544-550.

Haagensen CD. Diseases of the Breast. Philadelphia: WB Saunders Co.,1986.

Hoeffken W, Lanyi M. Mammography. Philadelphia: WB Saunders Co.,1977.

McDivitt RW, Stewart FW, Farrow JH. Breast carcinoma arising in solitary fibroadenomas, Surg Gynecol Obstet 1967;125: 572-576.

Nydick M, Bustos J, Dale HH, et al. Gynecomastia in adolescent boys, JAMA 1961;178: 449-451.

Rosen PP, Caicco JA. Florid papillomatosis of the nipple, Am J Surg Pathol 1986;10:87-101.

Wargotz ES, Norris HJ,Austin Rm, et al. Fibromatosis of the breast, Am J Surg Pathol 1987;11: 38-45.

Witten DM. The Breast: An Atlas of Tumor Radiology. Chicago: Year Book Medical Publishers, Inc.,1969.

Mastology - Breast Diseases
A.S.S. Figueira Fo et al., editors.

Benign breast disease: who and how to treat for mastalgia

I.S. Fentiman and H. Hamed
ICRF Clinical Oncology Unit, Guy's Hospital, London SE1 9RT

Introduction

The commonest breast symptom for which women consult their doctor is pain. For most this will be a mild and self limiting problem, but in a few this will have a major effect on their working, domestic and sexual life. Extensive data are available for clinical trials on the efficacy of the various treatments for cyclical mastalgia, but equally important is selection of appropriate patients. Additionally, the psychological profile of women with mastalgia and the impact of the treatment is of particular interest.

Which women require treatment?

For the majority of patients with cyclical mastalgia the condition lasts for only 2-3 months and then resolves spontaneously. Under these circumstances no treatment is necessary. Most trials have taken a history of 6 months of pain as being the minimum duration requiring treatment. Even under these circumstances up to 40% of patients will gain remission of symptoms in a 2 month lead in period before treatment [1].

The severity of the pain is difficult to assess objectively. Probably the best method is the 10 cm linear analogue scale and this does enable an assessment of individual response. It is only those patients with self-rated moderate or severe mastalgia who will wish to receive specific endocrine therapy.

A careful clinical examination is an important part of the selection in order to exclude extra-mammary causes of pain such as Tietze's syndrome. Patients who are most likely to seek treatment for mastalgia will be either divorced or separated, had a first baby at a young age, had a history of more than one termination of pregnancy and also have had a hysterectomy.

A recent study examined the psychosocial distress in 33 women who are participating in a study of goserelin for severe cyclical mastalgia [2]. Anxiety and depression were measured with the Hospital Anxiety and Depression Scale (HADS), and social functioning with the Psychosocial Adjustment to Illness Scale (PAIS). It was found that levels of anxiety and depression in these women was similar to those of patients with operable breast cancer on the morning of surgery. There was a significant improvement in both anxiety and depression in those whose pain was relieved. Additionally, in social scores there was an improvement in job performance, domestic life and sexual relations among those whose pain was relieved, but not in those who had had persistent mastalgia.

Which treatment for mastalgia?

At Guy's Hospital studies of treatment for mastalgia have mainly been concerned with blockade or inhibition of oestrogen, using tamoxifen and goserelin. In the first randomised trial women with moderate or severe mastalgia were given either tamoxifen 20 mg daily or placebo tablets (vitamin C) for three months [1]. At the end of that time those who had not responded to treatment were switched to the alternative arm. Breast pain was measured with a linear analogue scale and pain relief was achieved in 71% of the tamoxifen group and 38% of the placebo group. After crossover mastalgia was relieved in 75% of those receiving tamoxifen for a second course and 22% of those receiving placebo for a second course. The main side effects were menstrual irregularity and hot flushes, but the biggest problem was that after discontinuing the treatment the majority of patients developed mastalgia again.

Table 1.

Results of treatment with tamoxifen

Dosage (mg)	Duration (months)	Response (%)	Side Effects (%)	Relapse (%)
10	3	96	21	43
10	6	93	22	53
20	3	85	62	46
20	6	87	67	33

To try and reduce the incidence of side effects and of relapse of symptoms a second 2 x 2 factoral design trial was conducted. Women with mastalgia were given tamoxifen at a dosage of either 10 mg or 20 mg for either 3 months or 6 months [3]. Results are summarised in Table 1 which shows that dosages of 10 mg and 20 mg were equally effective, but the lower dose was associated with fewer side effects. Unfortunately relapse symptoms occurred with equal frequency after 3 months and 6 months of taking either dosage.

Because of this problem of relapse after cessation of treatment it was hypothesised that a more major endocrine intervention might so alter the breast tissue response to ovarian hormones the symptoms might be relieved long term. For this reason a study was conducted with women who had either refractory or relapsed mastalgia using the GnRh analgoue goserelin (Zoladex). Results of this study were encouraging with pain relief being achieved in 81% of patients [4].

Following this a second study was done on patients with previously untreated mastalgia who were given goserelin implants 3.6 mg every 4 weeks for a total of 24 weeks. Although the agent was successful in relieving the pain for most patients (90%) this was associated with substantial side effects such as flushes, headaches, nausea and vomiting, joint pain, depression, irritability, vaginal dryness and other oestrogen withdrawal symptoms. These were of such severity that some patients discontinued treatment. Unfortunately, after the prescribed course had been completed, mastalgia returned in 80% of the cases [5]. Finally, measurement of bone mineral density by dual photon absorptiometry revealed that there was bone loss during treatment which recovered partially on stopping, but had not returned to pre-treatment levels by 12 months after the end of the course of the treatment.

Thus at present at Guy's Hospital the standard treatment for women with cyclical mastalgia is tamoxifen at a dosage of 10 mg given for a 4-month course. A trial is underway to determine whether having relieved pain with tamoxifen this can be maintained using evening primrose oil.

REFERENCES

1. Fentiman, I.S., Caleffi, M., Brame, K. et al. Lancet (1986) i:287-288.
2. Ramirez, A.J., Jarrett, S.R., Hamed, H. et al. Recent Developments in the study of benmign breast disease. ed. R.E. Mansel. Parthenon 1993.
3. Fentiman, I.S., Caleffi, M., Hamed, M. et al. Br. J Surg (1988) 25:845-846.
4. Hamed, H., Chaudary, M.A., Caleffi, M. et al. Ann. Royal Coll. Surg (1990) 72 : 221-224.
5. Hamed, H., Fogelman, I., Smith, P. et al. Breast (1993) 2 : 79-72.

Mastology - Breast Diseases
A.S.S. Figueira Fo et al., editors.

New concepts in breast pain

Luiz Henrique Gebrim,

Geraldo Rodrigues de Lima,

Afonso C.P. Nazário

Claudio Kemp

Institute: Department of Gynecology and Obstetrics
Escola Paulista de Medicina - São Paulo - Brazil

Correspondence: Luiz Henrique Gebrim
Alameda Franca, 84 ap. 142
São Paulo - SP - Brazil
CEP 01422/000

Abstract: Breast pain is a frequent symptom among women, often associated with anxiety and cancerophobia. Clinical history and physical examination are sufficient to identify the origin and type of pain. Diagnostic methods should be used in a rational manner to rule out the presence of carcinoma. Hormone therapy should be used only in refractory forms of cyclic breast pain.

Introduction

Breast pain is a frequent symptom in gynecology and mastology, representing approximately 50.0% of breast complaints. It causes much anxiety especially in patients with cancerophobia, and should be considered a symptom rather than a disease. According to Preece [1], breast pain is classified as cyclic, non-cyclic, and non-breast.

Cyclic breast pain is a frequent symptom in women during menacme and should be considered normal or physiological. It starts three or seven days before menstruation and suddenly disappears at the beginning of the menstrual flow.

The synergistic action of estradiol, prolactin and progesterone promotes greater cell proliferation and edema in the mammary lobule during the premenstrual phase, increasing sensitivity and nodulations.

At times the pain is intense and limiting, and can be classified as cyclic pronounced. The persistence of the symptom throughout most of the menstrual cycle characterizes cyclic prolonged mastalgia [1, 2].

Non-cyclic breast pain is usually localized and unilateral and not associated with cyclic ovarian function. Approximately 10.0% of patients with carcinoma have this symptom. Most of the times, non-cyclic breast pain is due to benign changes such as duct ectasia, sclerosing adenosis, trauma, and pregnancy [2].

Painful syndromes (non-breast pain) originating in the rib cage (neuritis and costochondritis) and intrathoracically (pneumonia, angina, cervical rib, etc.) may simulate breast pain.

Diagnosis

The subjective nature of pain and the absence of an anatomopathological substrate reinforce the need for a detailed clinical examination [1-3]. Breast palpation should be preferentially performed on the eighth day of the menstrual cycle. When nodules are present, fine needle aspirative puncture is therapeutic for cysts and predictive of malignancy in solid formations. Mammography should be indicated for patients older than 35 years. Ultrasound may be useful when clinical examination is doubtful and when the breasts are dense to mammography. A biopsy should be indicated only in the presence of a tumor or of mammographic changes in order to exclude malignancy, and should be avoided in young women.

Treatment

Many patients with breast pain have a high degree of anxiety and cancerophobia. Reassurance has long been recognized as a necessary part of management.

Acyclic breast pain and non-breast pain are temporary and regress spontaneously. The use of massage, local heat or analgesic drugs may be useful. Hormone therapy should be avoided in these cases because of the low percentage of response [1, 4].

Cyclic breast pain usually is an exacerbation of premenstrual symptoms, which tend to regress spontaneously [1, 3, 4]. Audit of results has proved that reassurance alone was sufficient for 85% of cases, but medication has to be considered for the others [1, 5].

Although no variation in plasma hormones occurs in patients with cyclic breast pain, Peters [6] demonstrated a greater prolactin release after stimulation with TRH. However, stress and pain may secondarily cause these changes by increasing opioids and enkephalins.

Hormone therapy is used to reduce the synergism between estrogen and prolactin, and a response exceeding that of a placebo group is observed in more than 60% of patients. The limiting factors in the use of these drugs is their high cost and side effects. The period of administration ranges from 3 to 6 months and the symptoms recur after the end of treatment. Antiprolactinemic drugs (lisuride, 0.4 mg/day, or bromocriptine, 5 mg/day) significantly reduce pain in more than 70% of patients. The side effects observed in more than 40% of patients are vomiting, dizziness, and postural hypotension, and they can be reduced by reducing the dose [1, 7, 8].

Danazole (200 mg/day) acts as an antigonadotropic agent and promotes a significant improvement of pain and nodulations. Its most common side effects are amenorrhea and weight gain in approximately 30% of patients [1, 2].

Tamoxifen (10 mg/day) acts competitively with breast estrogen receptors, and also acts by inhibiting cell growth factors, relieving symptoms in more than 80% of patients. Its frequent side effects are well tolerated [1, 2, 9].

Studies on GNRH analogues have also shown a clinical response of more than 80%. However, the side effects of these agents prevent their clinical use [1, 10]. Gamma-linolenic acid presents results barely superior to those of placebo and studies currently underway may contribute to a better elucidation of the efficacy of this drug [1, 2, 5].

References

1. Preece PE. In: Smallwood JA, Taylor I (eds.) Benign breast disease. Baltimore: Urban & Schwarzemberg, 1990;44-55.
2. Maddox PR, Mansel RE. World J Surg 1989;13:699-705.
3. Jenkins PL, Jamil N, Gateley C, Mansel RE. Gen Hosp Psych 1993;15:55-57.
4. Kerin MJ, Williams NN, Cronin KJ, Dervan P, Ennis J. Dowling M, Fitzpatrick JM, Gorey TF. Br J Surg 1994;81:221-222.
5. Goodwing PJ, Neelam M, Boyd NF. Br J Surg 1988;75:837-844.
6. Peters F, Schuth W, Schurech B, Breckwoldt M. Obstet Gynecol 1984;64:381-385.
7. Mansel RE, Preece PE, Hughes LE. Br J Surg 1978;65:724-727
8. Durning P, Sellwood RA. Br J Surg 1982;69:248-249.
9. Fentiman IS, Caleffi M, Haned H, Chandary MA. Br J Surg 1988;75:845-846.
10. Haned H, Chandary MA, Caleffi M, Fentiman IS. Ann Roy Coll Surg Engl 1990;44:454-456.t

Mastology - Breast Diseases
A.S.S. Figueira Fo et al., editors.

MEDICAL TREATMENT OF BENIGN BREAST DISEASE

P. Sismondi, M. Giai, N. Biglia, R. Roagna, R. Ponzone, L. Sgro.

Department of Gynecological Oncology - University of Turin

SUMMARY

The benign disease of the breast (BBD) includes many clinical and anatomo-pathological pictures which, in the major part of the cases, can be considered simple aberrations or disorders of the normal processes of development and involution of the breast. In these cases, the indication for a medical treatment is limited and exclusively guided by the clinical symptomatology. Today, the substances of proved efficacy in the treatment of mastalgia and nodularity are bromocriptine, danazol, tamoxifen and LHRH analogs. Globally, about 70% of the patiens treated with hormonal drugs show an improvement of the symptomatology, but about half of these will have a recurrence in a short period after the suspension of the treatment. The possible correlations between BBD and breast cancer are still under discussion. New strategies are on study for women with clinical or anatomo-pathological condition of BBD associated with an increased risk of breast carcinoma; the treatment of BBD falls in these cases among the possible perspectives of chemoprevention.

INTRODUCTION

The benign disease of the breast (BBD) includes numerous clinical and histological pictures; fibrocystic mastopathy (FCM), a typical condition of the reproductive period, is the most frequent BBD. Many of the lesions generally described as "fibrocystic disease" can be considered simple aberrations or disorders either of the normal process of development or of the cyclic modifications or of the involutive phenomena that the breast gland undergoes in the course of the reproductive life.[1] The whole of these modifications can determine the appearance of nodules or thickenings which are completely physiological. The possible correlation between BBD and cancer is still the object of wide discussion; according to the classification of Dupont and Page, the BBD have been divided into 3 prognostic categories.[2] The lesions without proliferative activity and proliferative lesions, with or without atypia. The first group of women has not an increase in the risk of developing a breast carcinoma, the second group has a risk which is doubled, while the women with proliferative lesions with atypia have a risk which is 5 times greater with respect to the general female population. The presence of palpable breast cysts is another aspect of the correlation between BBD and breast cancer. Several epidemiological studies indicate that the women with type I apocrine cysts have an increased risk of developing a breast cancer: the relative risk varies between 1.73 and 4.15.[3,4] The concept of "disease", which in the past leads to treat however any type of breast pathology is overcome, and two main indications for the treatment emerge.[5,6] The first indication is the treatment of certain forms of serious mastalgia and nodularity; in these cases the therapeutic goal is only symptomatic and thus it must be the evaluation of the cost-benefit ratio to guide the choice of the drug.[6,7,8] The second indication is to avoid the evolution of the proliferative lesions considered as risk factors for a breast cancer. The treatment of the BBD falls then among the possible perspectives of chemoprevention of breast cancer.

SYMPTOMATIC THERAPY OF BBD

When a women asks a doctor about a breast problem the first effort of the clinician is to evaluate if a suspect of carcinoma exists. If the presence of a cancer is excluded, in the major part of the cases no therapy is necessary; it is sufficient to reassure the patient that her problem is a benign and not evolutive lesion. Today the hormonal therapies represent the most widely used drugs for the control of the symptomatology associated to BBD and include bromocriptine, danazol, tamoxifen and LHRH analogs.[9] Progesterone is no longer indicated in the treatment of mastalgia in such that two controlled clinical trials have not shown any difference between patients treated with a placebo or with topical progesterone or with oral medroxyprogesterone acetate.[10,11]

- Bromocriptine

Many controlled clinical trials have shown that bromocriptine can be used with benefit in the treatment of mastalgia.[12,14] A multicentric european study on 272 women with cyclic mastalgia randomised in two groups (bromocriptine 5 mg/day versus placebo) have confirmed the efficacy of the drug in reducing the mastodynia, the tension and the nodularity of the breast: 70% of the treated patients obtained an improvement of the breast symptomatology.[15] The incidence of nausea and vomit is about double in the group treated with bromocriptine (32% and 7%) compared to the placebo group and the suspension of the treatment because of the side effects occurs in 11% of the group treated with bromocriptine and 6% of the control group.

- Danazol

Danazol is at present the most effective drug for the treatment of mastalgia. In two clinically controlled studies the percentage of response varies from 70 to 80% at a daily dosage of 200 mg; the side effects are present in 22% of the treated patient, and in 6% of the cases they are of such an entity to require the suspension of the treatment.[16,17]

The side effects are represented by menstrual disorders, even reaching amenorrhea following the suppression of gonadotrophins; besides, the androgenic activity of the drug can cause weight increase, the appearance of acne, hirsutism and modifications in the tone of the voice.[18] As the side effects are dose-dependent, more recently the use of low doses of danazol has been proposed. A response is induced with 200 mg/daily, after 2 months the dosage is reduced to 100 mg/daily and after a further 2 months to 100 mg every other day or by limiting the treatment to the second half of the menstrual cycle. This scheme is also used in patients who relapse with mastalgia after the suspension of the treatment.

- Tamoxifen

Several studies have evaluated the use of tamoxifen in women with mastalgia; the response rate varies between 70 and 85%. In a double-blind controlled clinical trial tamoxifen, both at a daily dosage of 20 mg or 10 mg, resulted significantly more effective than the placebo in reducing the breast symptomatology evaluated by a pain chart.[19,20] However, about 50% of the patients, independently from the dosage used and the length of the treatment (3 or 6 months), show a relapse of the pain after 2-3 months from the suspension of the treatment.[20] The side effects, including hot flushes, menstrual irregularities or amenorrhea, nausea, weight increase, are significantly higher in the group treated with 20 mg compared to the group treated with 10 mg: 64% versus 21%; treatment of premenopausal women does not determine significant hormonal alterations.

- LHRH analogs

The LHRH analogs represent a new approach to the treatment of BBD, but the experience on the use of these drugs is still occasional and limited to few cases. In a pilot study De Vriese [21] reported the results obtained with goserelin depot administered s.c. every 28 days for 4 cycles to 15 women with FCM. After 3 months of therapy, the nodules and/or the thickenings and/or the cysts of the breast had completely disappeared in 12 patients. A reversible amenorrhea occurs in all the cases; however the side effects, above all hot flushes, did not cause the suspension of the treatment in any patient. In the study of Monsonego 22 on 66 women with breast mastopathy, 94% had mastalgia which disappeared in all the cases after 2 cycles of therapy with triptorelin administered i.m. every 28 days. After a median follow-up of 30 months the reappearance of pain occurs in 50% of the cases. The analogs of LHRH are effective even in women who have not responded to other hormonal treatments or who show a recurrence of mastalgia within a short term from the end of treatment. In this group Hamed [23] obtained, on 21 women, a complete response in 71% of the cases after 3 months and in 81% after 6 months of treatment with goserelin depot. The response to analogs is better in the patients who showed a relapse after the suspension of a previous treatment with bromocriptine, danazol, tamoxifen (100%), in respect to those who had not obtained any response to other drugs (56%). The use of LHRH analogs in premenopausal women is limited by the possible negative effects on the bone and lipid metabolism as a consequence of induced hypoestrogenism; short periods of treatment, 4 to 6 months, do not cause serious effects on the bone density.

CONCLUSIONS

Eventhough about 50% of western women in premenopause refer at least once in their life to the physician complaining mastodynia and/or nodules of the breast, only 4% then undergoes medical treatment. This should be reserved for those cases in which the symptomatology lasts for more than 6 months and interferes with the quality of life. The substances that today are considered effective in the treatment of mastalgia are bromocriptine, danazol, tamoxifen and LHRH analogs. Danazol is the drug that obtains the more rapid response, while bromocriptine gives less side effects. The use of tamoxifen and LHRH analogs must be limited to the patients included in clinically controlled trials and to the patients who do not respond to other previous drugs, because their long-term effects in premenopausal women have to be further evaluated. Globally, about 70% of the patients who undergo hormonal treatment present an improvement in the symptomatology, but about half of these, independently from the drug used, will present a recurrence of the symptoms in a short period after the suspension of the treatment. New prospectives are in phase of study for those women who show clinical and/or anatomo-pathological aspects of BBD associated with an increased risk of carcinoma.

References

1. Hughes L.E., Mansel R.E. and Webster D.J.T. Aberration of normal development and involution (ANDI): a new perspective on pathogenesis and nomenclature of benign breast disorders. Lancet 1987;2,1326.
2. Dupont W.D. and Page D.L. Risk factor for breast cancer in woman with proliferative breast disease. N Engl J Med 1985;312:146.
3. Ciatto S., Biggeri A., Rosselli del Turco M. et al. Risk of breast cancer subsequent to proven Gross Cystic Disease. Eur J Cancer 1990;26:555.
4. Bundred N.J., West R.R., Dowd J.O. et al. Is there an increased risk of breast cancer in women who have had a breast cyst aspiration?. Br J Cancer 1991;64:953.
5. Love S.M., Gelman R.S. and Silen W. Fibrocystic disease of the breast - a non disease_?. N Engl J Med 1982;307:1010.
6. Mansel R. Rationale for treatment of benign breast disease. In Current Controversies in the treatment of breast cancer. Howell A. (ed) 1991;159.
7. Gateley C.A. and Mansel R.E. Management of the painful and nodular breast. Br Med Bull 1991;47:284.
8. Andrews W.C. Hormonal managenent of fibrocystic disease of the breast. J. Reprod. Med. 1990;35:87.
9. Sismondi P., Giai M., Defabiani E. et al. Benign breast disease an update. Clin. Experimental Obstet Gynecol 1990;17:57.
10. Mc Fadyen I.J., Raab G.M., Macintyre C.C.A. et al. Progesterone cream for cyclic breast pain. Ibid 1989;298:931.
11. Maddox P.R., Mansel R.E., Harrison B.J. et al. A randomised controlled trial of medroxyprogesterone acetate in mastalgia. Ann R Coll Surg Engl 1990;72:71.

12. Mansel R.E., Preece P.E. and Hughes L.E. A double blind trial of the prolactin inhibitor bromocriptine in painful benign breast disease. Br J Surg 1978;65:724.

13. Blichert-Toft M., Nyboe Anderson A., Henriksen O.B. et al. Treatment of mastalgia with bromocriptine: a double -blind cross-over study. Br Med J 1979;1:237.

14. Durning P. and Sellwood R.A. Bromocriptine in severe cyclical breast pain. Br J Surg 1982;69:248.

15. Mansel R.E. and Dogliotti L. European multicentre trial of bromocriptine in cyclical mastalgia. Lancet 1990;1:190.

16. Pye J.K., Mansel R.E. and Hughes L.E. Clinical experience of drug treatments for mastalgia. Lancet 1985;2:373.

17. Mansel R.E., Wisbey J.R., Hughes L.E. Controlled trial of the antigonadotropin danazol in painful nodular benign breast disease. Lancet 1982;1:928.

18. Harrison B.J., Maddox P.R. and Mansel R.E. Maintenance therapy of cyclical mastalgia using low-dose danazol . J R Coll Surg Edinb 1989;34:79.

19. Fentinam I.S., Caleffi M., Brame K. et al. Double-blind controlled trial of tamoxifen therapy for mastalgia. Lancet 1986;1:287.

20. Fentinam I.S., Caleffi M., Hamed H. et al. Dosage and duration of tamoxifen treatment for mastalgia. A controlled trial. Br J Surg 1988;75:845.

21. De Vriese G., Bonte J. and Bossuyt A. Goserelin, an LHRH agonist, in the treatment of women with fibrocystic mastopathy. A pilot study. J Obstet Gynecol 1991;11:272.

22. Monsonego J., Destable M.D., De Saint Florent et al. Fibrocystic disease of the breast in premenopausal women: Histohormonal correlation and response to luteinizing hormone releasing hormone analog treatment. Am J Obstet Gynecol 1991;164:1181.

23. Hamed H., Caleffi M, Chaudary M.A. et al. LHRH analogue for treatment of recurrent and refractory mastalgia. Ann R Coll Surg Engl 1990;72:221.

Mastology - Breast Diseases
A.S.S. Figueira Fo et al., editors.

Physiopathology of the Benign Breast Disease

Dr. Román Torres Trujillo
Cirujano Oncólogo Hospital de México
Agrarismo 208 - 701 México, D.F. 11800

The physiopathology of Benign Breast Diseases (BBD) is determined by multiple factors such as estrogen predominance and progesterone deficiency, or inadequate corpus luteon function which may be secondary to an ovulation disorder. Also hyperprolactin secondary to hyperestrogen, lipid metabolic alterations mediated by prolactin and the exaggerated consumption of methylxanthines play a very important role in the appearance of BBD.

The Benign Breast Disease (BBD) includes a variety of disorders, which represent the same ailment in its different development and involution stages in the breast [5]. A common denominator in the BBD morphology is the proliferation of different breast tissues such as: cyst formation, fibrosis, cellular metaplasia and hyperplasia.

Estrogen predominance and progesterone deficiency are considered causative in the development of BBD [7]. Morphologically, estradiol is the hormone initially responsible for differentiation and development of the ductal epithelium and increase in the mitotic activity in the cylindric cells of the internal layer of the ducts. [6,7,8]. Progesterone acts, in the breast on the distal part of the duct, favoring differentiation in the acini. Therefore, it ensures the organization of the mammary gland for its secretory function; it is also an antiestrogen that can antagonize the action of estradiol on duct cells by changing the proliferative effect.

Almost 70 % of patients with BBD have either corpus luteum deficiency or anovulation [15]. If luteal progesterone secretion is deficient, hyperplastic changes occur in the breast, when estradiol levels are high. Nevertheless, there are some reports in which women with BBD have normal levels of estrogens and low plasma progesterone levels [9,14]. Additionally, other studies show elevated progesterone levels during the luteal phase in women with BBD [2]; and others in which the levels of progesterone are normal [3].

Prolactin

The possible role of prolactin (PRL) in the initiation and maintenance of BBD is still controversial, but many observations suggest that PRL is involved in mammary pathology [11]. The plasma prolactin level has been found slightly increased in approximately one third of women with cyclic mastalgia and nodularity. The increase in PRL levels has been explained by the predominance of estrogens and luteal deficiency of progesterone; estrogens enhance pituitary prolactin secretion [13].

Dilley and Kister [1] reported that human pituitary PRL, in combination with insulin, increased the mitotic index of organ cultures of normal breast tissues. There exists evidence that PRL influences lipid metabolism. These evidences postulate that cyclical mastalgia may be caused by a disorder of lipid metabolism. Goodwin et.al. [4] in randomized study of dietary fat reduction in women with cyclical mastopathy examined the effect of dietary fat reduction on the symptoms of cyclical mastopathy. The result of this study indicates that dietary fat reduction decreases the tenderness ($P=0.0001$) and swelling ($P=0.0002$) in contrast with the women control group. These changes in the breast were correlated with changes in plasma cholesterol, but not in serum hormone levels. This suggests that abnormalities in lipid metabolism, possibly mediated by PRL, can be part of the physiopathology of cyclical mastopathy. The role of PRL in lipid metabolism is not completely understood; apparently it may alter lipid metabolism by causing a diversion of lipid, particularly fat acid, from peripheral adipose tissue to the mammary gland.

Methylxanthines

Methylxanthines include compounds such as caffeine, theophylline, and theobromine, which are found in coffee, chocolate, colas and tea. These compounds inhibit the enzyme 3′ 5′ monophosphate phosphodiesterase, that degrades cyclic adenosine monophosphate (c AMP) to 5′ AMP which has greater importance in cell life cycle.

Minton et.al.[12] have promoted the hypothesis that the ingestion of dietary methylxanthines can alter the concentration of tissue cyclic adenosine monophosphate (c AMP) sufficiently to alter risk of BBD. The tissue levels of c AMP and c GMP (cyclic guanosine monophosphate) in BBD lesions are three times higher than those found normally [11] in epidemiology and endocrinology of BBD. Nevertheless other studies show different results [7]. Finally on an epidemiological basis, there is no clear evidence that women who present BBD have a higher caffeine consumption than those without BBD.

At the present time there does not exist a well-defined physiopathology of the BBD which affects women worldwide; this is due to the presence of many unknown factors in modern women lifestyle such as socio-economic status, alimentary habits, emotional and physical stress, and nicotine consumption. The outstanding aspect of BBD is its correct differential diagnosis from breast cancer.

References

1. Dilley, W.G. and Kister, S.J. In vitro stimulation of human breast tissue by human prolactin. JNCI;1975.

2. England P.C., Skinner L.G. et. al. Sex hormones in breast disease. Brit J Surg 1975;62:806-809.

3. Geller S, Grenier J, et.al.Insuffisance letuale et mastopathies benignes. Etude a la lumier des donnees de l'epreuve combinee LH-RH+TRH couplee a l'etude des steroides ovariens. Ann Endocrinol 1979:40:45-46.

4. Goodwin P.J., Neelam M., Boyd N.F. Cyclical mastopathy: A critical review of therapy. Br J Surg 1988;75:837-844.

5. Hughes L.E., Mansel R.E. Aberrations of normal development and involution. A new perspective on pathogenesis and nomenclature of benign breast disorders. Lancet,1987.

6. Jacobson D. Hormonal regulationn or mammry gland growth, milk. In: S.K. Kon and A.T. Cowie (eds) The Mammary Gland and its Secretion, New York: Academic Press 1961;127-160.

7. Mauvais-Jarvis P. De l'hormonologie des mastopathies á la prévention du cancer du sein. Nouv. Presse Med 1979;8:1817-1819.

8. Mauvais-Jarvis P. and Kuttenn F. L'insuffisance en progesterone est-elle cancerigéne? Nouv Presse Med. 1975;4:323-326.

9. Mauvais-Jarvis P., Sitruk-Ware R. et. al. Luteal phase insufficiency: A common pathophysiological factor in development of benign and malignant breast diease. In:Bulbrook R.D. and Taylor D.J. (eds.) Commentaries on Research in BReast Disease New York: Alan R. Liss, 1979:25-29.

10. Macguire W.L. Prolactin and breast cancer In:Crosignani P.G. and Robin (eds) Prolactin and human reproduction. New York: Academic Press 1977:143-151.

11. Minton J.P. Foecking M.K. et.al. Caffeine Cyclic nucleotides and breast disease. Surgery 1979;86:105-108.

12. Minton J.P. Matthews R.H. Wisenbaugh T.W. Elevated levels of 3'5'-cyclic monophosphate levels in human and animal tumours. J Nat Cancer Inst 1976;57:39-41.

13. Peters F., Schuth W. et.al. Serum prolactin levels in patients with fibrocystic breast disease. Obstet Gynecol 1984;64:381-385.

14. Reed M.J. Cheng R.W. et.al. Plasma levels of estrone sulfate and estradiol and the percentage of unbound estradiol in postmenopausal women with and without breast disease. Cancer Res 1983; 43:3940-3943.

15. Sitruh-Ware R., Sterkers N., Mouvais-Jarvis P. Benign breast disease I. Hormonal investibation. Obstet Gynecol 1979;53:450-457.

II Diagnosis

II.1 Mammography

Mastology - Breast Diseases
A.S.S. Figueira Fo et al., editors.

Optimizing the mammographic study

G.W. Eklund, M.D.

Abstract

Mammographic positioning

Failure to visualize a breast lesion mammographically can be due to numerous factors over which we have no control, such as the small size of the lesion or the absence of any radiographic alteration in normal breast architecture, or absence of calcifications in the case of ductal carcinoma in situ. Unfortunately, failure to visualize a breast cancer can also be due to errors in imaging technique. Two of the most common technical errors responsible for failure to detect breast cancer are related to deficiencies in mammographic positioning (1) Exclusion of the lesion, and (2) Superimposition (or masking) of the lesion. Attention to fundamental concepts in mammographic positioning can ensure maximum tissue visualization and virtually eliminate the problem of exclusion. Attention to supplemental or creative modified views in pursuing areas of clinical concern or incompletely visualized abnormalities can dramatically reduce the incidence of 'false negative' mammograms. Techniques which enhance our ability to expose subtle or clinically occult breast cancers can improve screening sensitivity and diagnostic specificity.

Technical considerations

High image contrast and high resolution are hallmarks of the technically ideal mammogram. Both high contrast and resolution are essential for the analytic process of detecting and characterizing subtle alterations from normal mammographic architecture that might be the earliest sign of a breast cancer.

Among the various factors affecting image quality, blurring or unsharpness, which may be relate to equipment or patient problems, requires perceptive skill on the part of the technologist and radiologist and the knowledge of technical factors required to resolve the problem.

Poor image contrast is unacceptable for modern film/screen mammography. The mammographer must understand the numerous factors influencing contrast and make every mammographic film part of the ongoing quality control program. A thorough understanding of the effects of kVp, mAs and alterations in the density control is essential to maintain consistent high contrast images. The effect of processing on single emulsion film is another important part of the equation for optimal contrast.

Nowhere in diagnostic imaging is the technologist and radiologists so dependant on an understanding of the technical factors used in the generation of images than in mammography.

Common imaging problems

Possible causes ... practical solutions

G.W. Eklund, M.D.

In spite of our best intentions and diligence to careful techniques, there seem to be a few recurring problems that present in every mammographic facility. Understanding their possible or probable causes will usually make a simple solution obvious. The following seem to be the most frequently recurring problems we see in our own practice and with outside films seen from time to time.

Problem: Underexposure (too light)

POSSIBLE CAUSES	SOLUTION
Photocell in wrong position (under fat rather than dense parenchyma)	Reposition photocell
Insufficient mAs (Density setting of phototimer set too low)	Increase density setting (when phototiming), or increase mAs (manual technique)
Suboptimal compression calling for more mAs than unit can deliver	Improve compression
Increase kVp to diminish mAs requirement	mAs requirement exceeds tube limit (mAs cutoff)
mAs tube limit exceeded (mAs cut off)	Increase kVp to decrease mAs needed to achieve prescribed density.

Problem: Poor contrast (too grey)

POSSIBLE CAUSES	SOLUTION
kVp too high	Lower kVp
Under development (insufficient time in developer or developer temperature too low)	Use extended developer processing with approximately 43 seconds of film contact with developer at 95 degrees F or 35 degrees C
Low contrast film (film type or defective film)	Use higher contrast film. Consult with manufacturer.
Low inherent contrast of breast tissue.	Assuming optimal film and processing, there may be no solution. Should use as low a kVp as possible without resulting prolonged exposure time that increases the risk of blurring.

Problem: Blurred or fuzzy images

POSSIBLE CAUSES	SOLUTION
MOTION Patient factors (tremor, agitation, mental impairment)	Make patient more comfortable. Do procedure with patient sitting. Consider rescheduling patient. Make exposure at the end of expiration, after two deep breaths.
Exposure factors (prolonged exposure, low kVp/high mAs)	Increase kVp to shorten exposure time
WIDE PENUMBRA Large focal spot with mag. views Subject/film distance Subject image distance	Use only 0.1 mm focal spot with mag views Keep area of interest close to film as possible Use small focal spot with areas of concern further from film. Use manufacturers recommended subject-film distance.
Film/screen factors (poor film/screen contact, or damaged screen or cassette)	Clean cassette. Replace damaged cassette
Double emulsion film	Use single emulsion film
Scatter radiation	Use grids or air gap (with magnification). Use optimal compression

Problem: Poor marginal definition

POSSIBLE CAUSES	SOLUTION
Superimposition	Change of angle. Spot compression view.
Scatter radiation	Use of grid. Lower kVp. Improved compression.
Large focal spot used for magnification	Switch to small focal spot
Underexposure	Increase mAs or density setting. If resulting mAs will be greater than 200 mAs, consider increasing kVp to reduce risk of motion from long exposure. If only dense parenchymal areas are overexposed, reposition the photocell to ensure photocell 'reading' of dense areas. If dense underexposed tissue is in the anterior portion of the breast, do anterior compression view.

Problem: Posterior abnormalities incompletely visualized

POSSIBLE CAUSES	SOLUTION
Improper MLO angle to achieve optimal separation of breast from underlying muscle.	Use gantry angle that allows compression parallel to pectoral muscle fibers.
Breast and pectoral muscle not moved medially and forward when doing MLO view.	Pull lateral breast and pectoral muscle medially and forward before positioning film holder along lateral margin of breast and engaging the compression paddle.
IMF not elevated when positioning for CC view.	Elevate IMF. Bring film holder up to maintain breast in elevated position.
Upper arm, axillary tissue or upper abdomen preventing posterior placement of the film holder.	Use small (18 × 24 cm) film holder. Consider spot compression paddle.

Problem: Lesion seen only on one view

POSSIBLE CAUSES	SOLUTION
Superimposition	Change aangle of X-ray beam. Roll tissue. Spot compression view.
Exclusion	Improved positioning to minimize tissue exclusion. Elevate IMF for CC views. Mobilize breast medially for MLO views. Pull lateral breast tissue into field with CC views. Do XCC views to include persistent exclusion of axillary tissue on the CC view.
Lesion not real	Spot compression views. Angled view.

Problem: Small breast wont remain compressed

PROBABLE CAUSE	SOLUTION
Unable to maintain breast in position until engaged by compression paddle.	Use narrow compression paddle. Use spot compression paddle. Tape breast in position.

Problem: Inadequate visualization of axillary breast in obese patient

PROBABLE CAUSE	SOLUTION
Large film holder limits ability to position cassette into axilla.	Use smaller film holder

Suggested readings

Positioning:

1. Bassett LW, Gold RH. Breast radiography using the oblique projection. Radiology 1983;149:585-587
2. Eklund GW, Cardenosa G. The art of mammographic positioning. In: Bassett LW (ed), Radiol Clin of North Am 1992; 30:21-53
3. Eklund GW, Cardenosa G, Parsons W. Assessing the adequacy of mammographic image quality. Radiology 1994; 190:297-307
4. Feig SA. Importance of supplementary mammographic views to diagnostic accuracy. AJR 151:40, 1988

5. Hall FM, Connaughton MA. Parallax technique in breast lesion localization (letter to the editor). AJR 1985; 145:653
6. Kopans DB, Waitzkin ED, Linetsky L, et al. Localization of breast lesions identified on only one mammographic view. AJR 1987; 149:39-41
7. Kopans DB. Breast imaging. Philadelphia: JB Lippincott, 1989:43-58
8. Logan WW, Janus J. Use of special mammographic views to maximize radiographic information. Radiol Clin North Am 1987; 25:953-959
9. Sickles EA. Magnification mammography. In Bassett LW, Gold RH, eds. Breast cancer detection: mammography and other methods in breast imaging, 2nd ed. New York: Grune & Stratton, 1987:111-117
10. Sickles EA. Practical solutions to common mammographic problems: Tailoring the examination. AJR 1988: 1512:31-39
11. Sickles EA. Combining spot-compression and other special views to maximize mammographic information. Radiology 1989; 173:571
12. Swann CA, Kopans DB, McCarthy KA. Localization of occult breast lesions: Practical solutions to problems of triangulation. Radiology 1987; 163:557
13. Tabar L. Microfocal spot magnification mammography. In Brunner S, Langfedt B, Anderson PE, eds. Early detection of breast cancer. Berlin: Springer-Verlag, 1984:62-68
14. Tabar L, Dean PB. Optimum mammographic technique: The annotated cookbook approach. Administrative Radiology 1989:54-56

Augmented breast

15. Eklund GW, Busby RC, Miller SH, Job JS. Improved imaging of the augmented breast. AJR 1988; 151:469-473
16. Eklund GW. Mammographic imaging of the augmented breast. Admin Radiol 1988; 12:42-43
17. Koides T, Katayama H. Calcification in augmentation mammoplasty. Radiology 1979; 130:337-340
18. Grant EG, Cigtay OS, Mascatello VJ. Irregularity of silastic breast implants mimicking a soft tissue mass. AJR 1978; 130:461-462
19. Smith DS. False-positive radiographic diagnosis of breast implant rupture: report of two cases; Ann Plast Surg 1985; 14:166-167
20. Argenta LC. Migration of silicone gel into breast parenchyma following mammary prosthesis rupture. Ann Plast Surg 1983; 7:253-254
21. Capozzi A, Dubou R, Pennisi VR. Distant migration of silicone gel from a ruptured breast implant. Plast Reconstr Surg 1976; 62:302
22. Leibman AJ, Kruse B. Breast cancer: Mammographic and sonographic findings after augmentation mammoplasty. Radiology 1990; 174:195-198

Technical:

23. Eklund GW, Cardenosa G, Parsons W. Assessing the adequacy of mammographic image quality. Radiology 1994; 190:297-307
24. Eklund GW, Pisano ED, McLelland R. Technical considerations in optimizing the mammographic Image. ACR symposium on mammography, Reston, VA:ACR, 1991:23-38
25. Haus AG. Recent advances in film-screen mammography. In: Sickles EA (ed), Radiol Clin of North Am 1987; 25:913-928
26. Hendrick RE. Requirements for quality breast cancer detection: Technical quality control. Cancer 1989; 64:(5)2710-2717

27. Hendrick RE. Standardization of image quality and radiation dose in mammography. Radiology 1990; 174:648-656
28. Hubbard LB. Mammography as a radiographic system. RadioGraphics 1990; 10:103-113
29. Kimme-Smith C, Bassett LW, Gold RH. Evaluation of radiation dose, focal spot and automatic exposure of new film-screen mammography units. AJR 1987; 149:913-918
30. Kimme-Smith C, Bassett LW, Gold RH. Workbook for Quality Mammography. Baltimore: Williams & Wilkins, 1992
31. Kimme-Smith C, Rothchild PA, Bassett LW, Gold RH, Moler C. Mammographic film-processor temperature, development time and chemistry. Effect on dose, contrast and noise. AJR 1989; 152:35-40
32. Law J, Finst P, Kirkkpatrick AE. Films, screens and cassettes for mammography. Brit J Radiol 1989; 62:163-167
33. Villafana T. Generators, X-ray tubes, and exposure geometry in mammography. RadioGraphics 1990; 10;539-554
34. Yaffe MJ, AAPM tutorial: Physics of mammography: Image recording process. Radiology 1990; 10:341
35. Radiologic technologist's manual. Hendrick RE (chair) ACR mammography quality control: Radiologic technologist's manual. Reston, VA: ACR; 1992
36. Tabar L, Haus AG. Processing of mammographic film: Technical and clinical considerations. Radiology 1989; 173:65-69

Mastology - Breast Diseases
A.S.S. Figueira Fo et al., editors.

INDIRECT MAMMOGRAPHIC SIGNS OF MALIGNANCY

Edward A. Sickles, M.D.

The great strength of mammography is its ability to detect breast cancers before they grow large enough to be palpable. With the current increased use of mammography to screen asymptomatic women, it has become more and more important for radiologists to recognize the earliest presenting features of carcinoma. Indeed, most nonpalpable cancers present with mammographic signs that are not characteristic of malignancy. To take full advantage of the capabilities of mammography, radiologists must search diligently not only for the classic mammographic features of malignancy but also for less specific signs, including those which indicate the presence of early-stage cancer only indirectly.

Masses and Clustered Microcalcifications.

Large-scale consecutive series show that fewer than 20% of nonpalpable (mammographically detected) breast cancers present as spiculated masses and that fewer than 25% present as clustered microcalcifications with linear and/or branching shapes. Therefore, more than half of early cancers do not demonstrate the classic mammographic features of carcinoma. Among those cancers that present with clustered microcalcifications, many are composed of calcific particles that are so tiny that their shapes cannot be clearly seen even with spot compression magnification mammography. Similarly, many screening-detected cancers that present as masses have indistinct (ill defined) but not spiculated margins. Both "indeterminate" calcifications and ill defined masses carry only about a 25% likelihood of malignancy, but tissue diagnosis should be obtained for all such lesions in order to identify those which are malignant at the earliest possible stage.

The most difficult of early cancers to find by mammography are those that contain no calcifications and also are surrounded by isodense fibroglandular tissue, impairing delineation of their tumor masses. To maximize detection of these subtle lesions, all mammographers should use techniques that include firm breast compression, for this practice not only increases the sharpness of the image by improving the imaging geometry, but also occasionally will spread apart islands of adjacent dense tissue sufficiently to permit visualization of the underlying cancers. However, despite the best mammographic technique, it is inevitable that there will be small malignancies that demonstrate neither masses nor calcifications. Some of these may be detected by recognizing one of several mammographic signs that indicate the presence of early cancer only indirectly.

Single Dilated Duct.

Mammographic demonstration of dilatation of a single retroareolar duct can be the only indication of an underlying intraductal carcinoma, since the cancer and the duct itself almost always are nonpalpable, and since these lesions often do not cause nipple discharge that is sufficiently worrisome for the patient to seek medical attention. The mammographic appearance of a dilated duct is characteristic, that of a tubular and branching structure, widest in caliber at the nipple, tapering as it proceeds distally into the parenchyma. Whether or not a duct remains dilated deep into the parenchyma, only its proximal part usually is seen. This of course is much more evident in a fatty breast than in one where the margins of the dilated duct are obscured by adjacent dense tissue. Some mammographers consider the demonstration of more than one adjacent dilated duct to have similar significance to that of a single dilated duct, but these broadened criteria are not universally accepted. In either case, the underlying cause much more often is benign than malignant, except in the unusual circumstance when the duct contains clustered calcifications characteristic of carcinoma. Furthermore, duct dilatation is only a rare presenting sign of carcinoma, accounting for the detection of only about 1% of nonpalpable cancers. Nonetheless, once dilatation of a single duct is discovered, subsequent management may include galactography (if nipple discharge is present), sonography (to determine whether the dilated duct is fluid filled), and cytology of aspirated fluid from the nipple. Occasionally, open surgical exploration and excision of the dilated duct(s) is done anyway, although in the absence of other suspicious radiographic or other signs, periodic mammographic surveillance is the preferred management alternative.

Asymmetry.

When an early carcinoma appears on mammograms as an indistinct (poorly defined) mass without microlobulated or spiculated margins, it still can be detected readily in a fatty breast. However, in breasts that contain substantial collections in dense fibroglandular tissue, especially if this dense tissue is distributed in discrete islands rather than in uniform sheets, detecting such a small cancer becomes an exercise in perception, even if it is possible to see the tumor mass in retrospect. It simply is difficult to identify a poorly defined malignant mass as being significantly different from the several other poorly defined benign densities elsewhere in the breast. One helpful perceptual aid in this situation is to view the mammograms of both breasts side by side, projection for projection, to facilitate recognition of a small cancer by the asymmetry with which it appears. One must realize that slight asymmetries in distribution of normal parenchyma occur frequently, and that even substantial asymmetry is seen in 3%-5% of normal breasts, so that the finding of asymmetry in and of itself is insufficient to prompt biopsy. Rather, the discovery of asymmetry should lead to a careful analysis of the other features of the asymmetric tissues, and the decision to suggest biopsy should be based primarily on these additional findings. Asymmetry has been found to be the major mammographic feature prompting biopsy in 3% of nonpalpable cancers. Most cases of substantial asymmetry are managed with periodic mammographic follow-up. Biopsy usually is reserved for those cases in which asymmetric density is palpable in retrospect in which the asymmetric density demonstrates convex margins (indeed representing a poorly defined mass), in which the absolute density of the asymmetric tissue is greater than that of other areas of dense tissue similar in size, or in which there is interval change in the asymmetric tissue.

Architectural Distortion.

Invasive carcinoma may distort the interfaces between fat and normal breast parenchyma due to the desmoplastic response of host tissues to the malignancy. In the fatty breast, there is no dianogstic dilemma, since this will result in the typical spiculated mass seen by mammography. However, in the very dense breast the tumor mass can be so obscured by adjacent benign tissues as to be invisible, leaving as the only indication of underlying malignancy an area of focal architectural distortion. Depending on the location of the cancer, the retractive phenomena producing architectural distortion will result in different mammographic appearances. Invasive cancers completely surrounded by a substantial mantle of dense parenchyma will be detected only if there is sufficient adjacent fat to permit visualization of some coarse retractive strands radiating from a central area. On the other hand, cancers in locations close to the interfaces between parenchyma and subcutaneous or retromammary fat will be identified, even if no coarse strands are visible, by the infolding of the interfaces themselves, caused by retractions from the tumors. Focal architectural distortion is the most commonly encountered "indirect" sign of malignancy, accounting for the detection of 9% of nonpalpable cancers. However, it should be noted that the presence of focal fibrosis, scarring or other benign retractive phenomena also produces coarse stranding and distortion of normal fat-parenchyma interfaces, in patterns that easily can be confused with the appearance of a malignancy. The result is that for cases of unexplained focal architectural distortion, several benign lesions must be biopsied to insure removal of each cancer.

Developing Density.

An early cancer may demonstrate mammographic features so subtle that it shows neither a poorly defined mass, nor asymmetry, nor focal architectural distortion. The only clue to its existence may be the *interval appearance* on mammograms of a small focus of increased density. One may ascribe significance to such a "developing density" because, except during puberty, pregnancy, lactation, and other periods of endogenous and exogenous estrogen stimulation, the breast is an involuting organ whose natural history involves progressive fatty replacement. It therefore is reasonable to consider as potentially malignant any newly apparent focus of increased mammographic density. Of course, the developing density sign is nonspecific, because benign lesions develop and grow just as cancers do; nonetheless, it is an important sign because it can be the earliest indicator of breast cancer. Developing densities account for 6% of nonpalpable cancers detected by mammography. They represent about one-third of all such cases that present only with "indirect" signs of malignancy. To identify a developing density, one must have previous mammograms available for comparison. Therefore, whenever feasible, one should locate and obtain prior mammograms before completing the interpretation of current examinations.

Summary.

Mammographic detection of nonpalpable breast cancer permits earlier diagnosis and reduces mortality from the disease. The increasing emphasis on using mammography to screen asymptomatic women for breast cancer is placing the responsibility for tumor detection more and more with the radiologist. While it has long been known that cancer occasionally presents mammographically with less than "textbook" features of malignancy, we now appreciate the great extent to which this occurs for nonpalpable neoplasms, just those tumors that we are expected to discover by screening. It is imperative that radiologists search carefully not only for spiculated tumor masses and linear/branching clustered calcifications, but also for indistinct (ill defined) masses, indeterminate clustered microcalcifications, and the even more subtle "indirect" signs of malignancy.

Selected Reading:

1. Kopans DB: Breast imaging. Philadelphia: Lippincott, 1989.

2. Martin JE, Gallagher HS: Mammographic diagnosis of minimal breast cancer. Cancer 28:1519-1526, 1971.

3. Martin JE, Moskowitz M, Milbrath JR: Breast cancer missed by mammography. Am J Roentgenol 132:737-739, 1979.

4. Moskowitz M: Minimal breast cancer redux. Radiol Clin North Am 21:93-113, 1983.

5. Sickles EA: Mammographic features of "early" breast cancer. Am J Roentgenol 143:461-464, 1984.

6. Sickles EA: Mammographic features of 300 consecutive nonpalpable breast cancers. Am J Roentgenol 146:661-663, 1986.

7. Sickles EA:Breast calcifications: mammographic evaluation. Radiology 1986;160:289-293.

8. Sickles EA: Detection and diagnosis of breast cancer with mammography. Perspectives Radiol 1988;1(2):36-65.

9. Sickles EA: Breast Masses: mammographic evaluation. Radiology 1989;173:297-303.

10. Sickles EA, Destouet JM, Eklund GW, Feig SA, Jackson VP. Breast disease (second series) test and syllabus. Reston, VA: American College of Radiology, 1993.

11. Tabar L, Dean PB. Teaching atlas of mammography. 2nd ed. New York: Springer-Thieme, 1985.

Mastology - Breast Diseases
A.S.S. Figueira Fo et al., editors.

MAMMOGRAPHIC FOLLOW-UP FOR PROBABLY BENIGN LESIONS

Edward A. Sickles, M.D.

Nonpalpable lesions that are judged to have a very low probability of malignancy are identified frequently at mammography. Periodic follow-up examinations usually are recommended for these lesions as an alternative to prompt excision (1-13). The purpose of this approach is to avert the morbidity and substantial cost of biopsies for lesions that almost certainly are benign. It also has been shown that careful mammographic surveillance (a) likely will identify by interval change those few lesions that actually are malignant, and (b) will do so while the tumors still have a favorable prognosis (5,12,13). It is preferable to categorize these lesions as "probably benign" rather than "minimally suspicious" or any other terminology implying suspicion of malignancy. The term "probably benign" conveys with greater confidence the overwhelming likelihood that these lesions indeed are benign and that management by observation is a reasonable, safe alternative to immediate biopsy.

The strongest evidence supporting management with periodic mammographic follow-up comes from two studies of prospectively identified, consecutive cases, each derived from a series of more than 20,000 mammography examinations (12,13). In these studies, from the University of California at San Francisco (UCSF) and the Hospital Pereira Rossell in Montevideo, Uruguay, as well as in other smaller and less well controlled investigations, the frequency of cancer among probably benign lesions ranges from 0.5% to 1.7%. Independent demonstration that probably benign lesions have such a low likelihood of malignancy justifies the now widespread practice of managing these lesions with mammographic surveillance.

It is important to distinguish from probably benign lesions those mammographic findings that are so clearly benign that subsequent imaging is limited to routine mammography at age-specific screening intervals. Such characteristically benign lesions include simple benign cysts diagnosed by aspiration or ultrasonography (14), sedimented calcium within tiny benign cysts (15), dermal calcifications even if clustered, characteristically calcified fibroadenomas, arterial calcification, dystrophic and/or sutural post-surgical calcification, intraductal or periductal calcifications of benign duct ectasia, discrete masses that are entirely or partially fatty in content, and masses that demonstrate the typical size, shape, and location of intramammary lymph nodes (16,17).

Mammographic findings interpreted as being probably benign with recommendation for periodic surveillance usually consist of two major categories, localized and generalized. The localized category is characterized by a focal distribution, occurring in one segment of one breast. This includes: (a) clusters of tiny calcifications (5 or more calcific particles per cm^3), if fine-detail images demonstrate that all of the particles are round or oval in shape; (b) noncalcified solid nonpalpable masses with round, ovoid, or gently lobulated contours and well defined margins where not obscured by adjacent fibroglandular tissue; (c) selected focal asymmetric densities (no size limitation, but nonpalpable), defined as discrete opacities readily visible on two orthogonal projection mammograms, with concave-outward margins and/or interspersed with fat; and (d) several miscellaneous focal findings, including single dilated ducts (especially if not associated with spontaneous nipple discharge), and subtle areas of architectural distortion without central increased density (when occurring at known biopsy sites).

The second major category of probably benign findings is characterized by a generalized distribution, demonstrating multiple (usually 3 or more) similar lesions,

either tiny calcifications or masses, randomly distributed in both breasts. Here the most important radiologic feature prompting
a "probably benign" interpretation is the similarity of the component parts of such scattered lesions. A distinction sometimes is made between two clearly different subtypes of widely distributed tiny calcifications: multiple discrete clusters of round or oval-shaped calcifications and numerous bilateral scattered and randomly clustered calcifications.

The likelihood of malignancy can be estimated for each of the mammographic findings that prompt a probably benign diagnosis. Table 1 lists the presenting mammographic findings of the 26 cancers that were detected during the course of mammography surveillance in the UCSF and Montevideo studies. Sixteen of these cancers presented as solitary noncalcified well defined solid nodules, indicating a positive predictive value of 1.8% for this mammographic finding. The remaining probably benign findings each had a positive predictive value of less than 1%. The positive predictive value for all probably benign lesions combined was 0.7%.

Finding	No. of Cases (n=3,719)	No. of Cancers (n=26)
Localized microcalcifications	1,338	5 (0.4)
Solid well defined mass	878	16 (1.8)
Focal asymmetric density	502	3 (0.6)
Generalized microcalcifications	619	1 (0.2)
Multiple solid well defined masses	329	1 (0.3)
Miscellaneous	53	0 (0)

Table 1. Specific Mammographic Findings in 3,719 Probably Benign Lesions and in the 26 Breast Cancers Detected among Them. (Note: numbers in parentheses are percentages.)

In general, the rendering of a probably benign interpretation requires additional imaging to supplement that provided by the conventional two-view-per-breast screening mammography examination. Ultrasonography should be done for the noncalcified mass, to establish or exclude the diagnosis of simple benign cyst. Solid masses, densities, and lesions involving microcalcifications all benefit from fine-detail imaging, especially spot-compression magnification mammography, to more clearly portray the shapes and marginal characteristics of these lesions, and also to serve as a baseline in case additional fine-detail images are obtained subsequently during the course of mammographic follow-up (18-20). At UCSF, we do not make probably benign interpretations directly from screening examinations; additional imaging always is required.

There is no universally accepted protocol of periodic mammographic surveillance for probably benign lesions. However, both patients and their referring physicians should be fully informed about the rationale for and timing of recommended follow-up mammography, specifically of its use as an alternative to biopsy. It also should be understood in advance that any interval change in the probably benign mammographic finding that raises even a slight suspicion of malignancy would prompt the suggestion of

immediate biopsy. The most widely used protocol calls for repeat mammography of the ipsilateral breast in 6 months, with orthogonal projection radiographs, using whatever technique most effectively portrayed the lesion on initial work-up. Subsequently, bilateral mammography is required 6 months later, followed by 1 or 2 additional bilateral annual mammography examinations. Thus, mammography surveillance involves a total of 3 or 4 follow-up examinations spanning a 2 or 3 year period, although this amounts to only one (unilateral) examination more than what ordinarily is recommended as routine annual screening.
When such a protocol is competently and confidently presented to patients and referring physicians, there will be overwhelming initial acceptance. At UCSF, less than 0.5% of women with probably benign lesions elect to have immediate tissue diagnosis instead of periodic mammographic surveillance (12). On the other hand, compliance with the full extent of the follow-up protocol is far less complete. In the UCSF series, although virtually all women underwent at least 1 follow-up examination, only 45% had all 4 recommended examinations (12).

The findings of the large-scale UCSF and Montevideo studies (12,13) support the hypothesis of Hall et al (5) that mammographic surveillance of probably benign lesions will correctly identify those lesions that are malignant, likely while the tumors remain curable. Indeed, 24 of the 26 cancers in these studies were biopsied because mammography showed interval progression prior to the development of palpable findings. In addition, prognostic factors are very favorable among all 26 of the malignancies detected during mammography surveillance. Four of the cancers were ductal carcinoma in situ, and all but one of the invasive cancers was a T1 lesion (2 cm or less in greatest dimension). Only 15% (4/26) of the cancers had axillary lymph node metastasis. All of the 17 UCSF cancer patients have been free of recurrent tumor, after a median follow-up period of more than 7 years; only 1 of the 9 patients in the Montevideo series has shown evidence of recurrence (distant metastasis from a T1,N0 cancer), after an average follow-up of 23 months. These various indicators of good prognosis are similar in fact to those found in large-scale *screening* programs using modern mammography (21,22). Therefore, there does not appear to be a clinically significant delay in diagnosis of cancer due to periodic mammographic follow-up of those few probably benign lesions that actually are malignant.

Hall et al also suggest on the basis of retrospective case review that the use of less aggressive interpretive criteria for mammography (i.e., managing probably benign lesions with mammographic surveillance) would increase the biopsy yield of cancer from the current United States average of 15%-30% up to approximately 40%, without a substantial reduction in the detection of small cancers (5). The results of prospective studies again support this estimate. During the periods of case accrual in the UCSF and Montevideo studies, the biopsy yield of cancer for nonpalpable lesions read as suspicious for malignancy indeed was 38% and 47%, respectively. These results were obtained during the same periods in which only 0.5% and 1.7% of probably benign interpretations eventually proved to represent malignant lesions.

Conservative management of probably benign lesions detected at mammography has several important advantages. Substituting mammographic surveillance for excisional biopsy will result in a substantial reduction in morbidity and induced monetary costs, thereby benefitting both patients and third-party payers. Similar benefits, primarily involving cost reduction, also will derive from using periodic mammographic follow-up instead of percutaneous imaging-guided tissue sampling procedures such as fine-needle aspiration and core biopsy (23). Another, perhaps more significant effect of widespread adoption of the follow-up approach for probably benign lesions is that by making screening mammography more cost-effective, this will help to remove a major remaining barrier to the utilization of screening (24).

In summary, two large-scale, independently conducted series of prospectively identified, consecutive cases establish the validity of managing probably benign lesions with periodic mammographic surveillance rather than immediate biopsy. Indeed, this approach to standard mammographic interpretation is now so widely accepted that the American College of Radiology includes "probably benign - short interval follow-up suggested" as one of the 5 allowable interpretations in the Breast Imaging Reporting and Data System which it encourages all radiologists to utilize (25).

As yet unresolved issues concerning probably benign lesions include whether to use patient age and lesion size (for masses) as additional criteria in choosing between the management alternatives of mammographic follow-up and immediate tissue diagnosis (26). However, there is general agreement that probably benign interpretations should involve: (a) cases restricted to nonpalpable lesions; (b) pre-interpretation comparison with prior mammograms, if available; (c) supplementary ultrasonography and spot-compression magnification mammography; and (d) use of the specific interpretive criteria described and illustrated previously.

References:

1. Homer MJ. Nonpalpable mammographic abnormalities: timing the follow-up studies. Am J Roentgenol 1981; 136:923-926.

2. Moskowitz M. The predictive value of certain mammographic signs in screening for breast cancer. Cancer 1983; 51:1007-1011.

3. Homer MJ. Imaging features and management of characteristically benign and probably benign breast lesions. Radiol Clin North Am 1987; 25:939-951.

4. Wolfe JN, Buck KA, Salane M, Parekh NJ. Xeroradiography of the breast: overview of 21,057 consecutive cases. Radiology. 1987; 165:305-311.

5. Hall FM, Storella JM, Silverstone DZ, Wyshak G. Nonpalpable breast lesions: recommendations for biopsy based on suspicion of carcinoma at mammography. Radiology 1988; 167:353-358.

6. Moskowitz M. Follow-up of benign mammographic lesions. JAMA 1988; 260:3669.

7. Moskowitz M. Impact of a priori medical decisions on screening for breast cancer. Radiology 1989; 171:605-608.

8. Brenner RJ, Sickles EA. Acceptability of periodic follow-up as an alternative to biopsy for mammographically detected lesions interpreted as probably benign. Radiology 1989; 171:645-646.

9. Hall FM. Mammographic second opinions prior to biopsy of nonpalpable breast lesions. Arch Surg 1990; 125:298-299.

10. Adler DD, Helvie MA. The "probably benign" breast lesion: work-up and management. In: Sickles EA, Kopans DB, eds. ACR Categorical Course Syllabus on Breast Imaging. Reston, VA: American College of Radiology, 1990:57-61.

11. Helvie MA, Pennes DR, Rebner M, Adler DD. Mammographic follow-up of low suspicion lesions: compliance rate and diagnostic yield. Radiology 1991; 178:155-158.

12. Sickles EA. Periodic mammographic follow-up of probably benign lesions: results in 3,184 consecutive cases. Radiology 1991; 179:463-468.

13. Varas X, Leborgne F, Leborgne JH. Nonpalpable probably benign lesions: role of follow-up mammography. Radiology 1992; 184:409-414.

14. Sickles EA, Filly RA, Callen PW. Benign breast lesions: ultrasound detection and diagnosis. Radiology 1984; 151:467-470.

15. Linden SS, Sickles EA. Sedimented calcium in benign breast cysts: the full spectrum of mammographic presentations. Am J Roentgenol 1989; 152:967-971.

16. Sickles EA. Breast calcifications: mammographic evaluation. State of the art. Radiology 1986; 160:289-293.

17. Sickles EA. Breast masses: mammographic evaluation. State of the art. Radiology 1989; 173:297-303.

18. Sickles EA. Microfocal spot magnification mammography using xeroradiographic and screen-film recording systems. Radiology 1979; 131:599-607.

19. Sickles EA. Magnification mammography. In: Bassett LW, Gold RH, eds. Breast Cancer Detection: Mammography and Other Methods in Breast Imaging. 2 ed. Orlando, FL: Grune & Stratton, 1987:111-117.

20. Sickles EA. Combining spot-compression and other special views to maximize mammographic information. Letter to the editor. Radiology 1989; 173:571.

21. Sickles EA. Quality assurance. How to audit your own mammography practice. Radiol Clin North Am 1992; 30:265-275.

22. Warren Burhenne LJ, Hislop TG, Burhenne HJ. The British Columbia Mammography Screening Program: evaluation of the first 15 months. Am J Roentgenol 1992; 158:45-49.

23. Sickles EA, Parker SH. Appropriate role of core breast biopsy in the management of probably benign lesions. Radiology 1993; 188:315.

24. Eddy DM, Hasselblad V, McGivney W, Hendee W. The value of mammography screening in women under age 50 years. JAMA 1988; 259:1512-1519.

25. American College of Radiology. Breast Imaging Reporting and Data System. Reston, VA: American College of Radiology, 1993.

26. Hall FM. Statistics, opinions, and controversies among expert mammographers. Breast Dis 1993; 6:173-175.

Mastology - Breast Diseases
A.S.S. Figueira Fo et al., editors.

PROBLEM-SOLVING MAMMOGRAPHY: USE OF ADDITIONAL VIEWS

Edward A. Sickles, M.D.

It is not uncommon for standard two-view-per-breast mammography to produce inconclusive results. Many of these cases are read as indeterminate simply because the imaging evaluation is incomplete. In such circumstances, additional views prove invaluable in solving the mammographic "problems" raised on standard examination. I will discuss several commonly encountered problems, concentrating on which extra views to obtain and when to obtain them.

Lesion Seen on Only One Standard Projection.

The basic decision to make in this situation is whether an abnormality indeed exists, or whether the "lesion" represents a fortuitous superimposition of otherwise innocuous overlapping shadows. One should always solve this problem before rendering an interpretation indicating suspicion of malignancy. If the lesion might not have been included on one standard view because it is located too deep in the breast, then an extra view or views should be obtained to image closer to the chest wall (see below). However, if you are convinced that the lesion was not cut off, then an extra view should be obtained in a projection only slightly different in obliquity from the one in which the lesion was seen. Spot compression and magnification techniques also can be utilized to enhance this additional exposure. If the lesion is real it will still be seen readily; on the other hand, summation shadows normally are no longer visible or appear much less worrisome with very minor changes in x-ray beam obliquity.

Lesion Not Included on Standard Views.

For deep lesions located far laterally or medially, try exaggerated craniocaudal views. Deep lesions within the upper outer quadrant are best seen using a mediolateral oblique (MLO) projection with beam obliquity adjusted so that breast compression is parallel to the plane of the pectoral muscle. Deep lesions in the lower inner quadrant are best shown by the superolateral-inferomedial oblique (SIO) view. Lesions located very high up on the chest wall require either caudocranial projection (equipment permitting) or a "lumpogram", which is a spot compression craniocaudal view that includes under the compression device only the uppermost breast tissues.

Further characterize an already detected abnormality.

For medial lesions, consider doing a true lateral view in lateromedial projection, to bring the lesion as close as possible to the film cassette. For lesions partially obscured by adjacent dense tissues, an additional oblique view or views with a nonconventional degree of beam obliquity may project the previously obscured portions of the lesion to overlie fatty tissue, where its border characteristics can be analyzed more readily. Tangential views are useful to establish (benign) dermal location for clustered calcifications and some superficially projected masses. Finally, spot compression and magnification techniques can be combined with any standard or nonstandard view to produce finer detail images.

References:

1. Sickles EA. Practical solutions to common mammographic problems: tailoring the examination. Am J Roentgenol 1988; 151:31-39.

2. Feig SA. The importance of supplementary mammographic views to diagnostic accuracy. Am J Roentgenol 1988; 151:40-41.

3. Logan WW, Janus J. Use of special mammographic views to maximize radiographic information. Radiol Clin North Am 1987; 25:953-959.

4. Kopans DB, Waitzkin ED, Linetsky L, et al. Localization of breast lesions identified on only one mammographic view. Am J Roentgenol 1987; 149:39-41.

5. Hall FM, Berenberg AL. Selective use of the oblique projection in mammography. Am J Roentgenol 1978; 131:465-468.

6. Sickles EA. Tailoring the mammogram: problem solving and special views. In Thrall JH, ed. Current practice of radiology. St Louis: BG Decker/Mosby, 1993:393-402.

Mastology - Breast Diseases
A.S.S. Figueira Fo et al., editors.

DIGITIZED MAMMOGRAPHY

B. GUERRIN - J.L. LAMARQUE - J. PUJOL - P. BOULET

Département d'Imagerie Médicale
Hopital Lapeyronie
Montpellier - France

Institut Montpelliérain d'Imagerie Médicale

For more than forty years, mammography has been improving, sometines through the quality of the image, sometimes through the reduction of the dose. It has proven its efficacy in screening and early diagnosis of breast pathologies.

Performance and Limitations :
The performance of present mammographic systems is very satisfactory with. for the best installations, mid-breast dose of 1 mGy, spatial resolution of close to 2O pairs of lines per millimeter when enlarged, with a mean gradient centered on 1.2 optical density and a value of 3.2 with an adapted development.

The major difficulty is obtaining, at the same time, visualization of contrast and spatial (subtle opacity and microcalcification) details, and this in a manner large enough to permit their visualization over the entire surface of the breast projection. A contrast-latitude of exposure compromise is indispensable, but this can't always be archieved, in which case it is necessary to take localized views, source of additional radiation, as well as an increase in the dose necessary for satisfactory spatial resolution through diminution of the thickness of the screens.

These difficulties have lead us to search for different solutions through digitization.

Constraint and advantages of digitization :
Whatever the system of digitization, it offers intrinsic solutions, computerized data storage, on-screen visualization, acquisition in which the parameters are no longer linked to the film and can be modified as the doctor wishes. The limits of the system are always the spatial and densitometrie resolution.

The spatial resolution should, to be equal to film taking into account the constraints of sampling, approach 25 μ per pixel. For an 18 x 24 film, we would have 7,200 x 9,600 pixels. At the present time, technological and financial restraints make it impossible to attain such resolutions.

It should be noted that a resolution equivalent to 20 pl/mm is only obtained with metallic 100% contrast test objects which do not exist in the breast. This remark is fundamental in justifying lesser spatial resolutions.

Thus, a disk 0.5 mm in diameter is visible with a contrast of 2% while in digitized mammography it is visible at 0.4%.

A satisfactory comprise is obtained with a size of 100 μm. The other factors correspond to the dose, to the signal to noise ratio quantum yield, linear response to radiant flux, flow intrinsic noise, to the size (18 x 24 cm) and to the time required to obtain the image.

A. MAMMOGRAPHIC DIGITIZATION SYSTEMS AT PRESENT AND IN THE NEAR FUTURE

1. Indirect digitization:

Systems in which the digitized image is obtained by using a mammographic film or, by extension, require an acquisition time of more than a few seconds, are considred as indirect digitization.

Digitization based on mammographic film:
This improves the visualization of certain zones within the limits of the exposure characteristics of the film. This technique is carried out with a camera, a scanner or a microdensitometer with variable resolutions of up to 10 μm for certain equipment.

Although limited, improvements can thus be obtained in the images, accentuation of contrasts, the fibers, storage, detection and analysis systems.

Digitizations with phosphorescent screen:
As opposed to radiographic screens, these screens remain in an intermediate state, fluorescence is triggered by an input of energy by a laser beam, the dimensions of this beam determine the spatial resolution of the system up to 100 μm minimum. This technique offers satisfactory latitude of exposure, the revelation of the latent image is comparable to the development time for a film, for a standard format.

2. Direct digitization:

Three research and development tracks:

Brilliance amplifier:
These systems present a disadvantage related to their dimensions, the amplifier and analyzer tube take up a large amount of space unadapted to this application.

CCD system : charge coupled device
The arrival of a photon brings about the production of a charge on the condenser register which is then read. This system is used in all of the cameras available to the public (camcorders). In order to be used in radiology, an intermediate fluorescent mechanism is needed. The size of these devices does not exceed 5 cmx5cm. A system of optical focalization (lens or optic fibre) is necessary. This system is presently used in stereotaxis and interventional breast stereoscopy. The physical or functional coupling of several elements permits a full field image to be obtained.

Physical coupling : the CCD plates are joined together or constituted of a single plate permitting overall mammography.

Functional coupling : an X-ray scans the breast simultaneously with a CCD receiver rod. This assumes that a mammographic scanning system has been installed. In all cases at the present time, spatial resolution never exceeds 100 μm in practice.

Amorphous selenium system :
This a numeric application of xerographic technique. The selenium is subjected to X-rays, modifies the electrostatic distribution of the surface charges, an electrostatic probe passes while the surface selenium can be subjected to an input of laser energy. There is amplification of electrosttic variations furnishing an image whose resolution can reach 50 μm.

NEAR FUTURE :

The two systems, CCD and amorphous selenium, will permit a global mammographic digitalization with spatial resolutions from 100 to 50 μm and with a density superior to all other mothods, the CCD technique permitting stereoscopic vision. The phosphorescent screen system approaches the selenium system.

B - APPLICATIONS OF DIGITIZATION

1 - Visualization and storage

- the images obtained can be modified as the user desires, luminosity, contrast, LUT (Look up Table), histogram equalization, contour enhancement, spatial filtering, convolution, subtraction, additiion, comparison. Depending on the case, search for opacity, architectural distortion, microalcification, computerized tools will facilitate their crystallization

- Interventional use under stereoscopic control with CCD systems.

- The images can be stored on computer supports with or without compressioin (GIPEG), transferred, treated by detection and analysis robots.

2 - Detection and analysis systems

These system will undergo considerable developement. In a recent study of detection of microcalcifications, we were able, with an automatic system, to surpass, in sensitivity, the capacities of human detection in current reading.

Moreover, we have developed an analysis robot which permits a significant reduction in the number of suspicions of malignancy. Other work on comparison, detection of opacities, is also very encouraging. The analysis and detection robots will thus become our most attentive assistants.

CONCLUSION

The development of mammographic digitization permits, with an increase in quality and a reduction of dose, computerized tools to be obtained which will allow the development of diagnostic assistance robots.

References

1. Bunch PC, Huff KE, Van Metter R. Analysis of the detective quantum efficiency of a radiographic screen-film combinaison. J. Opt. Soc. Am. 1987;4:902-909.
2. Chan HP, Doi K, Galhotra S, Vyborny CJ, MacMahon H, Jokich PM. Imagae feature analysis and computer-aided diagnosis in digital radiography. I. Automated detection of microcalcifications in mammography. Med. Phys. 1987;14:538-548.
3. Chan HP, Doi K, Vyborny CJ et. al. Improvement in radiologists' detection of clustered microcalcifications on mammograms: the potential of computer-aided diagnosis. Invest. Radiol. 1990;25:1102-1110.
4. Chan HP, Cheng SN, Ikeda DM, Niklason L, Adler D. Computerized detection of microcalcifications on mammograms: effects of data compression (abstr). Radiology 1991;177(P):311.
5. Cook HM, Fox MD. Apllication of expert systems to mammographic image analysis. Am. J. Physiol. Imaging 1989;4:16-22.
6. Doi K, Giger ML, MacMahon H, Hoffmann KR et. al. Computer-aided diagnosis: development of automated schemes for quantitative analysis of radiographic images. Semin Ultrasound CT MR 1992;13:140-152.
7. Fam BW, Olson SL, Winter PF, Scholz FJ. Algorithm for the detection of fine clustered calcifications on film mammograms. Radiology 1988;169:333-337.
8. Giger ML, Yin FF, Doi K, Metz CE, Schmidt RA, Vyborny CJ. Investigation of methods for the computerized detection and analysis of mammographic masses. Proc SPIE 1990;1233:183-184.
9. Grimaud M, Muller S, Meyer F. Automated detection of microcalcifications in mammogramms (abstr.). Radiology 1990;177(P):288.
10. Holdsworth DW, Nishikawa RM, Mawdsley GE, Yaffe MJ, Fenster A. Slot-beam digital mammography using a time-delay integration (TDI) CCD. Proc SPIE 1989;1090:306-313.
11. Jiang Y, Nishikawa RM, Giger ML, Doi K, Schmidt RA, Vyborny CJ. Method of extracting signal area and signal thickness of microcalcifications from digital mammograms. Proc SPIE 1992;1778:28-36.
12. Jin HR, Matsumoto K, Kobatake H. Automatic diagnosis of breast cancer with structural line analysis and mathematical morphology. Radiology 1990;177(P):319.
13. Karssemeijet N. A stochastic method for automated detection of microcalcifications in digital mommograms. In: Colchester ACF, Hawkes DJ. Information processing in medical imaging. New York: Springer-Verlag 1991;227-238.
14. Kato H. Photostimulable phosphor radiography design considerations. In Seibert JA, Barnes GT, Gould RG, eds. Specification, acceptance testing and quality control of diagnostic x-ray imaging equipment. Proceedings of the 1991 summer school. American Association of Physicists in Medicine, Santa Cruz, CA, July 15-19, 1991.
15. Nishikawa RM, Doi K, Giger ML et al. Use of morphological filters in the computerized detection of microcalcifications in digital mammograms (abstr). Med. Phys. 1990;17:524.
16. Nishikawa RM, Giger ML, Doi K, Vyborny CJ, Schmidt RA, Yin FF. Effect of case selection on the performance of computer-aided etection schemes (abstr). Med. Phys. 1992;19(P):803.

17. Nishikawa RM, Mawdsley GE, Fenster A, Yaffe MJ. Scanned projection digital mammography. Med. Phys. 1987;14:717-727.
18. Nishikawa RM, Yaffe MJ. Signalo-noise properties of mammography film-screen systems. Med. Phys. 1985;12:32-39.
19. Nishikawa RM, Yaffe MJ. Effect of various noise sources on the detective quantum efficiency of phosphor screens. Med. Phys. 1990;17:887-893.
20. Patrick EA, Moskowitz M, Mansukhani VT, Gruenstein El. Expert learning system network for diagnosis of breast calcifications. Invest. Radiol. 1991;16:534-539.
21. Rowlands JA, Hunter DM, Araj N. X-ray imaging using amorphous selenium: a photoinduced discharge readout method for digital mammography. Med. Phys. 1991;18:421-431.
22. Shtern F. Digital mammography and related technologies: a perspective from the National Cancer Institute. Radiology 1992;183:629-630.
23. Winsberg F, Elkin M, Macy J, Bordaz V, Weymouth W. Detection of radiographic abnormalities in mammograms by means of optical scanning and computer anslysis. Radiology 1967;89:211-215.
24. Wolfe JN. Breast patterns as an index of risk for developing breast cancer. AJR 1976;126:1130-1139.

Mastology - Breast Diseases
A.S.S. Figueira Fo et al., editors.

Digitalization of mammograms: state of the art in equipment, and computer aided diagnosis

C. Frouge[1-2], H. Benali[2], H. Guillemet[2], E. Kahn[2], R. Di Paola[2], M. Bléry[1]

[1]Department of Radiology, Hôpital de Bicêtre. 78, rue du Général Leclerc. 94275 Le Kremlin Bicêtre. France

[2]INSERM U 66

Abstract

Digital mammography will be available in routine practice in the years to come, but for the moment, indirect digitalization is the only way to analyze mammograms with a computer. In the first part of the paper, different types of digitizers will be compared, since there is a wide range of cost and performance. We will also try to determine which device is more suitable for the different applications of indirect digitalization. In the second part of the paper we will look at the stat the art of computer aided diagnosis and look on the hope and limits for the fut

The different kinds of digitizers

The different configurations to digitalize the analogic information contained in mammograms are roughly summarized in table 1. The least expensive digitizer is a simple camescope associated to a microcomputer with a video entry (such as Mac Intosh AV). The lens of the camescope has to be set on the 'macro' position and directly put on the mammogram and a view box. This allows a good analysis of a 2,5 × 3 cm field of view (FOV). The interest of a CCD camera is the high speed of acquisition allowing a direct feed-back of the image on a video monitor. The interactive settings of the luminance and the optical zoom are very easy to use after a short training period. The major limitation of the CCD camera is the big loss of information when it is used for a large FOV like a whole mammogram. It is a good diagnostic tool when used as a numeric magnifying glass. One important point is the quality of the lens allowing magnification without distortion.

Scanners are much more expensive, but allow a better spatial resolution. The digitalization takes more time and the settings are more difficult. The microdensitometer can be considered as the reference for indirect numerization, but is only a research tool. It allows a very high spatial resolution, but the scan time is too long to be used in routine practice. When the digitalization is performed, the grayscale needed depends of the FOV. There is not a big lost of information with 256 gray levels (8 bits) when the study is limited to a small part of the mammogram.

Table 1
Characteristics and applications of the main types of digitizers

	Camescope	CCD Camera	CCD Scanner	Micro-densitometer
manufacturers	Sony	Cohu	Vidar VXR 12	Almaworks lambda
resolution (DPI)	150	300	(60 to 300)	1500
pixel size μm	170	85	(425 to 85)	15-20
pixel number	512 × 512	1024 × 1024 840 × 1200 to 4200 × 5100	15000 × 15000	
field of view (cm)	(2,5 × 3) Zoom	(2,5 × 3) Zoom	(36 × ∞)	(25 × 25)
optical density	0 to 1.5	0 to 2.5	0 to 3	0 to 4,5
grayscale	8 bit (256)	8 or 12 bits	8 or 12 bits	12 bits (4096)
scan speed (seconds)	1/25	1/25	51	400
applications	multimedia, teaching tool	diagnosis, small office	archiving, hospital department	research
recommended hardware	PC or Mac intosh AV	PC or Mac intosh AV	PC or Mac intosh AV	PC + Silicon graphics, Sparc
Price (US $)	1000	4000 (+ lens)	30000	50000

However, 4096 gray levels (12 bits) are mandatory when the whole mammogram is numerized.

Computer aided diagnosis

Computer aided diagnosis can be defined as a diagnosis made by a radiologist who takes into consideration the results of computerized analysis of radiographic images and uses the analysis as a second opinion in detecting lesions and in making a diagnosis [1]. In mammography, this help would be very important since 5 to 10% of false negative mammograms are due to a failure of detection of abnormalities that were obvious retrospectively. [2].

Detection of focal lesions

Many publications used digitalization to increase the detection rate of microcalcification clusters during mass-screening [3, 4, 5, 6, 7, 8]. To detect microcalcifications, the pixel size has to be around 0,1 mm. A smaller pixel size is neede to properly analyze the shape of microcalcification , but the spatial resolution of the mammogram is always limited by the size of the focal spot. Chan proposed a preprocessing with two spatial filterings: one to enhance the signal to noise ratio and the second to suppress the ratio. The difference between the two resulting images yields an image in which the variations in background density are largely removed. Many other methods have been proposed to increase the signal prior to feature extraction like median, contrast reversal, box rim filters or wavelets. The rate of detection is generally around 80 to 90% with one false positive detection per image [9].Wu et al used an artificial neural network to extract microcalcification image data from digital mammograms and was able to eliminate 50% of the false positive results [10, 11]. Computer aided diagnosis has already demonstrated its value in routine practice for microcalcifications [3, 12]. The detection of stellate lesion, architectural distortion and mass is much more difficult and is usually based on deviation from the symmetry of normal left and right breast.

Characterization of focal lesions

Clusters of microcalcification are a highly sensistive sign of minimal breast cancer, but their specificity is low: under 20% [13]. Since the works of Lanyi [14, 15, 16, 17, 18] and Le Gal [19, 20], the microcalcification shape has been known to be highly suggestive of the nature of the underlying lesion. Digitalization of mammogram allows a better analysis of microcalcifications and morphometrical analysis gives quantitative information about shape, distribution and density of microcalcifications.

The characterization of microcalcifications is very difficult since there is an important overlap between their appearance on mammography in benign and malignant lesions. [21] This is easily explained by radio-histological studies which demonstrated that irregular microcalcifications due to intraductal necrosis are highly suggestive of cancer, but regular round calcification due secretion can either be found in benign lesions or non comedo intraductal carcinoma. In 1989, a retrospective blind study was performed in 80 microcalcifcation clusters to determine the best morphometrical parameter [22]. There were 36 breast cancers, 8 border-line lesions, and 36 benign lesions.

The number of microcalcifications ranged from 4 to 40. Clusters associated with other mammographic or clinical signs were excluded. The age of the patients ranged from 40 to 70, with an homogeneous distribution of cancer but more mastosis before 45. 60 plain mammograms and 20 radiographies of biopsy specimens (one view by cluster) were digitalized with a high resolution CCD camera (512 or 1024 matrix). Optical magnification (x10) increased the spatial resolution to a pixel size of 0.07 mm. The digitalized images were processed with various algorithms to increase the signal to noise ratio of microcalcifications and binarized to allow morphometrical analysis. The most difficult step was the manual thresholding. When the threshold was too high, close microcalcifications were melting, giving wrong numbers and when the threshold was too low there was a loss of information.

The morphometrical analysis was performed by a microcomputer, and for each microcalcification, the area, the perimeter, the number of pixels, the barycenter, the Feret diameters in X and Y were analyzed. Only two parameters were studied in a statistical analysis: compactness and eccentricity. Compactness ($4\pi \times$ area/perimeter^2) reflects the irregularity of the shape. A perfect circle has a compactness of one and this value decreases when the shape is irregular. Eccentricity is an average of the distance of the barycenter from the periphery, this value increases with irregularity. A diagram was done for every cluster. The only parameter with a significant difference (a = 0,05) between benign and malignant lesions in biopsy specimen was compactness. There was a threshold of 0.35, if only the lowest value of compactness in the cluster was considered, and of 0.46 for the average of the five lowest compactness of the cluster. The average on 5 microcalcifications was a little more specific, but with a big loss in sensitivity. The lowest compactness was the most reliable parameter to quantify the microcalcification shape. After this study performed on biopsy specimen, its value for decision on mammogram had to be detemined. This was done in a second study with an other software allowing individual thresholding of every microcalcification.

To determine the modification in decisions due to digitalization of mammograms, 220 clusters of microcalcifications were retrospectively studied. Three observers gave their decision (surgery or follow-up) with their level of confidence (7 levels) before and after digitalization to realize ROC analysis. In 147 benign lesions (including 11border line lesions) and 73 carcinomas (23 invasives, 50 in situ) including 20 non-comedo DCIS, the Malignant to Benign ratio was 0.33. The 3 observers had a good concordance. They all increased sensitivity after digitalization by higher detection of cancer (74% vs 65%) but with a big loss in specificity (66% vs 75%). These results are bad if we consider intraductal carcinoma as a whole, but they are much better if we make a difference between comedo and non-comedo carcinomas. Thus if we change our minds and admit that there is no consequence for patients to delay diagnosis of a LCIS or a non-comedo DCIS until other signs appears (new irregular microcalcifications or small density) during a close follow-up, then we can significantly decrease the number of unnecessary biopsies. There is no other alternative and the best computer will not further reduce this overlap, because microcalcification clusters in the biopsy specimen have the same appearance.

Hope for the future

The digital image can be archived and retrieved efficiently and simultaneously in multiple locations.This could be very interesting for a mass screening, affording a distant mammographic interpretation by experts (telemammography). Intelligent mammographic workstations will be available very soon to allow a second opinion and to increase the detection rate of focal lesions. It will also be a help in the decision-making, since intraobserver variations are quite significant in mammogram interpretation.

Conclusion

There is a wide range of equipment enabling digitalization of mammograms for every application: teaching files, diagnostic help as magnifying glass, computer aided diagnosis. This last application is a work in progress but is very promising. For the microcalcifications, the rate of detection is already satisfying, but the task is much more complex for architectural distortion and assymetry of density. The major interest of the caracterization of focal lesion is its role in he decision-ma when microcalcifications are found. Computers will help and have an important place in the detection of focal lesions in mass screening, but the diagnosis in senology will continue for a long time to be a synthesis of the different data coming from the clinical examination, ultrasounds, mammograms and cytology.

Aknowledgements: The authors thanks M. Hittinger for her critical reading of the manuscript.

References

1. Giger M. Computer-aided diagnosis. RSNA categorical course in physics 1993; 283-298.
2. Martin J, Moskowitz M, Milbrath J. Breast cancers missed by mammography. AJR 1979; 132:737-739.
3. Chan H, Doi K, Vyborni C, Lam K, Schmidt R. Computer-aided detection of microcalcifications in mammograms. Methodology and preliminary clinical study. Invest Radiol 1988; 23:664-671.
4. Chan HP, Galhotra S, Vyborny CJ, MacMahon H, Jokich PM. Image feature analysis and computer-aided diagnosis in digital radiography. Automated detection of microcalcifications in mammography. Med. Phys. 1987; 14:538-548.
5. Chan HP, Doi K, Vyborny CJ, Metz CE, MacMahon H, Jokich PM, Galhotra S. Digital mammography: development of a computer-aided system for detection of microcalcifications. SPIE Medical Imaging 1987; 767:367-370.
6. Doi K, Chan H, Vyborni C, Schmidt R, Metz C, Lam K, Ogura T, WU Y, Mac Mahon H. Improvement in radiologist detection of clustered microcalcifications on mammograms. The potential of computer-aided diagnosis. Invest Radiol 1990; 25:1102-1110.
7. Fam B, Olson S, Winter P, Scholtz F. Algorithm for the detection of fine clustered calcifications on film mammograms. Radiology 1988; 169:333-337.
8. Olson S, Fam B, Winter P, Scholz F, Lee A, Gordon S. Breast calcifications : analysis of imaging properties. Radiology 1988; 169:329-332.
9. Vyborny C, Giger M. Computer vision and artificial intelligence in mammography. AJR 1994; 162:699-708.
10. Wu Y, Doi K, Giger M, Nishikawa R. Computerized detection of clustered microcalcifcations in digital mammograms: aplications of artificial neural networks. Med phys 1992; 19:555-560.
11. Wu Y, Giger M, Doi K, Vyborny C. Artificial neural networks in mammography: application to decision making in the diagnosis of breast cancer. Radiology 1993; 187:81-87.
12. Chan H, Doi K, Vyborni C, Schmidt R, Metz C, Lam K, Ogura T, Wu Y, Macmahon H. Improvement in radiologists' detection of clustered microcalcifications on mammograms: The potential of computer aided diagnosis. Investigative Radiology 1990; 25:1102-1110.
13. Sickles EA. Breast calcifications : mammographic evaluation. Radiology 1986; 160:289-293.
14. Lanyi M. Formanalyse von 153 mikroverkalkungsgruppen maligner genese. Das 'Dreieck prinzip'. Radiologe 1977; 17:123-125.

15. Lanyi M, Neufang K. Mögligkeiten und grenzen der differential diagnostik gruppierter intramammärer mikroverkalkungen. ROEFO 1984; 141:4-6.
16. Lanyi M. Microcalcifications in the breast: a blessing or a curse? Diagn imaging Clin Med 1985; 54:126-145.
17.
18. Lanyi M. Diagnosis and differential diagnosis of breast calcifications. Springer-Verlag 1986; 35-36.
19. Le Gal M, Chavanne G, Pellier D. Valeur diagnostique des microcalcifications groupées découvertes par mammographie. Bull Cancer Paris 1984; 71:57-64.
20. Le Gal M, J.C. D, Laurent M, Pellier D. Conduite à tenir devant une mammographie révélatrice de microcalcifications groupées sans tumeur palpable. Nouv Presse Med 1976; 1623-1637:
21. Bremond A, Magnin I. Traitement d'image appliqué à la mammographie: Exemple des microcalcifications. Progrès en pathologie mammaire. Masson 1989; 12-18.
22. Frouge C, Bousser P, Goumot PA, Blery M. Morphometry of breast microcalcifications. 70 th Congress of the R.S.N.A 1989; pp 50 (abst).

Mastology - Breast Diseases
A.S.S. Figueira Fo et al., editors.

BREAST microcalcifications: a histo-radiological correlation

J-M. GUINEBRETIERE

Histopathologie C Institut Gustave ROUSSY Villejuif FRANCE

The screening mammograms used to detect non palpable breast cancer have led to an increasing number of biopsies for isolated clusters of microcalcifications (MC). The management of this kind of biopsy is an irksome task for the pathologist. Usually, there is an absence of any palpable or visible lesion at gross examination of the surgical specimen. The pathologist is concerned about the accuracy of sampling and can easily fail to select the suspicious area for the microscopic examination. We have elaborated at the Institut Gustave Roussy (IGR) a special device, based on preexisting devices, designed to improve the accurate localization of the area corresponding to the mammographic abnormality. It is composed of two radiotransparent plexiglass plates, one of which is riddled with 1 mm holes, 1 cm apart, and marked by a letter for the Y axis and with numbers for the abcissa. The surgical specimen is placed between the two plates, with the one with the numbers and the letters above the specimen. The whole apparatus and biopsy is then X-rayed, and the holes and the different letters and numbers clearly identified on the X-ray allow the accurate localisation of the abnormality. With the help of these co-ordinates, the pathologist is able to pinpoint the suspicious area accurately on the specimen and verify the adequacy of sampling. Such a device is quite important for a proper examination of the specimen and can allow historadiological correlations. Moreover, radiographs of the paraffin blocks are sometimes needed to select the blocks containing the MC which require further slicing. The use of orthogonal views, as proposed by some authors, is helpful in locating deep-seated MC in the blocks.

Benign lesions:

One of the lesions most frequently associated with MC is the cyst, which contains MC in about two thirds of cases. Microscopically, MC are most typically found in the lumen of cysts, suspended in the secretory material, and may be sedimented depending on their position. Usually they are not numerous, are large and regular in shape. Sometimes they are smaller in size. This is difficult to identify microscopically, but can be clearly seen with the help of special staining. They can also be found inside the wall of the cysts, under the epithelial border.

The presence of sedimented calcium, responsible for the tea-cup appearance, is one of the best radiographic signs of cysts. Typically they are multiple, bilateral and scattered, but occasionally they can be unilateral with a clustered distribution. When in doubt, ultrasonography will demonstrate the presence of a cyst.

Another type of MC, found in approximately 15% of cysts, is the Weddellite.This cristal, recently discovered in the breast by L Frappart [1, 2], is composed of a special calcium salt, calcium oxalate. For a long time, these MC were completely overlooked by pathologists because they cannot be detected with the usual stains, but can be identified because of their birefringence under polarized light. Their microscopic appearance is quite typical: translucid with the usual staining agents, large >200μm, polyhedric in shape, and always located inside a benign lesion, especially apocrine cysts. In less than 10% of cases, malignant lesions can be associated with Weddellites, which are at a distance from them and the lesions mainly consist of lobular carcinoma in situ. As the presence of Weddellite calcification is associated in numerous cases with benign lesions, it would be particularly interesting to be able to spot them on mammograms. It is the study of C Frouge and M Meunier which demonstrated that mammographically detected polyhedric shaped MC correspond to Weddellites. It is noteworthy that when a malignant lesion was associated with a polyhedric MC there were typical suspicious MC at a distance from them. Radiologists should be aware of their presence and use a magnifying glass to be detect them.

The other lesion which frequently contains MC is adenosis, found in about 70 % of cases. Adenosis stems from an increase in the size of a lobule due to an increase in the connective tissue or in its epithelial component. MC are usually numerous, with a variety of sizes found together in the same lesion, and regular in shape. They are found in the lumen, and in the wall or even in the connective tissues.The mamographic appearance is sometimes characteristic with a few MC packed closely together in a " diplococcus-like pattern ", but the MC are sometimes numerous and smaller and the cause of a non specific " sand-like " pattern. Inversely, in cases of hyperplasia of the ductal and lobular epithelium, MC are rarely found. They occur in less than 15% of cases. The rate is greater when atypical features are present (35%), but in all the cases MC are smaller than 100μm, and undetectable on mammograms. Thus it is the associated lesions, (adenosis, cysts...) where are present the largest MC, which lead to the detection of these hyperplastic lesions. Since Page [3] found that patients with these lesions have an increased relative risk of breast cancer, 5 or even 10 times the rate of the general population, their presence lead to a regular and strict follow-up of the patient. The mammographic appearance seen here is inconsequential.

Adenofibroma is a tumor rarely discovered as a result of the presence of MC. They are small and have a hyaline connective component.MC are large in size, and located along the epithelial structures and follow their irregular architecture.

Malignant lesions:

Among the malignant lesions, lobular carcinoma in situ is the least likely to be associated with MC, (found in 25% of the lesions). MC are scarce and smaller, consequently their detection is due to the associated lesions containing the larger MC. The mammographic appearance is not striking and it is well known that lobular carcinoma in situ is generally found fortuitously.

Intraductal carcinomas with or without micro-invasion is the lesion most frequently associated with MC, of all the lesions, be they benign or malignant, but their characteristics differ according their particular histologic type.

First, there is the non comedo type which groups together, cribriform, micropapillary, clinging carcinoma... MC are frequently (82%) associated and numerous and exhibit a slight irregular shape. Although a few MC are present in necrotic material and are large in size, most of them are smaller, and occasionally undetectable on mammograms. They occur within the cystic spaces and cleftlike openings, and are considered to be the result of a secretory mechanism. Moreover the variety in the sizes of MC would account for the discrepancies between the size of the cluster on mammograms and the extent of the lesion determined at microscopic examination. Holland [4] found variations of several centimeters! The mammographic appearance of MC is usually regular with a linear arrangement.

The other group of intraductal carcinoma, the comedo-type, is characterised by a large amount of necrosis and large, irregular cells. MC are always present, not numerous, but large in size, irregular in shape and found inside the necrotic material. This suggests that necrosis may be the mechanism responsible for the induction of the calcification. Unlike the non comedo-type, the difference between the mammographic and microscopic size is smaller, about one centimeter according to Holland [4]. These lesions have a typical mammographic appearance. MC form casts of the duct and exhibit an elongated, rod-shaped, branching pattern. Radiologists must be able to recognize these patterns even in small clusters.

Some MC are not located inside the entire spectrum of malignant lesions but rather in the benign associated lesions located around or at a distance from the cancer [5]. Most of these lesions are lobular carcinoma in situ but also comprise intraductal carcinoma of the non comedo type and even invasive carcinoma. Such MC may be considered an indirect sign of cancer. The main implication of this finding for the pathologist is that he/she will have to sample, not only the area corresponding to the mammographic abnormalities, but also the surrounding breast tissue [6].

Conclusion:

Histo-radiologic correlations are important for a better understanding of the different radiologic features and may help the radiologist and the surgeon in the management and the selection of patients with an isolated cluster of MC. However the management of these biopsies implies great care on the part of the pathologist, first to detect the area corresponding to the abnormalities and to sample it entirely, and also to sample the surrounding breast tissue additionally in order to avoid overlooking some cancer and underestimating their extent. This is why this type of surgical biopsy must be appropriately sampled with a greater number of blocks than the other biopsies.

References :

1. Frappart L, Boudelle M, Boumendil J, et al. Structure and composition of microcalcifications in benign and malignant lesions of the breast. Hum Pathol 1984;15:880.

2. Frappart L, Remy I, Hu Chi L, et al. Different types of microcalcifications observed in breast pathology.
Virchows Archives 1986;314:53.

3. Page DL, Dupont WD, Rogers LW, Rados MS. Atypical hyperplastic lesions of the female breast. A long term follow-up study. Cancer 1985;55:2698.

4. Holland R, Hendricks JH, Verbeek AL, Mravunac M, Steckhoven JH. Extent, distribution, and mammographic-histologic correlations of breast ductal carcinoma in situ. The Lancet 1990;335:519.

5. Homer R, Safaii H, Smith T, Marchant DJ. The relationship of the mammographic microcalcifications to histologic malignancy: radiologic-pathologic correlation. AJR 1989;153:1187.

6. De Mascarel I, Trojani M, Bonichon F, Coindre JM. Histological examination of 2859 breast biopsies. Analysis of adequate sampling. Pathological Annual 1993;part1:1.

Mastology - Breast Diseases

A.S.S. Figueira Fo et al., editors.

MAMMOGRAPHIC ANALYSIS OF BREAST CALCIFICATIONS HISTOPATHOLOGICAL CORRELATION

J.L. LAMARQUE - F. DI RUGGIERO
B. GUERRIN - J. PUJOL - P. BOULET

DEPARTEMENT IMAGERIE MEDICALE
HOPITAL LAPEYRONIE
MONTPELLIER
FRANCE

INSTITUT MONTPELLIERAIN D'IMAGERIE MEDICALE

The mammary gland can be divided into three compartments : the interior environment composed of conjunctivo-adipose tissue, the exterior environment represented by the ductal galactophorous light, and, finally, the interface epithelium bordering the galactophore.

For BALDET, the formation of breast microcalcifications proceeds according to the model of osseous mineralization and therefore requires an organic phase (type 1 collagen fibers, collagenic proteins) and an osseous mineral phase (calcium phosphate).

Most breast microcalcifications are due to the secretion or to altered cells. The formation of breast microcalcifications can, therefore, be linked to inflammatory, degenerative, metabolic or traumatic processes.

Other authors have proposed an histological and biochemical classification of microcalcifications (Frouge - Frappart 86) wich distinguishes two types depending upon their structure and their chemical composition. Type 1, also called Weddelite, and type 2 composed of calcium phosphate. This physiochemical classification is commonly accepted at the present time.

Type 1 or Weddelite calcifications have a polyhedral form under optical microscopy. Most authors associate this type of calcification with benign pathologies.

Type 2 microcalcifications (calcium phosphate) are, in general, avoid or fusiform. Their surfaces are irregular in electron microscopy. They correspond more to cellular deposits, debris or necrosis.

However, this study is not of immediate practical interest as mammographic resolution is only 50 microns and the Mach effect can deform a polyhedral form into a spherical form.

The study of clusters shows characteristic foci of benignity (arterial, annular, curvilinear,calcifications, iatrogenic, cutaneous and subcutaneous calcifications of fibroadenomas).

For other clusters which are not formally benign, morphological criteria have emerged through several classifications (Legal, Lanyi, Sigfusson).

In 1990 based on 1,000 cases of microcalcifications, LAMARQUE and colleagues established a relative risk of cancer according to 12 morphological criteria.

The criteria retained are :

- number of microcalcifications > $20/cm^2$
- number between 10 and $20/cm^2$
- irregularity in size
- irregularity in density
- size of the cluster > 2 cm^2
- aligned arrangement
- arborescent arrangement
- vermiform aspect (type V of Legal)
- type IV Legal microcalcifications
- type III microcalcifications
- the number of clusters

Diffuse microcalcifications are disseminated, without clusters, most often in all quadrants and bilaterally.

There exist two groups of diffuse microcalcifications.

The first group is composed of typically benign calcifications.

The second group includes mixed diffuse microcalcifications of small size, variable, elongated round, vermiform, regular or irregular forms.

Nearly one in three cases of mixed diffuse microcalcifications is correlated to a high-risk histological state.

BIBLIOGRAPHIE

AHMED A.
Calcifications in human breast carcionmas : intrastructural observations
J. Pathol. 1975 : 117 : 247-251

BALDET P.
La minéralisation tissulaire normale et pathologique.
Le Sein 1991, 2 : 91-1O1

D'ORSI Carl S, REALE F., DAVIS M. BRAWNT
Breast specimen microcalcifications : radiographic validation and pathologic radiologic correlation
Radiology 1991, 180 : 397-401

EYNIUS F.
Les critères mammographiques de distinction des regroupements micro-calciques en foyer (A propos de 400 cas)
Thèse Médecine, Montpellier, 1990

FRAPPART L., REMY I., HUDRI L.
Different types of microcalcifications observed in breast pathology.
Virchow Arch. 1986, 314 : 53-55

FROUGE C.
Diagnostic précoce des cancers du sein. Corrélations radio-cliniques
Thèse de Doctorat, 1993, Paris XI

GOING J.J., ETERSON TJ, CROCKER J R, LEVISON D.A.
Weddelite calcifications in the breast : eighteen cases with implications for breast cancer screening
Pathology 1990, 16 : 119-124

LAMARQUE J.L. et coll.
Differential diagnosis of microcalcifications X-Rau analysis of 60 intraductal carcinoma.
Radiology 1977, 17, 213-216

TAVASSOLI F.A.,
Pathology of the breast
Saunders New York 1992, 132-139

II.2 Ultrasonography

Mastology - Breast Diseases
A.S.S. Figueira Fo et al., editors.

Diagnosis by color Doppler and contrast agents

H. Madjar*, A. Pfleiderer*, R. Schürmann and R. Schlief

* Gynecology Department, University of Freiburg, Germany
Clinical Research and Development Diagnostics, Schering Berlin

Adress for correspondence:

Helmut Madjar
University of Freiburg
Department for Gynecology and Obstetrics
Hugstetterstr. 55
D 79106 Freiburg, Germany

Abstract

Recent developments of sensitive color Doppler equipment allow for flow detection in microscopic small vessels. An analysis of multiple flow parameters was performed in a group of 390 patients at the University of Freiburg. An Ultramark 9 - HDI (ATL/USA) was used with a broadband linear transducer L 10-5. NUMBER OF TUMOR VESSELS, AVERAGE, MAXIMUM AND TOTAL FLOW VELOCITY showed significant differences ($p < 0.0001$) between 98 cancers and 292 benign lesions. Flow spectrum analysis (RI-values and AB-ratio) did not show significant differences. Due to a number of low vascularized cancers and benign lesions with increased blood flow, the sensitivity and specificity was only 90%.

In order to improve tumor differentiation by doppler, we used a new ultrasound contrast agent SHU 508 (Schering/Berlin) to analyse flow enhancement in 22 lesions with inconclusive findings. Quantitative flow parameters showed enhancement in all carcinomas (n=14). In contrast only 2 of 8 benign lesions with an increased vascularity showed further flow increase. These results were obtained from a small number of patients. However, it seems that contrast agents allow a better differentiation.

Introduction

High resolution ultrasonic imaging has improved the accuracy of breast diagnosis. With transducer frequencies at 7 - 10 MHz and advanced signal processing, this technique allows for the detection of tumors below 1 cm in diameter. In combination with mammography this allows for better differentation of small lesions. Furthermore, measurement of tumor size and detection of multifocal growth is highly accurate and allows improved preoperative management (1). However, there are still a number of lesions where differentiation must be improved to reduce the rate of unnecessary biopsies.

Doppler techniques allow the assessment of physiological and biological changes by blood flow measurements. It is well known, that malignant growth is associated with an increased vascularity (2, 3). Therefore, angiography has been used to differentiate tumors by their abnormal vascular pattern (4, 5). However, the vascular anatomy requires selective and invasive diagnostic procedures.

Doppler ultrasound allows noninvasive and direct flow measurements of breast lesions. Due to the small size of tumor vessels below 1 mm in diameter, standard Duplex systems are not sensitive enough for flow detection. Therefore most studies have been performed with continuous-wave (CW) Doppler equipment at 8 - 10 MHz transducer frequency (6, 7). This method is sensitive, but combination of CW-Doppler and B-mode imaging is technically difficult (8). Therefore CW Doppler is mainly useful for flow detection in palpable lesions.

New developments of sensitive Color Doppler equipment allow for flow detection in microscopic small vessels and, in combination with high resolution imaging techniques, vascularity in subclinical lesions can be measured. In a previous study we compared different systems and found that this method depends on equipment, transducer selection and tuning (9).

Methods

In order to establish the role of color Doppler we evaluated different flow parameters using an ATL Ultramark 9 HDI,L 10/5 MHz broadband linear-transducer.

A) Tumor differentiation:

390 patients with abnormal clinical or mammographic findings were examined by B-mode imaging followed by a color Doppler survey for vascularity in the abnormal area. Maximum systolic and diastolic flow velocity were measured in each vessel after angle correction. Resistance index and AB-ratio were also calculated. All flow data were computed for a statistical comparison of 292 benign lesions and 98 cancers.

The most important criteria were:

- Number of tumor arteries (ART)
- average of all flow velocities measured in each tumor (Vav)
- maximum flow velocity detected in each tumor (Vmax)
- sum of all flow velocities in each tumor (Vsum)
- average resistance index in all tumor vessels (RI)
- minimum resistance index detected in each tumor (RImin)
- average A/B-ratio measured in all tumor vessels (AB)
- minimum A/B-ratio detected in each tumor (ABmin).

B) Contrast agents:

Echo contrast agents have been used to improve the signal to noise ratio for vascular Doppler examinations and mainly in echocardiography. Recently, a new transpulmonary contrast agent has been developed (SHU 508 A, Schering/Germany) which, after intravenuous injection leads to a strong increase of backscatter from blood even in small vessels of the peripheral vasculature. The contrast agent was provided as dra galactose granules which were suspended in water immediately before injections. The standard dose for the first injection was 10 ml of 300 mg/ml solution. AT least 2 injections were made after an interval of more than 15 minutes with a higher concentration of 8 ml with 400 mg/ml.

Intravenuous injections of SHU 508 A were made in 22 lesions with suboptimal Doppler signal intensity in the baseline Doppler examination. 14 carcinomas with low tumor vascularity and 8 benign lesions. The baseline study was performed under video-control. With continuous time registration intravenuous bolus injections were given. The time interval for signal enhancement was measured in color Doppler and Duplex mode. Additionally the amount of signal enhancement was estimated in color Doppler mode on a continuous scale from 1 - 100. This parameter was called the "confidence level" (CL).

Results

A) Tumor differentiation:

Quantitative blood flow measurements in 292 benign and 98 malignant tumors showed significant differences ($p < 0.0001$). Flow spectrum analysis (RI-values and AB-ratio) did not show significant differences. Average flow resistance in carcinomas was increased compared to benign tumors. Due to low vascularized cancers and benign lesions with increased blood flow, the sensitivity and specificity was only 90% (Table 1).

B) Contrast agents:

After intravenuous injection of SHU 508 contrast enhancement was found after an average time interval of 21.91 seconds. Signal enhancement disappeared slowly after 5.35 minutes on average. The Quantitative flow parameters showed enhancement in all carcinomas (n=14). The average confidence level (CL) was only 29.6, as these lesions were preselected and low vascularized cancers. Injection of SHU 508 improved the CL to an average of 88.1. The 300 mg/ml solution was sufficient in 10 cases. In 4 lesions the higher dose

Table 1 Mean flow values (+/- standard deviation) obtained in 390 patients with breast abnormalities.

	BENIGN (n=292)	MALIGNANT (n=98)
ART	2 (s.d. 2)	12 (s.d. 10)
Vav (cm/s)	11 (s.d. 7)	20 (s.d. 18)
Vmax (cm/s)	13 (s.d. 10)	37 (s.d. 20)
Vsum (cm/s)	29 (s.d. 18)	285 (s.d.147)
RI	0.68 (s.d.0.1)	0.74 (s.d.0.1)
RImin	0.64 (s.d.0.1)	0.62 (s.d.0.1)
AB	3.64 (s.d.1.7)	5.52 (s.d.2.7)
ABmin	3.10 (s.d.1.5)	3.01 (s.d.1.3)

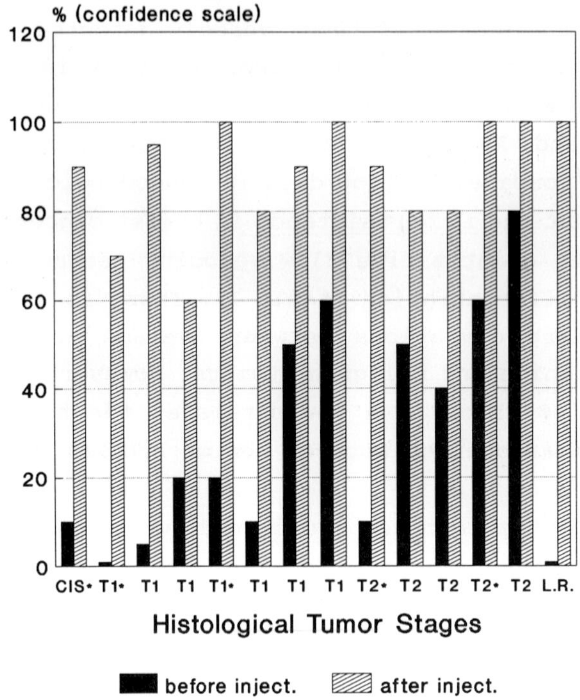

Dosage: 300mg/ml (10ml), *400mg/ml (8ml)

Figure 1 Enhancement of tumor vascularity. Measurement of the confidence level after intravenuous injection of SHU 508 A.

of 400 mg/ml allowed for a better differentiation. The findings in 14 cancers, one carcinoma in situ (CIS), one local recurrence and 12 T1 - T2 lesions are shown in figure 1.

Flow increase was not found in any of the 8 benign lesions when the lower dose of 300 mg/ml was used. After injection of the 400 mg/ml solution, only 2 of the 8 benign lesions showed further flow increase.

Discussion

Color Doppler imaging allows flow detection in nonpalpable tumors and improves the differentiation of solid lesions. Different criteria can be used to describe tumor vascularity. The easiest parameter is the number of tumor vessels detected by color flow mapping with an average of 12 tumor arteries in 98 carcinomas and 2 arteries in 292 benign lesions ($p < 0.0001$). The flow indices RI and AB ratio failed to demonstrate significant differences. Compared to flow data in gynecological tumors it is surprising that the flow resistance in breast cancers is slightly increased. The quantitative flow velocity measurements allowed an accurate differentiation (table 1). There is a small overlap of the standard deviations between average and maximum flow velocity in benign and malignant tumors. However, the sum of all flow velocities which is a new parameter for total tumor flow does not show an overlap between benign and malignant.

The results of the contrast agent study were only obtained from a small number of patients. However, it seems that ultrasound contrast agents allow a better differentiation of lesions. This needs further evaluations in larger clinical studies.

Acknowledgement

This study was supported by a research grant of the DFG (Deutsche Forschungsgemeinschaft), Bonn, Germany.

References

1. Madjar H, Ladner HA, Sauerbrei W, Oberstein A, Prömpeler H, Pfleiderer A (1993) Preoperative staging of breast cancer by palpation, mammography and high-resolution ultrasound. Ultrasound Obstet Gynecol 3: 185-190

2. Folkman J (1986) How is blood vessel growth regulated in normal and neoplastic tissue? Cancer Res 46: 467-473

3. Natzuki S, Yamazaki K (1988) A study on the vascular proliferation in tissues around the tumour in breast cancer. Jpn. J Surg 18: 235-242

4. Feldman F (1969) Angiography of cancer of the breast. Cancer 23: 803-810

5. Maeda M (1979) Die weibliche Brust - Neue angiographsche Kenntnisse. Fortschr Röntgenstr 130: 711-715

6. Wells PNT, Halliwell M, Skidmore R, Webb AJ, Woodcock JP (1977) Tumour detection by ultrasonic Doppler blood-flow signals. Ultrasonics 15: 231-232

7. Madjar H, Sauerbrei W, Münch S, Schillinger H (1991) Continuous-wave and pulsed doppler studies of the breast: clinical results and effect of transducer frequency. Ultrasound Med Biol 17: 31-39

8. Jellins J (1988) Combining imaging and vascularity assessment of breast lesions. Ultrasound Med Biol 14 (Suppl 1):121-130

9. Madjar H (1992) Breast examinations with continuous wave and color Doppler. Ultrasound Obstet Gynecol 2: 215-220

Mastology - Breast Diseases
A.S.S. Figueira Fo et al., editors.

High-frequency (10-15 MHz) ultrasound of the breast

Giorgio Rizzatto, Roberta Chersevani

Department of Radiology, General Hospital, via Vittorio Veneto 171, 34170 Gorizia, Italy. fax 39 481 535346

Abstract

High-frequency breast ultrasound improves spatial, contrast and vascular resolution. New technologies permit to produce dedicated probes that allow better definition of normal and pathologic patterns; at the same time more than 95% of the breasts can be studied with a frequency of 10 MHz or higher.

High-frequency breast ultrasound imaging increases sensitivity and specificity of this technique. More anatomic structures can be defined; the visualization of the ductal system offers unique informations in benign duct ectasia and in important pathologies like inflammations and cancers.

High-frequency Doppler analysis opens the possibility to evaluate normal breast vascularity and to refine the informations related to nodular pathology.

A correct ultrasound examination of the breast requires an appropriate equipment. To-day we can work with instruments that make use of high-frequency transducers, sophisticated focalization and computing capability; the same instrument may allow high quality B-mode imaging and sensitive Doppler analysis.

High frequency, real-time, hand-held specific transducers ranging from at least 10 MHz up to 15 MHz and more, and focused in the near field, may allow enough resolution to discriminate the very subtle differences of acoustic impedance among the breast soft tissues and their pathology. High frequency probes, when compared to those of lower frequency, can improve both spatial (axial and lateral) and contrast resolutions.

They provide better definition of normal as well as pathologic features; consequently they increase the diagnostic possibilities and clinical precision of this technique [1].

The superficial location of the breast also makes it possible to increase the frequency of the Doppler signal that is used both for spectrum analysis and color flow mapping; as a result also the vascular resolution may increase. High-frequency Doppler analysis opens the possibility to evaluate normal breast vascularity and to refine the informations related to nodular pathology.

On ultrasonic images, the **spatial resolution** varies within every image and among the three directions defined by the scan plane.

The main factor that determines axial resolution is the length of the ultrasound pulse which is closely correlated with the transducer's frequency. For a constant number of cycles as the frequency is increased, the shortened wavelength decreases the spatial pulse length and improves the axial resolution; as a trade off ultrasound waves of higher frequencies will be absorbed more rapidly. In order to overcome this limitation many probes use new composite ceramics with a wider bandwidth; they improve axial resolution up to the values of wavelength, still avoiding to expose the tissue to a too high peak acoustic intensity. These ceramics offer multiple frequencies in a single transducer and in broad band arrays; this allows to maximize the sensitivity at various depths. Resolution in the near field is improved and, at the same time, there is enough penetration in the far field; actually, more than 95% of the breasts can be studies with the 10 MHz transducers. Broad band technology is also useful for Doppler analysis: the low-frequency component optimizes flow evaluation, while the higher frequency component allows an adequate study of morphology and structure through gray scale imaging.

The principal determinant of lateral resolution is the width of the ultrasound beam; consequently the lateral resolution increases with thin beams and is maximum in the focal zone of the ultrasonic beam. The most valid technical solution is that offered by the higher frequencies and the more advanced technology of liquid-path dedicated probes, that have an improved focalization because the transducer has been moved inside the probe and there is a fluid path between the transducer and the skin surface. Such transducers, annular arrays or single crystal, consist of wide diameters, higher frequency and oscillating movement which produce high intensity and correctly focused signals, introducing a very homogeneous resolution.

An increase in frequency results in a deeper near field and a less diverging far field; as a result the region of best lateral resolution is extended. A broad bandwidth transducer will produce many frequencies that tend to make the near field more uniform. At the same time the lower frequencies are used to produce the far field and to reduce the gain settings. The large diameter of these transducers is responsible of higher intensity signals that can go deeper into the tissues; this depth is also favoured by very particular liquids used in the fluid path inside the probe. Palpation is easily done while scanning with liquid-path probes and there are no limitations to interventional procedures whatsoever.

Recent dramatic increase in computing capability allows to provide good focalization also to linear arrays, still maintaining adequate frame rates. Using these powerful focusing configurations, some 10-13 MHz linear arrays are now producing high quality diagnostic images; due to the inherent complexity of the signal processing they are still of lower definition when compared with those obtained with liquid-path transducers.

Contrast resolution defines the ability to discriminate the differences of acoustic impedance among tissues. It is affected by echo amplitude and tissue attenuation. If the echoes arising from a definite tissue are weak, it will be impossible to detect them without increasing the receiver gain and, therefore, the noise.

All the techniques that increase the signal-to-noise ratio, enhancing spatial resolution as well as beam penetration, will also increase contrast. For superficial scanning, the use of higher frequencies results in better contrast resolution within the near field; appropriate preprocessing techniques are used to further enhance the contrast between tissues and microcalcifications.

Vascular resolution defines the diagnostic capability of the color flow mapping (CFM) systems (with superimposition of flow information as colors on a gray scale image) to recognize the presence of flow. One determining factor in Doppler performance is that the intensity of the scattered wave increases with the fourth power of frequency; as a consequence, doubling the frequency will result in an echo from the blood that is 16 times stronger. At present, the ability to localize low-flow superficial structures has increased without critical expense of spatial resolution and frame rate. New broad band linear array probes allow to image relatively deep areas of interest (up to 4-6 cm) with peak frequencies ranging from 7.5 to 13 MHz; at the same time they use the 4.5 to 7 MHz frequency to optimize the Doppler analysis of the lower flow.

The final result of a CFM image mostly depends on the choice of the highest ultrasonic frequency that can be employed at the depth of the structure of interest; the correct use of beam focalization avoids exaggerated attenuation and increases the efficiency of scattering at higher frequencies.

Recently many manufacturers have developed a technique that encodes the amplitude of the returning Doppler signal in color (Power Doppler, Ultrasound Angio, Color Doppler Energy, Color Intensity Doppler, etc.). In power Doppler the amplitude of the signal is always larger than that of noise. To each signal is assigned a different color from noise; therefore, the differentiation is clear even at the weakest levels.

This technique does not provide information about the speed or direction of flow. On the other hand power Doppler has many advantages: it avoids aliasing, is three to five times more sensitive than the mean frequency shift, and does not loose sensitivity at quite perpendicular incidence. The use of power Doppler associated to higher frequency transducers, actually allows to define the presence of rich vascularity also in normal breasts.

References

1. Rizzatto G, Chersevani R, Solbiati L. High-resolution ultrasound assists in breast diagnosis. Diagnostic Imaging Int 1993; 5: 42-45

Mastology - Breast Diseases
A.S.S. Figueira Fo et al., editors.

Current concepts in breast ultrasound: Developments in technology and quality assurance

Jack Jellins, International Breast Ultrasound School, P O Box 479, Double Bay NSW 2028, Australia

Abstract

Ultrasonic image quality has improved substantially with high frequency, high resolution scanning equipment, and breast images demonstrate more accurately the subtle features found in breast anatomy and pathology. Improvements in spatial and contrast resolution of the imaging system have significantly enhanced the display of small tissue detail and breast structures. Different transducer configurations are available, and both linear array and mechanical sectoring transducers can be used for high quality breast imaging. Quality assurance programmes need to be implemented to ensure consistent high quality imaging, and to validate the diagnostic accuracy of the examination technique.

Ultrasonic imaging equipment with high resolution transducers can be used to display breast anatomy and pathology [1]. For the successful display of small lesions, transducers in the range of 7 to 10 MHz must be utilized, and even higher frequency transducers better demonstrate ductal anatomy [2-4]. Whilst higher frequencies are more suitable to resolve the smaller structures, the upper limit is restricted by the frequency-dependent attenuation of tissues, and the need to image the deeper portions of the breast. The development of transducer materials with improved acoustic matching reduces acoustic noise, and the improvement in dynamic range enhances the ability to display subtle tissue variations. Modern transducer materials function over a wide range of frequencies, and thus the newer transducers designed for breast imaging at 7 MHz are effective from 5 to 10 MHz [5].

High frequency transducers inherently have small footprints which are convenient for good coupling to the breast surface but which display only a portion of the breast volume in any one image. The whole breast can be examined by moving the transducer over the total breast surface in a number of different scanning planes, and with experience the total breast volume can be imaged in a few minutes. Image interpretation relies on understanding the variations of normality with the ability to recognize the changes resulting from benign and malignant disease processes.

For the assessment of early breast disease and to delineate small lesions, the ultrasonic equipment should incorporate the minimum characteristics described in Table 1.

Spatial resolution is a 3-dimensional quantity which consists of axial, lateral and elevational components, and determines the ability to distinguish two structures of similar echo strengths. Contrast resolution determines the ability to distinguish the presence of tissues with small amplitude echoes adjacent to tissues with much larger amplitude echoes (high-contrast resolution), as well as the differentiation of adjacent tissues with only minimally different echo amplitudes (low-contrast resolution).

The need for good spatial resolution is widely accepted as being a prime requirement of a high-resolution scanner, and is critical to the accurate interrogation of small normal structures (such a ducts) as well as small solid lesions. However the more important parameter for effective breast imaging is contrast resolution which determines the ability to display the subtle variations between normal tissue and breast pathology. Contrast resolution depends significantly on transducer characteristics, signal processing parameters, and background electrical and acoustical noise. Developments in transducer technology have improved contrast resolution so that ultrasonic breast images better demonstrate the presence of disease processes.

Transducer frequency of 7.5 MHz or higher

Good spatial and contrast resolution (uniform characteristics throughout the field of view are desirable)

An electronic linear array transducer or mechanically driven sector transducer (single element or annular array) can be used, and should have a penetration depth better than 4 cm at 7.5 MHz

Good near field resolution should be provided either by using an acoustic stand-off or by signal processing methods which may include variable aperture and variable frequency techniques

Table 1. Desirable equipment characteristics for high quality breast imaging to display the subtle variations between normal tissue and breast pathology. Contrast resolution depends significantly on transducer characteristics, signal processing parameters, and background electrical and acoustical noise. Developments in transducer technology have improved contrast resolution so that ultrasonic breast images better demonstrate the presence of disease processes.

Different transducer configurations are available for breast imaging, and these are either linear arrays or mechanically driven sector (single element or annular array) transducers. All transducers provide their best resolution in the imaging plane, where the lateral resolution may approach the maximum potential value [6,7]. However single element or annular array transducers maintain the same resolution in the elevational plane as these transducers have the same physical dimensions in both planes since their construction is symmetrical. Thus at right angles to the imaging plane, the resolution of single element and annular array transducers is the same as in the imaging plane, and the resolution cell is symmetrical. Linear array electronic transducers have an asymmetrical resolution cell as these transducers cannot optimize the beam profile in the elevational plane to the same degree as in the imaging plane. The asymmetrical resolution cell of linear array transducers can degrade the overall spatial resolution but overall may not adversely affect image interpretation severely as in practice other equipment-related factors contribute to the diagnostic value of the image.

The successful elucidation of relevant ultrasonic features is critically dependent on the optimisation of acquired ultrasonic data and signal processing parameters. Ultrasonic imaging equipment has a large number of variables which affect image quality, and these include transducer type, transducer frequency, acoustic output, receiver gain, TGC control, preprocessing, dynamic range, post-processing, and video/hard-copy display controls. Uniformity of field is paramount to high quality breast imaging, and can be achieved with multiple transmit zones and dynamic focussing on reception. These techniques are in common use with multi-element (linear and annular) array transducers. Single element fixed-focus transducers cannot maintain uniformity over the penetration range since the beamwidth varies over the field of view.

The fields of view obtained with the three different transducer configurations are shown in Figure 1. The hatched areas represent the regions where acceptable resolution is achieved with each configuration. The linear array has uniform lateral spatial resolution over its field of view but the poorer elevational resolution can degrade the image at both extremities of the field. The single element transducer has symmetrical spatial resolution over its field of view but only has a limited focal zone due to the fixed curvature of the transducer element. The annular array transducer also has symmetrical spatial resolution, and with its ability to dynamically focus the beam provides optimum focus over the entire field of view. Of all the transducer configurations, the annular array provides the best resolution in the elevational plane, and therefore the narrowest slice thickness which a vital parameter for maximum contrast resolution.

Typical images obtained with high resolution ultrasonic imaging equipment are shown in Figures 2 and 3. Graticule markers representing one cm intervals are shown on the vertical axes. Good spatial and contrast resolution demonstrate the subtle textural differences inherent in the component tissues of the breast, and the images clearly display the low level echogenicity of the subcutaneous adipose tissues compared to the higher level echoes of the glandular tissues. The presence of pathology is recognized by applying the accepted grey-scale diagnostic criteria to regions of disturbed breast architecture.

The need to maintain equipment performance is a foremost requirement to ensure consistent high quality imaging [8,9]. A tissue-mimicking phantom, designed for small parts imaging, is appropriate for monitoring system performance, but the composition of phantoms does not adequately duplicate the complex nature of breast tissues. Phantom images show the equipment's ability to display small liquid filled areas and interfaces in the phantom material, but do not reliably predict the scanner's performance with breast lesions where the ultrasonic characteristics between the normal tissues and the pathology may only be small.

Regular monitoring of equipment performance should be undertaken on at least a monthly basis to ensure that high quality imaging is maintained. The following parameters can be included in a quality assurance programme: measurement accuracy, relative system sensitivity, relative dynamic range, geometric distortion, and hardcopy performance such as stability of the settings for brightness and contrast. Small parts tissue-mimicking phantoms are appropriate for monitoring system parameters, but cannot completely assess the scanner's ability to differentiate tissues as the composition of phantoms does not adequately duplicate the complex nature of breast tissues. Scanning a suitable body part can be employed for this purpose, such as a limb or a thyroid gland. It is essential that the same part and person are

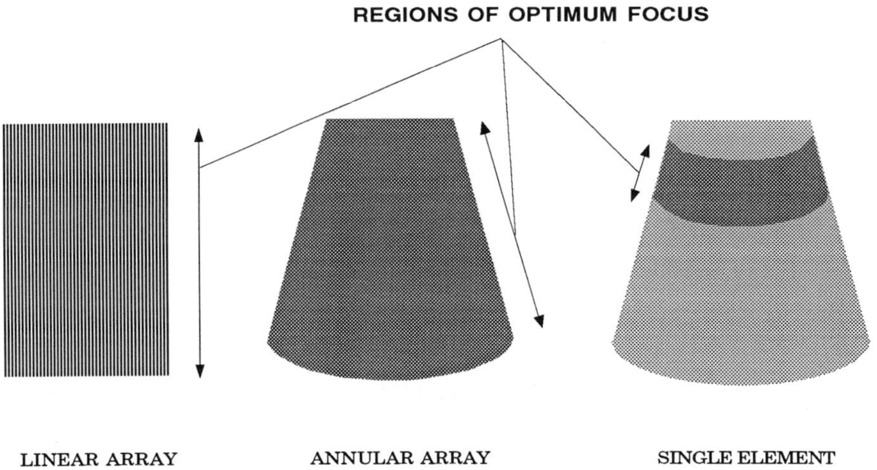

Figure 1. Fields of view for different transducer configurations suitable for breast imaging. The limited optimal focal zone of the single element transducer is shown by the darker region.

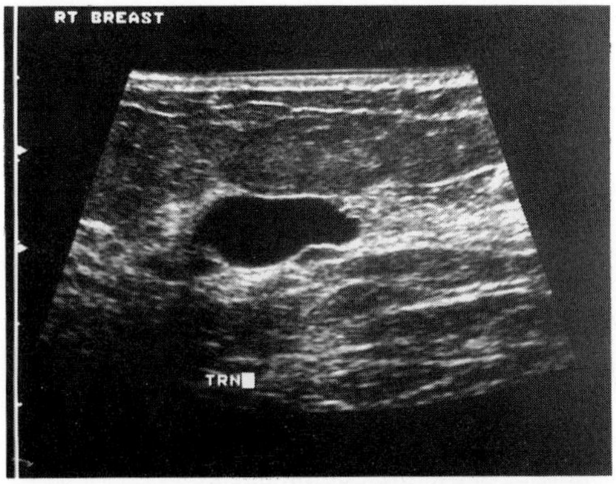

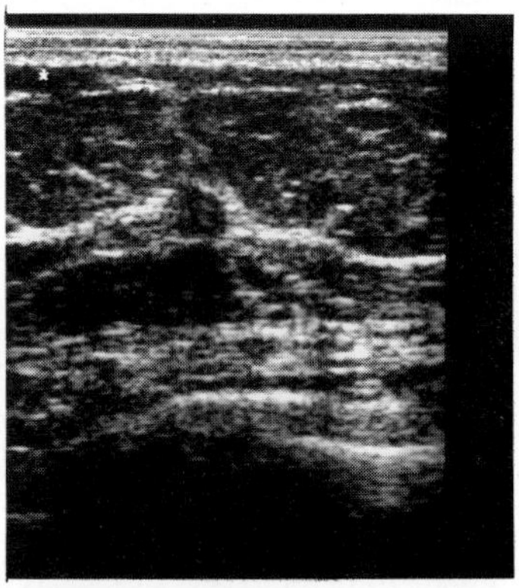

Figure 2 (left). An image obtained with a high resolution 7.5 MHz, 36 mm diameter, 12 ring annular array showing an elongated lesion with well-defined margins and echo-free internal content. The appearance is consistent with a cyst measuring 20 x 9 mm. On one side of the posterior margin of the cyst, there is a protrusion resulting from a small region of intramammary fatty tissue.

Figure 3 (right). An image obtained with a high resolution 10 MHz linear array demonstrating a 6 mm solid lesion with ultrasonic features consistent with an invasive carcinoma. The lesion is clearly defined by its low echogenicity and irregular margins. There is disruption of the surrounding parenchyma and Cooper's ligaments.

available for monitoring, and that the images and records of the equipment settings are carefully documented for later comparison. The ultrasonic scanner should be serviced on a regular basis according to the recommendations of the manufacturer, and accurate records of the image quality kept for each service period.

Conclusion

Developments in technology have significantly contributed to the improvements in spatial and contrast resolution, and the better display of breast anatomy and pathology has established ultrasound as a suitable imaging modality for the evaluation of early breast disease. The accurate interpretation of ultrasonic images not only relies on considerable clinical expertise but also on substantial knowledge of the physical interaction of ultrasound with soft tissues. Significant improvements in equipment design have resulted in high quality breast images being available from different types of ultrasonic equipment, but further improvements in image quality may occur in the future as a result of better understanding the physical basis of ultrasonic image acquisition [10-13].

References:

1. Jellins J. Developments in Ultrasonic Breast Imaging Techniques: Water-Bath and Real Time. In: (eds) J. Gebhardt, B. J. Hackelöer, G. v. Klinggräff, et al. Ultraschall-Diagnostik '89, Heidelberg, Springer-Verlag, 1990: 33-36.
2. Rizzatto G. et al. Sonography. In: (ed) L. Gandolfi. Breast Ultrasound. Italy, Diagnostic Ultrasound Books, 1992: 15-20.
3. Teboul M. Ductal Echography: A new Ultrasonic Imaging and Sampling Tecnic For Breast Malignancies. In: (eds) F. Kasumi, E. Ueno. Topics in Breast Ultrasound. Tokyo, Shinohara Publishers Inc, 1991: 48-57.
4. Kamio T. et al. Significance of Ductal Findings in Ultrasonic Examination of the Breast: Diagnosis of Intraductal Tumour and Intraductal Spreading of Breast Cancer. In: (eds) F. Kasumi, E. Ueno. Topics in Breast Ultrasound. Tokyo, Shinohara Publishers Inc, 1991: 200-205.
5. Goldstein A. Broadband transducers improve image quality. Diagnostic Imaging, May 1993: 89-93 & 100.
6. Bamber JC. Trends in Ultrasonic Instrumentation and Research: Future Possibilities for Breast Investigations. In: (eds) F. Kasumi, E. Ueno. Topics in Breast Ultrasound. Tokyo, Shinohara Publishers Inc, 1991: 35-41.
7. Hykes DL, Hedrick WR. Real-Time Ultrasound Instrumentation: An Update. JDMS 1990; 5: 257-268.
8. Maslak SH. Computed Sonography. In: (eds) R. C. Sanders, M.C. Hill. Ultrasound Annual. New York, Raven Press, 1985: 1-16.
9. Alasaarela E, Koivukangas J. Evaluation of Image Quality of Ultrasonic Scanners in Medical Diagnostics. J Ultrasound Med 1990; 9: 23-34.
10. Hill CR et al. What Might Echography Learn From Image Science. Ultrasound in Med & Biol 1991; 17(6): 559-575.
11. Harris RA et al. Ultimate Limits in Ultrasonic Imaging Resolution. Ultrasound in Med & Biol 1991; 17(6): 547-558.
12. Beach KW. 1975-2000: A Quarter Century of Ultrasound Technology. Ultrasound in Med & Biol Vol 1992;18(4): 377-388.
13. Wells PNT et al. The Envelope That Tissue Imposes On Achievable Ultrasonic Imaging. J Ultrasound Med 1992; 11: 433-439.

II.3 Biopsy

Mastology - Breast Diseases
A.S.S. Figueira Fo et al., editors.

FINE NEEDLE BIOPSY
MICROBIOPSY
STEREOTATIC BIOPSY

J.L. LAMARQUE - K. EL M'RINI
F. DI RUGGIERO - J. PUJOL - B. GUERRIN
P. BOULET - J. CHERIFCHEIKH - J.C. LAURENT

DEPARTEMENT D'IMAGERIE MEDICALE
HOPITAL LAPEYRONIE
MONTPELLIER - FRANCE

INSTITUT MONTPELLIERAIN D'IMAGERIE MEDICALE

Mass screening campaigns can bring about a 20 to 40 % reduction in mortality for certain age groups, through the diagnosis of very small non-infiltrating or non-invasive breast cancers of less than one centimeter.

Thus, the frequency of radiological anomalies found through screening is increasing regularly and it is necessary to evaluate thom correctly in order to prevent a large increase in the number of unnecessary biopsies.

Since 1989, we have been carrying out, to this effect, cytological biopsies guided by stereotaxis. This mode of localization has the advantage of being precise to within one millimeter. We rapidly became aware of the limitations of cytoaspiration, which are essentially a large rate of insufficient samples and an absence of information concerning the degree of tumoral invasion.

As a result, since 1990 we have systematically combined microbiopsy done with an automatic needle gun with cytoaspiration ; a retrospective study carried out over two years was set up to evaluate the efficacy of the method on diverse breast lesions.

From October, 1990 to November, 1992, 321 double cytohistological breast biopsies were performed in the department of medical imaging at the Lapeyronie Hospital (Professor J.L. LAMARQUE - Montpellier, France).

724 of the biopsies were guided by stereotaxis and the others were done either by classical methods or with echography.

On the pratical level, the quasi-totality of the needle biopsies were carried out with a 600T mammograph combined with a Stereotix 1 - General Electric Medical System ; towards the end of 1992, a certain number were carried out with a DMR combined with a Stereotix 2.

The microbiopsy was performed first (as opposed to other teams), in order to obtain the best possible "carrot" ; the tissular deterioration provoked by the microbiopsy further increases the quality of the cytological samples.

The first needle biopsies were done using 16 and 18 G needles, and guns with small and large strokes from 12,5 to 25 mm (Bard Biopty Cut), then in 1992 only with large caliber needles (14G) using the large stroke, thus considerably improving the quality of the fragments.

All of our samples were analyzed by four confirmed cytologists, and, more particularly, by two accustomed to breast pathology. In order to facilitate statistical calculations, the results were regrouped as insufficient samples, normal tissue or moderate hyperplasia without atypism, A.E.H., and cancers.

When the "quartet" C.R.C.H. (clinical-radiology-cytology-histology) was unanimous in its diagnosis of benignity, no surgical histological control was performed. This group included 191 cases with 163 needle biopsies carried out with stereotaxis and 28 without. The images which were biopsied were submitted to a simple follow-up varying from 6 to 24 months (12 months on average). 161 controls were purely radioclinical, 30 required a new needle biopsy for security.

In the case of an unanimously malignant quartet or discord, a surgical control was carried out, except in special cases. This group included 130 cases with 111 stereotactic needle biopsies, 18 biopsies without, and 1 with echography. The exeresis took place in the month following the needle biopsy after location by large needle in the great majority of cases.

In our study, tests were considered positive where cytohistological results favored A.E.H. or cancer, and as negative in normal, dystrophic samples or those with moderate regular hyperplasia without atypism (R.E.H.).

Non-contributory samples were not considered as negative tests, but more as a diagnostic failure, not entering into the various statistical calculations.

Concerning the group of women not undergoing surgery, no cellular atypism was notable for contributory samples ; radioclinical follow-up revealed no progressive pathology.

For the group of cases with surgical intervention, among the 111 stereotactic needle biopsies performed, 11 were insufficient (or 10 % of all cases). The biopsy sample furnished sufficient material in 90 % of cases. This figure went up to 98 % when cytoaspiration was added.

The evolution of rates over time revealed that with 16 and 18 G needles, 9 samples out of 47 were judged non-significant, or 19 % of cases ; with 14 G needles, only 2 samples out of 64 were insufficient, or 3 % of cases.

The malignant samples numbered 46, with 45 true positives. One relative false positive corresponded to a cluster of A.E.H. with type B opacity.

The tumors detected were essentially infraclinical, of which 57 % were smaller than 1 cm. The dimensions varied from 3 to 30 millimeters with a mean diameter of 14 millimeters.

The sensitivity of microbiopsies done in an isolated manner was 96 % and its specificitywas 94 %.

The results of cytoaspiration revealed 8 % of insufficient samples in a relatively consistent manner from 1990 to 1992 with a sensitivity of 82 % and a specificity of 95 %.

Combining the results of cytoaspiration with those of microbiopsy, we obtained 98 % of samples contributory to diagnosis, a sensitivity of 94 % and a specificity of 95 %.

The two methods combined distinctly improved the performance of cytology, especially concerning sensitivity.

Present development in screening and the progress of imaging are considerably multiplying the number of patients for whom surgical exploration can be discussed faced with a "doubtful" lesion. there is unquestionably a very great risk of surgical inflation with all the excesses and disadvantages which that engenders. At the same time, interventional imaging in the form of cytopunctures and stereotactic microbiopsy is developing with success. Microbiopsies are becoming more and more reliable at the price of a simple gesture, less traumatic for the patient, but also more economical for society.

With the result that finally it appears that traditional surgery and microbiopsy should no longer be presented as being in competition, but, on the contrary, in terms of being complementary. In this spirit, microbiopsies would be used essentially to lower the rate, still much too high, of benign lesions being surgically explored.

Mastology - Breast Diseases
A.S.S. Figueira Fo et al., editors.

PERCUTANEOUS NEEDLE BIOPSY OF THE BREAST

Bruno D Fornage
Department of Diagnostic Radiology
The University of Texas M. D. Anderson Cancer Center, Houston, Texas

Percutaneous needle aspiration biopsy of palpable breast masses was popularized in the 1970's in Sweden. Today, mammography and sonography (US) can be used to guide the insertion of fine or large-core needles into nonpalpable breast lesions. Because a hematoma may interfere with subsequent imaging, any attempt at percutaneous biopsy of the breast should be performed after completion of mammographic and US examinations.

Fine-needle aspiration biopsy

FNA is a quick, accurate, safe, and low-cost procedure. It causes very little discomfort and can be repeated, if necessary. Experience in every step is needed to yield optimal results. Whatever the guidance technique employed, the success of FNA depends on (a) the skills of the operator in hitting the target, (b) successful tissue extraction (which depends on the operator's technique and the cellularity of the tumor), (c) adequate preparation of the smears, and (d) interpretation by an expert cytopathologist.

Standard, hypodermic, 20- to 22-gauge, 1.5-inch (3.8-cm) needles are used. The "no-aspiration" sampling technique has proved to work as well as the conventional suction technique. Local anesthetization is usually unnecessary for FNA. After the needle has penetrated the lesion, the needle is moved to and fro and rotated in a corkscrew maneuver to detach some of the tumor tissue. With the rapid Papanicolaou stain, a diagnosis can be obtained within 15 minutes.

Complications of FNA are virtually inexistent. At most a local hematoma may develop, usually in the surrounding fat.

FNA is highly accurate in the diagnosis of breast cancer and it can further characterize certain special forms of malignancy and metastases to the breast. The hormonal receptor status of the tumor is now routinely assayed in fine-needle aspirates using various techniques. Other new cytologic studies include the evaluation of proliferation markers (DNA ploidy, Ki-67). Cytology can also establish the diagnosis of many benign conditions, including fibroadenomas, fat necrosis, and intramammary lymph nodes with reliability, if rigorous cytologic criteria are used.

Inadequate specimens include acellular or insufficient smears or smears contaminated with excessive blood. They have no diagnostic value at all, and no assumption should be made regarding the tumor they were obtained from; the procedure must be repeated. Inadequate specimens usually result from a deficient aspiration technique (whatever the guidance technique employed) and are also more likely to occur with firm, fibrous tumors. The widespread practice of excluding inadequate specimens when calculating the sensitivity and specificity of FNA should be abandoned because the flattering results obtained do not reflect the actual performance and usefulness of the technique in everyday practice.

Cutting needle biopsy

Large-bore (18-14 gauge) guillotine (Tru-cut®) needles have been favored by some clinicians because they reliably yield a tissue core that can be readily interpreted by any pathologist. Recently, various automatic spring-loaded biopsy devices known as biopsy guns (Biopty®, Argovac®), which activate a cutting needle automatically in a fraction of a second have been commercialized. Disadvantages of Tru-cut® needle biopsies include the need for local anesthetization, more discomfort to the patient, and the limitation of sampling along a single axis, thus requiring multiple passes. Also, exceptional cases of malignant seeding along the needle tract have been observed.

Stereotaxic guidance

Until recently, because only pairs of orthogonal mammographic projections were available for guidance, the placement of a biopsy needle in small lesions was not reliable. The interest of radiologists in mammographically guided needle biopsy of nonpalpable breast lesions has been revived through the development of the stereotaxic method.

The general principle of stereotaxic guidance is that the three-dimensional coordinates of a given point in the volume radiographed can be calculated from two stereoradiographs taken at an angle of ±15° in relation to the central beam direction. First, the breast is positioned so that the target lesion projects through the window of the compression plate. Then, two stereoradiographs are exposed on the same film, after shifting of the cassette. The scales on the sides of the two views allow measurement of the coordinates of the target along the X and Y axes on both views. These values are processed by a microcomputer, which calculates the third coordinate (depth) of the target. Knowing the overall length of the biopsy needle to be used, the operator can then adjust the needle guide's position in such a way that the needle tip will lie at the selected point within the target after full insertion of the needle. The use of large-core needle biopsy has become the standard with stereotaxic guidance, primarily because this technique is mostly applied to calcifications and because only a core can allow the pathologist to determine whether a carcinoma is invasive.

Stereotaxic guidance is highly accurate, with the needle tip being placed usually within a distance of 1-2 mm from the selected target point. Despite the recent advent of near-real-time digital mammographic display and image manipulation, stereotactically guided needle biopsy remains a long procedure (30 minutes on average), during which the compression is maintained and the patient should not move at all. Another limitation is that the technique cannot be applied to extramammary lesions, e.g., lymph nodes and peripheral lesion, which cannot be included in the mammographic projection.

US guidance

Recent mammograms should be carefully examined before the US procedure is undertaken to make certain that the lesion seen on US correlates perfectly with the suspicious mammographic abnormality. High-frequency (7.5-MHz) hand-held transducers are required to delineate small lesions. Linear-array transducers are superior to sector scanners because of their higher resolution in the near-field and their wider field of view. The probe is soaked in alcohol for a few minutes. Depending on the location of the tumor, the patient is placed in a dorsal decubitus or oblique position, to spread the breast on the chest wall. Alcohol is used to cleanse the skin and also serves as an acoustic coupling medium. The probe is then placed in direct contact with the skin and the lesion is localized.

The needle is inserted along the scan plane, obliquely from one end of the transducer. Both the tip and the distal portion of the needle are continuously displayed, which results in utmost accuracy and safety. Real-time guidance is instrumental in confirming needle penetration into mobile targets such as fibroadenomas embedded in loose fat, which often move away from the needle and represent a known source of failure of stereotaxic guidance.

With FNA, when the needle has reached the target, sampling is begun as described above. The no-aspiration technique leaves one hand available to hold the transducer and thus allows continuous monitoring of both the needle insertion and sampling. US-guided aspiration of a cyst takes a few seconds. Sampling of solid masses takes about 30 to 40 seconds.

With automatic cutting needle devices, the most horizontal position of the needle is chosen to exclude any risk of hitting the chest wall after the needle has been fired. For safety purposes, it is crucial to always keep in mind the length of the needle's throw and project it on the scan to have an accurate estimation of where the needle tip will lie on the post-fire scan. In the case of masses—US cannot be used for isolated microcalcifications—3 to 5 cores are taken. With the 18-gauge full-cylinder (punch) cutting needle (Argovac®) that we use, there is no need for a skin nick and the throw can be conveniently adjusted from 1 to 4 cm. Satisfactory cores are consistently obtained with this full cylinder core cutting needle (compared with the half-cylinder core of the guillotine-type needles).

US versus stereotaxic guidance for nonpalpable masses. Which technique to use?

Whatever the guidance technique, cytologic results must be correlated with the mammographic and/or US appearances and any discrepancy carefully

reevaluated.
Advantages of US guidance include real-time monitoring of the needle, which guarantees accuracy and safety; the shortest needle pathway; low cost; rapidity; a limited number of passes; and therefore an excellent tolerance by the patient. US guidance is applicable to lesions that are poorly seen or not visible on mammograms and well demonstrated on US, such as lesions in dense or augmented breasts. It is also ideal for FNA of nonpalpable masses in the axilla or infraclavicular region. Disadvantages include the inapplicability to isolated microcalcifications and to very small masses and the operator dependence of the procedure.
Isolated microcalcifications, focal areas of architectural distortion, and minute masses cannot be visualized on US scans and require stereotaxic guidance. On the other hand, in our experience, the vast majority of masses detected on mammograms can be visualized on sonograms and US-guided needle biopsy is preferred because of its accuracy, rapidity, and remarkable tolerance by the patient. Not infrequently in dense breasts, indeterminate focal lesions ranging from atypical cysts to small carcinomas are detected by US alone. In such cases, needle biopsy can be performed only under US guidance.

Although they overlap, the indications for the two guidance techniques also show complementarity. It would be beneficial for radiologists who have an interest in breast biopsy to become expert in both techniques so that in any given patient they could use the most appropriate technique in terms of cost-effectiveness (in particular, time consumption) and patient tolerance.

Suggested reading

Zajdela A., Zillhardt P., Voillemot N.: Cytological diagnosis by fine needle sampling without aspiration. Cancer, 1987, 59, 1201-1205.

Wanebo H.J., Feldman P.S., Wilhelm M.C., Covell J.L., Binns R.L.: Fine needle aspiration cytology in lieu of open biopsy in management of primary breast cancer. Ann. Surg., 1984, 199, 569-579.

Flowers J.L., Burton G.V., Cox E.B., et al.: Use of monoclonal antiestrogen receptor antibody to evaluate estrogen receptor content in fine needle aspiration breast biopsies. Ann. Surg., 1986, 203, 250-254.

Shabot M.M., Goldberg I.M., Schick P., Nieberg R., Pilch Y.H.: Aspiration cytology is superior to Tru-Cut® needle biopsy in establishing the diagnosis of clinically suspicious breast masses. Ann. Surg., 1982, 196, 122-126.

Fornage B.D., Faroux M.J., Simatos A.: Breast masses: US-guided fine-needle aspiration biopsy. Radiology, 1987, 162, 409-414.

Fornage B.D.: A simple phantom for training in ultrasound-guided needle biopsy using the freehand technique. J. Ultrasound Med., 8, 701-703, 1989.

Fornage B.D.: Interventional ultrasound of the breast. In: McGahan J.P. (ed). Baltimore, Williams & Wilkins, 1989, pp. 71-83.

Fornage BD, Coan JD, David CL. Ultrasound-guided needle biopsy of the breast and other interventional procedures. Radiol Clin North Am 1992;30:167-185.

Fornage BD, Sneige N, Singletary SE. Masses in breasts with implants: Diagnosis with US-guided fine-needle aspiration biopsy. Radiology (in press).

Sneige N, Fornage BD, Saleh G. Ultrasound-guided fine-needle aspiration of nonpalpable breast lesions: Cytologic and histologic findings. Am J Clin Pathol (in press).

Gordon PB, Goldenberg SL, Chan NHL. Solid breast lesions: Diagnosis with US-guided fine-needle aspiration biopsy. Radiology 1993;189:573-580.

Parker SH, Jobe WE, Dennis MA, Stavros AT, Johnson KK, Yakes WF, Truell JE, Price JG, Kortz AB, Clark DG. US-guided automated large-core breast biopsy. Radiology 1993;187:507-511.

Liberman L, Evans WP III, Dershaw DD, Hann LE, Deutch BM, Abramson AF, Rosen PP. Radiography of microcalcifications in sterotaxic mammary core biopsy specimens. Radiology 1994;190:223-225.

Lovin JD, Sinton EB, Burke BJ, Reddy VV. Stereotaxic core breast biopsy: Value in providing tissue for flow cytometric analysis. AJR Am J Roentgenol 1994;162:609-612.

Schackmuth M, Harlow CL, Norton LW. Milk fistula: A complication after core breast biopsy. AJR Am J Roentgenol 1993;161:961-962.

Meyer JE, Lester SC, Frenna TH, White FV. Occult breast calcifications sampled with large-core biopsy: Confirmation with radiography of the specimen. Radiology 1993;188:581-582.

Sickles EA, Parker SH. Appropriate role of core breast biopsy in the management of probably benign lesions. Radiology 1993;188:315.

Parker SH, Lovin JD, Jobe WE, Burke BJ, Hopper KD, Yakes WF. Nonpalpable breast lesions: Stereotactic automated large-core biopsies. Radiology 1991;180:403-407.

Harter LP, Swengros J, Ponto G, Craig PH. Malignant seeding of the needle track during stereotaxic core needle breast biopsy. Radiology 1992;185:713-714.

Elvecrog EL, Lechner MC, Nelson MT. Nonpalpable breast lesions: Correlation of stereotaxic large-core needle biopsy and surgical biopsy results. Radiology 1993;188:453-455.

Ciatto S, Catarzi S, Morrone D, Rosselli Del Turco M. Fine-needle aspiration cytology of nonpalpable breast lesions: US versus stereotaxic guidance. Radiology 1993;188:195-198.

Mastology - Breast Diseases
A.S.S. Figueira Fo et al., editors.

Guided needle biopsy of nonpalpable breast masses

Bruno D. Fornage, M.D.

Department of Diagnostic Radiology, The University of Texas M. D. Anderson Cancer Center, 1515 Holcombe Blvd., Houston, Texas 77030 USA.

Abstract

Indications for percutaneous needle aspiration biopsy of nonpalpable breast lesions have increased because of the widespread use of screening mammography and the concomitant desire to reduce the number of unnecessary surgical biopsies for these lesions. The techniques of fine-needle aspiration biopsy and large-core cutting-needle biopsy guided by stereotaxic mammography and real-time high-frequency sonography are discussed. Stereotaxy is the only technique applicable to microcalcifications and minute masses that cannot be seen on sonograms. With few exceptions, discrete masses larger than 0.7-0.8 cm can be visualized on high-frequency sonograms. Because of the continuous real-time monitoring of the needle's position and of the sampling procedure, sonographically guided needle biopsy has proved to be highly accurate and safe in experienced hands. The procedure is expeditious and well accepted by patients. Percutaneous needle biopsy of breast lesions requires teamwork, and its success also relies heavily on the expertise of the pathologist. With stereotaxic or sonographic guidance, there is a learning curve before optimal results will be achieved and training on phantoms is therefore recommended.

Because of the overlap between the imaging characteristics of benign and malignant lesions in the breast, a biopsy is required not infrequently. Needle biopsy of nonpalpable lesions with guidance by mammography or sonography (US) is expected to reduce the number of unnecessary open biopsies (1). The two most popular techniques are fine-needle aspiration biopsy (FNA) and large-core needle biopsy (LCNB). Because a hematoma may interfere with subsequent imaging, any attempt at percutaneous biopsy of the breast should be performed after completion of mammographic and US examinations.

Fine-needle aspiration biopsy

FNA is a quick, accurate, safe, and relatively inexpensive procedure. It causes very little discomfort and can be repeated if necessary. Experience is needed to yield optimal results. Whatever the guidance technique employed, the success of FNA depends on (a) the skills of the operator in hitting the target, (b) successful tissue extraction (which depends on the operator's technique and the cellularity of the tumor), (c) adequate preparation of the smears, and (d) interpretation by an expert cytopathologist.

Standard, 20- to 22-gauge, 1.5-inch (3.8-cm) hypodermic needles are used. Local anesthetization is usually unnecessary for FNA. For several years, we have been using the "no-aspiration" sampling technique, which has proved to work as well as the conventional suction technique. After the needle has penetrated the lesion, the needle is moved to and fro and rotated in a corkscrew maneuver to detach some of the tumor tissue. The capillarity force drives the dissociated material into the lumen spontaneously (2). Then a syringe is used to expel the material onto slides. With the rapid Papanicolaou stain, a diagnosis can be obtained within 15 minutes. Complications of FNA are virtually nonexistent. At most, a local hematoma may develop, usually in the surrounding fat.

FNA is highly accurate in the diagnosis of breast cancer, and it can further characterize certain forms of malignancy and metastases to the breast. The diagnosis of malignancy is often obtained with a single pass (3, 4). The estrogen- and progesterone-receptor status of the tumor is now routinely assayed in fine-needle aspirates (5). Other new cytologic studies include the evaluation of proliferation markers (DNA ploidy, Ki-67). Cytology can also establish the diagnosis of many benign conditions, including fibroadenomas, fat necrosis, and intramammary lymph nodes with reliability if rigorous cytologic criteria are used (6).

Inadequate specimens include acellular or insufficient smears or smears contaminated with excessive blood. These have *no* diagnostic value, and no assumption should be made regarding the tumor from which they were obtained; the procedure must be repeated. Inadequate specimens are usually due to a deficient aspiration technique (whatever the guidance technique employed) or to the presence of firm, fibrous tumors. The widespread practice of excluding inadequate specimens when calculating the sensitivity and specificity of FNA should be abandoned because the flattering results obtained do not reflect the actual usefulness of the technique in everyday practice (7).

Large-core needle biopsy

Biopsy using large-core (14- to 18-gauge), guillotine-type (Tru-cut®) needles has been favored by some clinicians because it reliably yields a tissue core that can be interpreted by any pathologist. Recently, various automatic spring-loaded biopsy devices known as biopsy guns (e.g., Biopty®, Argovac®), which activate a cutting needle automatically in a fraction of a second, have become commercially available. When large-core needles are used, local anesthetization is mandatory. Disadvantages of LCNB include the inability to aspirate or inject fluid or air, the difficulty in controlling the pathway of the needle in the case of a minute, mobile mass, and the limitation of sampling along a single axis, thus requiring multiple passes. Also, complications such as malignant seeding along the needle track and milk fistula have been observed (8, 9). Advantages og LCNB include the recovery of a large amount of material and the ability to perform histopathologic analysis, thus enabling differentiation of invasive from in situ carcinomas. Because expert cytopathologists are available at our institution, LCNB is reserved for cases in which FNA previously failed (most commonly with fibroadenomas) and knowledge of the tumor's invasiveness will affect management.

US guidance

As a rule, US cannot visualize isolated microcalcifications. Therefore, US guidance can be used for masses only. Recent mammograms should be carefully examined before the US procedure is undertaken to make certain that the lesion seen on US correlates perfectly with the suspicious mammographic abnormality (10). High-frequency (7.5- or 10-MHz) linear-array transducers are required to delineate small lesions. The probe is first soaked in rubbing alcohol for a few minutes. Depending on the location of the tumor, the patient is placed in a dorsal decubitus or oblique position to spread the breast on the chest wall. For FNA, alcohol is used to cleanse the skin and also to serve as an acoustic coupling medium (11). For LCNB with large (14-gauge) cutting needles, the skin should be prepared with an iodine solution (Betadine) and local anesthetics given.

The probe is then placed in direct contact with the skin and the lesion is localized. The needle is inserted along the scan plane, obliquely from one end of the transducer. This can be done "freehand" or with the use of a needle guide that clips to the transducer. Both the tip and the distal portion of the needle are continuously displayed, which results in utmost accuracy and safety in the placement of the needle. Real-time monitoring is instrumental in confirming needle penetration into mobile targets such as fibroadenomas embedded in loose fat; such lesions often move away from the needle and are a well-known source of failure of stereotaxic guidance. US guidance is also ideal for performing FNA of a mass lying near a breast prosthesis (12).

With FNA, when the needle has reached the target, sampling is begun as described above. The no-aspiration technique leaves one hand available to hold the transducer and thus allows continuous monitoring of both the needle insertion and sampling (3). Sampling of solid masses takes about 30 to 40 seconds. US-guided aspiration of a cyst takes only a few seconds.

For LCNB with automatic cutting needle devices, the most horizontal needle path is chosen to exclude any risk of hitting the chest wall after the needle has been fired (13). It is critical to always keep in mind the length of the needle's throw and project it mentally on the monitor to provide an accurate estimation of where the needle tip will lie on the post-fire scan. In the case of solid masses 3 to 5 cores are taken. With the 18-gauge full-cylinder (punch) cutting needle (Argovac®) that we use, there is no need for a skin nick, and the throw can be conveniently adjusted from 1 to 4 cm depending on the size of the lesion and of the breast. Satisfactory cores are consistently obtained with this full-cylinder core cutting needle (compared with the half-cylinder core of the guillotine-type needles).

Stereotaxic guidance

Until recently, because only pairs of orthogonal mammographic projections were available for guidance, the placement of a biopsy needle in small lesions was not reliable. However, the interest of radiologists in mammographically guided needle biopsy of nonpalpable breast lesions has been revived with the development of the stereotaxic method (14, 15). The general principle of stereotaxic guidance is that the three-dimensional coordinates of a given point in the volume radiographed can be calculated from two stereoradiographs taken at angles of ±15° in relation to the central beam direction. First, the breast is positioned so that the target lesion is seen through the window of the compression plate. Then, two stereoradiographs are exposed on the same film, after shifting of the cassette. The scales on the sides of the two views allow measurement of the coordinates of the target along the X and Y axes on each view. These values are processed by a microcomputer, which calculates the third coordinate (depth) of the target. By knowing the overall length of the biopsy needle to be used, the operator can then adjust the needle guide's position so that the needle tip will lie at the selected point within the target after full insertion.

Stereotaxic guidance is highly accurate, with the needle tip being placed usually within 1 to 2 mm from the selected target point. In the case of isolated microcalcifications, it is recommended that radiographs of the cores be obtained to determine the presence or absence of the suspicious calcifications in the specimen, as is done for surgical specimens (16, 17). Despite the recent advent of near-real-time digital mammographic display and image manipulation, stereotaxically guided needle biopsy remains a long procedure (30 minutes on average), during which breast compression is maintained and the patient should not move. Another limitation is that the technique cannot be used for extramammary lesions, e.g., lymph nodes and peripheral lesions, which cannot be included in the mammographic projection.

US versus stereotaxic guidance for nonpalpable masses: Which technique to use?

Needle biopsy of the breast is a team effort that involves the radiologist, the pathologist, and the surgeon. Whatever the guidance technique, pathologic results must be correlated with those of the physical, mammographic, and/or US examinations and any discrepancy carefully reevaluated.

Advantages of US guidance include real-time monitoring of the needle, which guarantees accuracy and safety; the shortest needle pathway; low cost; rapidity; a limited number of passes; and, therefore, excellent tolerance of the procedure by patients (18, 19). US guidance is applicable to lesions that are poorly seen or not visible on mammograms but well demonstrated on US, such as lesions in dense or augmented breasts. It is also ideal for FNA of nonpalpable masses in the axilla or infraclavicular region. Disadvantages of US guidance include its inapplicability to isolated microcalcifications, focal areas of architectural distortion, and minute masses (all of which require stereotaxic guidance, and the dependence of the procedure's success on operator skill.

Radiologists who have an interest in breast biopsy should become expert in both techniques so that in any given patient they can use the most appropriate technique in terms of type of lesion, cost-effectiveness, time consumption, and patient tolerance. Both stereotaxy and US guidance require proper training, for which phantoms are available (20).

References

1. Wanebo HJ, Feldman PS, Wilhelm MC, Covell JL, Binns RL: Fine needle aspiration cytology in lieu of open biopsy in management of primary breast cancer. Ann Surg 1984;199:569-579.

2. Zajdela A, Zillhardt P, Voillemot N: Cytological diagnosis by fine needle sampling without aspiration. Cancer 1987;59:1201-1205.

3. Fornage BD, Coan JD, David CL. Ultrasound-guided needle biopsy of the breast and other interventional procedures. Radiol Clin North Am 1992;30:167-185.

4. Gordon PB, Goldenberg SL, Chan NHL. Solid breast lesions: Diagnosis with US-guided fine-needle aspiration biopsy. Radiology 1993;189:573-580.

5. Flowers JL, Burton GV, Cox EB et al. Use of monoclonal antiestrogen receptor antibody to evaluate estrogen receptor content in fine needle aspiration breast biopsies. Ann Surg 1986;203:250-254.

6. Sneige N, Fornage BD, Saleh G. Ultrasound-guided fine-needle aspiration of nonpalpable breast lesions: Cytologic and histologic findings. Am J Clin Pathol (in press).

7. Fornage BD. Guided fine-needle aspiration biopsy of nonpalpable breast lesions: Calculation of accuracy values (letter). Radiology 1990;177:884-885.

8. Harter LP, Swengros J, Ponto G, Craig PH. Malignant seeding of the needle track during stereotaxic core needle breast biopsy. Radiology 1992;185:713-714.

9. Schackmuth □M, Harlow CL, Norton LW. Milk fistula: A complication after core breast biopsy. AJR Am J Roentgenol 1993;161:961-962.

10. Fornage BD: Interventional ultrasound of the breast. In: McGahan JP (ed). Interventional Ultrasound. Baltimore, Williams & Wilkins, 1989, pp 71-83.

11. Fornage BD, Faroux MJ, Simatos A: Breast masses: US-guided fine-needle aspiration biopsy. Radiology 1987;162:409-414.

12. Fornage BD, Sneige N, Singletary SE. Masses in breasts with implants: Diagnosis with US-guided fine-needle aspiration biopsy. Radiology (in press).

13. Parker SH, Jobe WE, Dennis MA, Stavros AT, Johnson KK, Yakes WF, Truell JE, Price JG, Kortz AB, Clark DG. US-guided automated large-core breast biopsy. Radiology 1993;187:507-511.

14. Parker SH, Lovin JD, Jobe WE, Burke BJ, Hopper KD, Yakes WF. Nonpalpable breast lesions: Stereotactic automated large-core biopsies. Radiology 1991;180:403-407.

15. Elvecrog EL, Lechner MC, Nelson MT. Nonpalpable breast lesions: Correlation of stereotaxic large-core needle biopsy and surgical biopsy results. Radiology 1993;188:453-455.

16. Liberman L, Evans WP III, Dershaw DD, Hann LE, Deutch BM, Abramson AF, Rosen PP. Radiography of microcalcifications in sterotaxic mammary core biopsy specimens. Radiology 1994;190:223-225.

17. Meyer JE, Lester SC, Frenna TH, White FV. Occult breast

calcifications sampled with large-core biopsy: Confirmation with radiography of the specimen. Radiology 1993;188:581-582.

18. Fornage BD. Percutaneous biopsies of the breast: State of the art. Cardiovasc Intervent Radiol 1991;14:29-39.

19. Ciatto S, Catarzi S, Morrone D, Rosselli Del Turco M. Fine-needle aspiration cytology of nonpalpable breast lesions: US versus stereotaxic guidance. Radiology 1993;188:195-198.

20. Fornage BD: A simple phantom for training in ultrasound-guided needle biopsy using the freehand technique. J Ultrasound Med 1989; 8:701-703.

Mastology - Breast Diseases
A.S.S. Figueira Fo et al., editors.

Fine needle aspiration biopsy: importance of the cytologist during the removal of the material and analysis of the samples. A study of 1938 cases.

Cláudio Kemp, Geraldo Rodrigues de Lima.
(1) Assistant and (2) Titular Professors at the Discipline of gynecology of the Escola Paulista de Medicina.

Address for correspondence: Rua Dr.Bacelar, 333 - Vila Clementino - 04026001, São Paulo/SP, Brazil.

Abstract - The present study reports the experience of our cytology Unit concerning the utilization of the fine needle aspiration biopsy since 1985, reaching a total of 1938 cases. The method demonstrated a 91.7% sensibility, 99% specificity and 95.7% accuracy. The respective predictive values for positiveness and malignancy were 98.7% and 93.5%. When suspicious results (10%) and insufficient material (17.6%) were included; the specificity, sensibility and accuracy dropped to 68%, 70% and 78% respectively. These data suggest that the disparity in the results is due to the cytologist's inexperience in removing or reading the samples, and that the method is of high predictivity.

Text - The fine needle aspiration biopsy is a widely accepted method that has also achieved increasingly support in our sphere. Several publications have praised its precision and given prominence to its value as the favourite method for the preoperative diagnosis of mammary tumors (1,3,5,7). This method has been ordinarily applied by the Mastology Unit of the discipline of gynecology of the Escola Paulista de Medicina since 1985 and the correlation between the positive and negative cytological results and the histopathological findings in 261 initial cases is presented in table I. The analysis of these results generated a specificity of 99%; 91.7% of sensibility and 95.7% of accuracy, therefore being in agreement with the existent literature. The inclusion of the suspicious results and inadequate material gave rise to a wide variability of figures. The specificity was reduced to 68%, the sensibilty was of 70% and the accuracy, 68%. Among the main reasons for these unequal results are the inaccurate collection of the material, reading of the slides by various cytologists, mainly when the latter were not used to the method (1,2,3,7,10,11). The value of these statements are exposed in tables II, III and IV. The evaluation of the fluctuations in the percentage of inadequate material whenever one or more examinators were involved in the collection can be visualized in table II. The amount of insufficient material increased from 5.1% to 22.9%, owing to the fact that the collection of the samples by a single examinator during an initial period was subsequently performed by various examinators, which in our case can be explained by the execution of this service by medical students under constant recyding. The cytological results from July/1985 to April/1994 are presented in table III. These results, converted into percentage and separated year by year (Table IV) give clear evidence of the increase in the amount of insufficient material (44%) and suspicions results in 1990. Moreover, there was a reduction in the number of positive and negative cytological reports. This period coincides exactly with that of the cytology Unit's chief's severe illness and decease. Thereafter, we could observe a tendency to the normalization of the cytological reports during subsequent years, revealing the gain of experience by the new examinator in charge. Although this technique is relatively simple, we could verify that the skillfulness to perform it, i.e., the readiness of movements, needle guidance, maintenance of a constant and sufficient negative pressure as will as the examinator's sensibility on choosing the best site for the aspiration and the macroscopic judgement of the aspirate were of major importance during the obtention of samples. The lesions in study also influence the attained specimens through the supply of insufficient material, as in those with massive fibrosis, which could be benign or malignant, e.g., the fibrocystic alterations and the scirrhous carcinoma; in addition to other entities such as lipoma and infections processes (5,7,10). Another cause of divergence is the percentage of suspicious results, which ranges from 0.5 to 12.4% (1,5,8,10,11). The suspicious report may result from the cytologist's inexperience (table IV), little cellularity and the histological differentiation degree (4). Another possibility to be considered is the problem of false results. In our series, only one false positive result was reported (during the initial phase) from a total of 1938 cases. It was a lump sited in the intersection of the lateral quadrants of which an anatomopathological investigation revealed a lymphonodal hyperplasia. False negative findings may derive material insufficiency and the high degree of cellular differentiation of tumors. The evaluation of these data allows us to consider the utilization of the method as a valuable propedeutic tool for the diagnosis of mammary tumors. It also reveals the major importance of the examinator's experience for the adequate obtention of material and subsequent analyses of the samples. The high predictive value obtained through this method for malignancy (98.7%) is of prime importance for clinical use, enabling the selection of patients who need internation, supplementary examinations for the staging of the tumor, preparation and previous discussion about the treatment. This method also makes possible the use of techniques that have already been initiated in the cytology Unit.; e.g., the immunocytochemical technique, which allows the determination of the hormonal status (10) and parameters of proliferative activity (6) in a preoperative stage;

enabling the guidance of the neo-adjuvant systemic therapeutics.

Table I
Correlation between results of 261 cases of F.N.A. and histopathological findings

cytology		Histopathology Malignant	Histopathology Benign
Positive	79	78	1
Negative	109	7	102
Suspicious	27	15	12
Insufficient	46	11	35
TOTAL	261	111	150

Analisys of Positive and Negative results
Sensibility = 91,7% Specificity = 99,0%
Predictive value + = 98,7% Predictive value - = 93,5%
Accuracy = 95,7%

Table II
Comparison of Insufficient cytological material results between single and various examinators.

Examinators	Period	No.cases	Insuff.	%
Single	July/85 July/86	78	4	5.1
Various	August/86 August/88	183	42	22.9
TOTAL		261	46	17.6

Table III
Cytological Results from 1985 to 1994

	85	86	87	88	89	90	91	92	93	94	TOTAL
P	9	6	35	43	25	42	31	26	36	13	266
N	51	60	115	103	68	67	65	83	113	61	766
S	1	6	19	28	16	46	35	50	32	10	243
I	20	32	47	56	47	96	90	109	117	49	663
T	81	104	216	230	156	251	201	268	298	133	1938

Table IV

see annex

Cytologic Results. Period 1985 to 1994

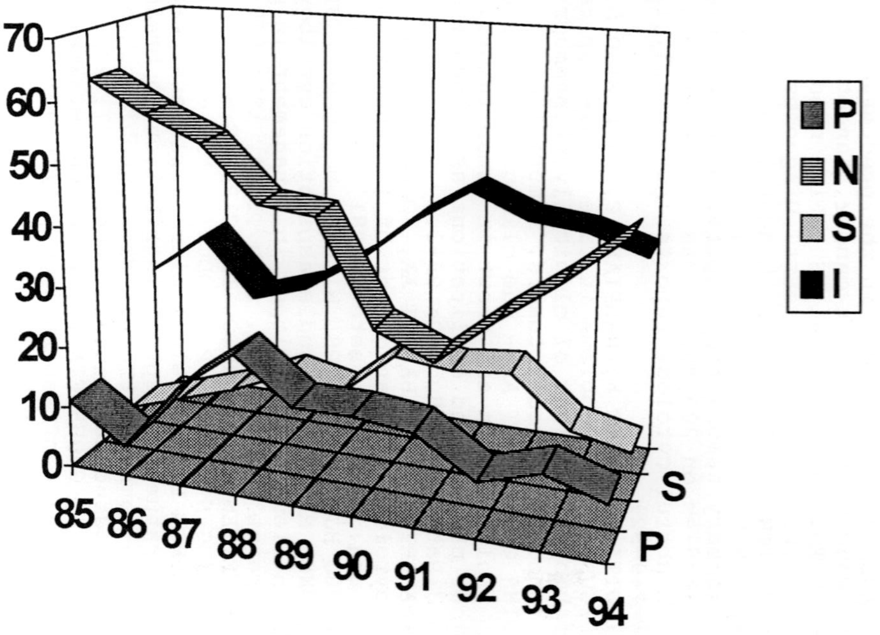

Value in % / Total 1.938 cases

Breast Unit Gynec. Disc. E.PM. Brazil

References

01 - DIXON JM, ANDERSON TJ, LAMB J, NIXON GJ, FORREST APM - Fine needle aspiration cytology, in relationship to clinical examination and mammography in the diagnosis of a solid breast mass. Br. J. surg.,1984, 179: 593-6.

02 - GARDECKI TIM, HOGBIN BM, MELACHER DH, SMITH RS - Aspiration cytology in the preoperative management of breast cancer. Lancet,1980, 2: 790-2.

03 - KLINE TS, JOSM LP, NEAL HS - Fine needle aspiration of the breast. Diagnoses and pitfalls: a review of 3545 cases. Cancer,1979, 44: 1458-64.

04 - KREUZER G & ZAJICEK J - Cytological diagnosis of mammary tumors from aspiration biopsy smears. III. Studies on 200 carcinomas with false negative or doubtful cytology reports. Acta cytol.,1972, 16: 249-52.

05 - PILOTTI S, RILKE F, DELPIANO C, DI PIETRO S, GUSSON A - Problems in fine needle aspiration biopsy cytology of clinically or mammographically uncertain breast tumors. Tumori,1982, 68: 407-12.

06 - QUINN CM, WRIGHT AN - The clinical. Assessment of proliferation and growt in human tumors: Evolution of methods and applications as prognostic variables. J.Pathol.;1990, 160: 93-1.

07 - STRAWBRIDGE HTG, BASSET AA, FOLDES I, - Role of cytologic in management of lesions of the breast. Surg. gynecol. Obstet.,1981, 152: 1-7.

08 - WANEBO HJ, FELDMAN PS, WILHELM MC, COVELL JL, BNNS RL - Fine needle aspiration cytology in lieu of open biopsy in management in primary breast cancer. Ann. Surg.,1984, 199: 569-79.

09 - VAN NETTEN JP, THORNTOU IG, CARLYLE SJ, BRIDGEN ML, COY P, GOODCHILD NL, GALLAGHER, S, GEORGE ES - Multiple microsample analysis of intratumor receptor distribution in breast cancers by a combined prochemical/imunohistochemical method. Eur. J. cancer. Clin. Oncol.,1987, 23: 1337-42.

10 - ZAJDELA A, GHOUSSEIN NA, PILLERON JP, ENNUEYER A - The value of aspirations cytology in the diagnostic of breast cancer: experience at the fundation curie. Cancer,1975, 35: 499-506.

11 - ZAJICEK J, FRANZEN S, JAKOBSSON P, RUBIO C, UNSAGRD B - Aspiration biopsy of mammary tumors in diagnosis and research: a critical review of 2200 cases. Acta cytol.,1967, 169-75.

II.4 Special Aspects

Mastology - Breast Diseases
A.S.S. Figueira Fo et al., editors.

THE ROLE OF THE COMPUTER IN BREAST IMAGING

Edward A. Sickles, M.D.

A conventional desktop microcomputer can be programmed to carry out a wide variety of activities that are useful in the operation and management of a mammography screening practice. These include entry, storage and retrieval of the records of screening examinations, direct entry of film interpretation data by the radiologist, automatic printing of boilerplate-text "normal" and "abnormal" examination reports, scheduling of screening appointments, tracking of follow-up procedures (including the generation of reminder letters to clients and referring physicians), and the conduct of medical audits of screening results.

Menu-driven turnkey software is widely available in the United States to perform some or all of these functions. Modern computer systems are highly reliable, but hardware breakdowns, software malfunctions, and power outages do occur, any of which can result in irretrievable loss of data, potentially crippling all operations. To ensure against the possibility of data loss, it is absolutely essential to make frequent (at least daily) back-up copies of all mammography data.

In general, computer-based activities can be completed more rapidly, more reliably, and at lower cost than the conventional operations they are designed to replace. All mammography screening practices can benefit from computer support.

The various computer functions described to support screening also can be adapted to work for a diagnostic mammography practice or for a practice that does not segregate screening from problem-solving examinations. In either circumstance, software will have to be adapted to record, store, display, and report the more complex findings and more varied management recommendations that are encountered in symptomatic patients. An extensive diagnostic coding system may be used, in which case specially tailored word-processing capabilities will be required to expand these codes into readily understandable text. Several commercially available applications already have been developed.

Additional roles for computer management have great promise but are not yet ready for general use. Digital imaging eventually may provide superior image quality and less expensive image archiving than current silver halide film recording systems; and software programs ultimately may be created that reliably identify and characterize undetected mammographic lesions, simultaneously instructing radiologists in image interpretation. However, these techniques are still not fully developed, their roles being experimental in nature.

References

1. Bates BF: A personal-computer reporting system for mammography. AJR 1988;151;1237-1239.

2. Chan H-P, Doi K, Vyborny CJ, Schmidt RA, Metz CE, Lam KL, Ogura T, Wu Y, MacMahon H. Improvement in radiologists' detection of clustered microcalcifications on mammograms: the potential of computer-aided diagnosis. Invest Radiol 1990; 25:1102-1110.

3. D'Orsi CJ, Getty DJ, Swets JA, Pickett RM, Seltzer SE, McNeil BJ. Reading and decision aids for improved accuracy and standardization of mammographic diagnosis, Radiology 1992; 184:619-622.

4. Frank MS. Computerized mammography data bse systems. Am J Roentgenol 1993; 161:287-290.

5. Haug PJ, Tocino IM, Clayton PD, Bair TL. Automated management of screening and diagnostic mammography.. Radiology 1987;164:747-752.

6. Monticciolo DL, Sickles EA. Computerized follow-up of abnormalities detected at mammography screening. AJR 1990;155:751-753.

7. Shtern F. Digital mammography and related technologies: a perspective from the National Cancer Institute. Radiology 1992; 183:629-630.

8. Sickles EA, Weber, WN, Galvin HB, Ominsky SH, Sollitto RA. Mammographic screening: how to operate successfully at low cost. Radiology 1986;160:95-97.

9. Sickles EA. The use of computers in mammography screening. Radiol Clin North Am 1987;25:1015-1030.

10. Sickles EA, Ominsky SH, Sollitto RA, Galvin HB, Monticciolo DL. Medical audit of a rapid-throughput mammography screening practice: methodology and results of 27,114 examinations. Radiology 1990;175:323-327.

11. Sickles EA. Usefulness of computers in managing the operation of a mammography screening practice. Am J Roentgenol 1990; 155:755-761.

12. Sickles EA. Current status of digital mammography. In Ioannidou-Mouzaka L, Agnantis NJ, Karydas I, eds. Senology. Amsterdam, Elsevier, 1992, pp 23-28.

13. Wu Y, Giger ML, Doi K, Vyborny CJ, Schmidt RA, Metz CE. Artificial neural networks in mammography: application to decision making in the diagnosis of breast cancer. Radiology 1993; 187:81-87.

Mastology - Breast Diseases
A.S.S. Figueira Fo et al., editors.

Combined diagnosis in breast cancer: Role of anatomic pathology

Marcelo Alvarenga, M.D.

State University of Campinas, Pathology Institute of Campinas,
Adress: Av. Francisco Glicério, 1867 13021.000 Campinas – SP Brazil

Abstract

Modern senology, like all medical subespecialty, must be practiced by a multidisciplinary group composed by surgeons, senologists, clinical oncologists, radiologists, radiotherapists, pathologists, cytopathologists and molecular biologists. For a complete pathologic diagnosis in breast biopsies, several requirements must be fulfilled: experienced pathologist and cytopathologist, careful gross and microscopic examinations, trained pathologists in frozen sections, multidisciplinary approach, diagnostic and prognostic information, active participation of all members of the multidisciplinary group in treatment decisions and continuous medical education.

Introduction

Examining breast biopsies, the anatomic pathologist must answer the main question: is it cancer or not? If the answer is 'no', it is not a cancer, the pathologist must especify if the benign lesion has or not some risk to develop into invasive breast carcinoma. Dupont and Page [1] and Tavassoli and Norris [2] assessed the relative risk for some histologic lesions. Women having proliferative lesions without atypia (moderate and florid ductal hyperplasia and sclerosing adenosis) had a risk of cancer that was 1,9 times and 1,7 times respectively, the risk in women with nonproliferative lesions (cyst, ductal ectasie, mild ductal hyperplasia and fibrosis). The risk in women with atypical hyperplasia was 5.3 times that in women with nonproliferative lesions. A family history of breast cancer, as well as calcification detected by mammography, elevated the cancer risk in patients with proliferative epitheliol lesions.

If the answer is 'yes', it is a cancer, the pathologist must evaluate all the prognostic factors, such as: tumor size, histologic type, histologic grade, nuclear grade, vascular invasion, lymph node status, invasion of skin, nipple and/or muscle, multicentricity, estrogen receptor status, oncogen analyses (c-erb-2) and ploidy of tumor cells.

Pathologic prognostic factors

There are several histologic types of breast carcinomas related with favorable prognosis: tubular, mucinous, papillary, medullary, adenoid cyst, invasive cribriform carcinoma, invasive ductal carcinoma with predominantly intraductal component and in situ carcinomas. The histologic types of breast carcinomas related with poor prognosis are: inflammatory carcinoma (dermal lymphatic carcinomatosis), lipid rich carcinoma, signet ring carcinoma, sarcomatoid carcinoma and neuroendocrine carcinoma ('oat cell type').

Histological documentation of metastasis to regional lymph nodes remains the most valuable currently accepted determinant of prognosis in breast cancer, according to Fisher et al [3]. The pathologist must specify the total number of lymph nodes involved by cancer, the level of metastatic axillary lymph nodes, the size of largest metastatic lymph nodes, the presence of solitary micrometastasis, the extranodal extension of tumor cells and the patterns of reaction in lymph nodes.

Value of deferred excision biopsy

There are several methods for pathologic diagnosis in breast cancer: fine needle aspiration cytology, needle biopsy for histologic examination, frozen section, incision biopsy and deferred excision biopsy. The deferred excision biopsy allows a complete study of the specimen with examination of multiple areas of the tumor and adjacent breast tissue, diagnosis of histologic type, histologic grade and nuclear grade. It also allows the exact measurement of the size of the invasive component of the primary tumor excluding the size of in situ component. This may change the clinical stanging of the tumor. Example: a 5,5 centimeter tumor (T3) with 5 centimeter of in situ component changes the postsurgical stage to pT1a.

The deferred excision biopsy allows the detection of microscopic skin invasion in superficial tumor as well as the detection of lymphatic vascular invasion by tumor cells. Examples: 1) a 2 centimeter tumor (T1) with skin invasion = pT4b; 2) a 3,5 centimeter tumor (T2) with dermal lymphatic carcinomatosis = pT4d. These informations given by the pathologist may change the extension of the patient surgical treatment.

Ductal carcinoma in situ and local recurrence

The pathologist play an important role in the diagnosis and treatment of ductal carcinoma in situ by given the following information: size of the tumor, number of involved ducts by cancer cells, histologic subtypes (comedo and non-comedo), microscopic evaluation of ressected margins and careful examination of ductal basement membrane to ruled out microinvasion.

It is also the pathologist's role to mention in the report all the factors related with influence in local recurrence after conservative treatment for breast cancer, such as: size of the invasive component of the primary tumor, involvement of ressected margins by in situ or invasive carcinoma, extensive in situ carcinoma within or adjacent to the primary invasive tumor and extensive vascular (lymphatic) invasion by tumor cells.

Diagnostic pitfalls in breast biopsies

To accomplish this important role in senology, the pathologist as well-all members of the multidisciplinary group, must be aware of several diagnostic pitfalls in breast biopsies:

1) Failure of the multidisciplinary mechanism. The pathologist ignores the reason for breast biopsy, particulary when suspicious calcifications were detected by mammography.
2) Inadequated gross specimen examination.
3) Frozen section difficulties.
4) Limited number of sections taken for microscopic examination.
5) Inadequated quality of histologic preparations.
6) Difficulty differential diagnostic problems:
   - atypical hyperplasia or in situ carcinoma
   - sclerosing adenosis or tubular carcinoma
   - intraductal papilloma or papillary carcinoma
   - phyllodes tumor: benign or malignant

References

1) Dupont WD, Page DL. N. Engl.J.Med. 1985; 312: 146-151
2) Tavassoli FA, Norris HJ. Cancer 1990; 65: 518-529.
3) Fisher ER, Sass R, Fisher B et al. Cancer 1984; 53: 712-723.

Mastology - Breast Diseases
A.S.S. Figueira Fo et al., editors.

QUALITY CONTROL TODAY IN BREAST PATHOLOGY

Geneviève Contesso, Christian Nezelof and Eric Peltier

Institut Gustave-Roussy, Villejuif, France

Abstract

Today, quality control in anatomic pathology is a necessity because the responsability of the pathologist is uppermost. The pathologist is the guardian of the sometimes unique specimen which must be used advisedly without being dilapidated.

Quality control in AP should comprise two steps : a type of internal quality assessment should be instituted in each laboratory. This review should address technical adequacy time required to report information, the contents and compilation of the report as well as the accuracy of the diagnosis itself. The second step, which is on a national and external level, is setting up a *"Committee of Wisemen"* responsible for establishing quality "norms". Each AP laboratory could be assessed for technical adequacy and the accuracy of diagnosis, by periodically sending a set of slides, randomly selected for control purposes to a voluntary service. Laboratories tested thus could pride themselves on this control and consider it a stamp of quality vis a vis their colleague clinicians or pathologists.

It is in the United States that Quality Control in Anatomic Pathology was first mentioned. As of 1940, the College of American Pathologists started to become interested in this question, and has, since the last 20 years, been relayed by the Association of Directors of Anatomic and Surgical Pathology and QA/QC Committee [1-7] In Great Britain the implementation of directives has also gained momentum. The same has not occurred in other European countries [8-15] and especially in France where the quality has only been initiated in cytology.

General considerations

The evaluation of the quality of a product or a service has proven necessary in recent years under the influence of consumer associations, health and safety committees , ethical committees and leaders responsable for the reputation of a profession, a corporation, a craft industry.

Medicine cannot escape this general law. This evaluation is desired, for patients in search of a greater margin of safety, by the medical association, responsible for medical ethics, by financial agencies , the National Health Insurance scheme, mutual benefit insurance schemes , private and public heath systems.

Today, Quality Control in anatomic pathology (AP) is becoming a necessity since the pathologist's responsability is uppermost. The entire orientation of the patient's treatment will depend on his diagnosis [16]. Now treatment protocols have become very diversified during recent years, so much so that the details in the final report are becoming increasingly numerous. Moreover, the reliability of the diagnosis of breast cancer , and in particular borderline lesions, in the framework of screening campaigns, is directly linked to this quality [17-18].

But a particular problem arises in anatomic pathology since the histopathological procedure comprises 2 separate parts : a technical part, namely the production of an objective document and a strictly medical part which is interpretative, clearly intellectual and more subjective.

1-The technical part of the document

First of all it is important to note that the pathologist is the guardian of samples, specimens which are sometimes unique, a sort of precious object . He must oversee specimen adequacy in terms of fixation and preservation. It must be used advisedly without being dilapidated. This is all the more important since samples are more and more reduced in size. For example, needle biopsies under sterotaxic guidance are becoming widespread.

The quality of the documents resulting from these specimens can be evaluated because this is permanent material which can be sent to others and submitted to complementary investigations. In particular :

a- in certain cases, such as that of samples obtained during screening of occult breast lesions, confronting histologic lesions and modifications discovered on mammograms involves a radiograph of the operative specimen [19] ;

b- the number of blocks is usually linked to the volume of the specimen and above all to the lesion. However, for all occult lesions, the average number of blocks included is significantly higher than that required for infiltrating carcinomas and run of the mill benign breast disease. Indeed, a complete slice must be included in "grid" pattern, with further sectioning of the suspicious area, i.e. on average 15 blocks per case [20] ;

c- the orientation of the specimen is crucial for , it will allow further sectioning if judged necessary. The number of blocks should be specified in the histologic report ;

d- labelling of specimens, using letters or numbers on a diagram sent to the surgeon allows a better comparison of clinical/radiologic signs and histologic findings ;

e- the status of the margins of an operative specimen, using indian ink, has now become mandatory due to an increase in "conservative" treatments. The tumor extent can be better evaluated and a specific area towards the invaded margin could eventually undergo further resection by the surgeon ;

f- the quality of the evaluation of lymph node involvement is appraised at several levels. The number of nodes dissected by the pathologist must be adequate, average, currently 15 per axilla, for a de-escalation has occurred in relation to the extensive axillary dissection during the sixties when the average number was more like 30. Nevertheless, if only 3 to 5 nodes are mentioned on the histologic report, then the quality of the dissection is questionable, unless it was done by a surgeon who was zealously economical ! Furthermore, the reliability of axillary assessment depends on the number of slices examined per node : in a study at the IGR, it was demonstrated that the inclusion of serially macroscopic slices of each node, increased the number of N+ nodes by at least 5 % [21] ;

g- the quality of fixation is a crucial step which conditions subsequent steps and can definitively render a slice illegible, more than the quality of the fixative itself. The amount of fixative used in relation to the volume of samples must at least respect a ratio of 2:3 as opposed to 1:3. Further cutting of certain bulky samples before fixation is indispensible. The duration of fixation is a function of the volume of the fragment undergoing fixation. The fixative solution must in certain cases be changed... Any error or negligence at this stage, be it precipitation or economy, will cause irreparable damage ;

h- the quality of cutting must avoid any scratching and/or folds ;

i- the quality of standard staining must be verified and staining solutions must be renewed or readjusted daily ;

j- storage of documents must be adequate for its conditions their retrieval.

The whole of this technical part can be easily and rapidly assessed. It is clear that apart from a few cases, it faithfully reflects the technical performance, technical competence and thus the quality of the laboratory. It is in fact more linked to the number of staff members and the conscientiousness of the histotechnologists than to the number and price of the various machines present in the laboratory which only provide secondary elements of appreciation.

In fact, all these different elements should appear on the histologic report as well as the clinical details accompanying the specimen.

Recently, new techniques such as immunohistochemistry, in situ hybridization, flow cytometry and others have burst upon the scene in anatomic pathology laboratories giving rise to, often for reasons of profitability, either excess complementary examinations which are not always justified or at the other end of the spectrum, penalisation of smaller laboratories, due to their cost. Furthermore, the control of quality of some of these new techniques has not been formulated nor has the incidence of these analyses on the prognosis and treatment [22]. Hence the very uncertain appraisal that can be offered and which has slowed down the development of quality control in anatomic pathology in France until now.

2-The medical, intellectual part

It concerns the interpretation of the document and proposing a diagnosis. Indeed, the cyto or histopathologic diagnosis is, like every medical procedure, a highly individual act, putting into the balance the observer's experience, alertness and wisdom. These are non tangible qualities which are difficult to assess and even more so to evaluate.

In addition, we should be aware that today, no consensus has been reached regarding the diagnosis of borderline lesions, as we realize when comparing the photos in the book of John Azzopardi to those of David Page. This variability in the interpretation of epithelial hyperplasia of the breast has been well demonstrated by the studies by Macartney and Beck and Rosai's and Schnitt's tests [11][23-25].

How to conduct quality control ?

Quality control in anatomic pathology must comprise two steps, as is the case in certain American Hospitals :

1- First of all a type of internal quality self-assessment should be implemented in each AP laboratory. In units of a certain size a small group composed of 2 histotechnologists, a secretary and a senior pathologist should be designated, who meet once a month and randomly select for control purposes cases that have been stored during the month.

This review should refer to a checklist which will vary according to the type of disease. It should include items concerning :

- the quality of the technical procedure (number of blocks, slice thickness, spreading and standard and special stain adequacy..) ;
- on the content and clarity of the written report ;
- as well as on the diagnosis itself, including that of the frozen section.

This first step will not only permit an improvement, if technical problems are discovered but additionally, reports can be rendered uniform based on the needs of clinicians and young pathologists can be educated.

With regard to the interpretation of the document, and proposing a diagnosis, the appraisable elements are only, in reality, indirect and evaluate :

- the rejection and multiplication of samples (number of blocks), ;

- the search for complementary biological or clinical information from clinicians ;

- requesting the opinion of colleagues who are more familiar with a particular disease, for which there is tangible evidence in the report or through the exchange of letters ;

- regularly frequenting post-graduate teaching staff, etc.

Obviously, these data are imperfect and lacking but they bear witness to a desire, on the part of the pathologist, to do the best that is possible. Furthermore, they are objective and relatively easy to demonstrate.

2- The second step, concerning national external quality assessment consists in setting up a committee of experts comprising both pathologists and histotechnologists recognized for their experience, based on the number of cases seen annually (in the past or currently) in a disease or a given technique and for their integrity, neutrality and independence. These experts could be enjoying early retirement or have just started their retirement. For histotechnologists, a period of training will be requested before their selection. This committee will be responsible for :

- establishing a uniform terminology for the diagnosis ;

- establishing quality "norms" : number of blocks, a minimal checklist for each disease which should be given with the final report [27] ;

- it could revise the national health fee schedule, which is ill-adapted to breast pathology in France. This would allow a more judicious breakdown of the fee schedule so that Anatomic pathology laboratories can work in better conditions.

As concerns the pratical implementation of the evaluation of AP laboratories, it will only be possible after completing the first step. Sets of randomly selected slides from the laboratory under examination will be sent to experts along with the corresponding histologic reports. The experts will only intervene in cases of divergent opinions whereupon, if need be, they may go to the laboratory concerned. This system will obviously require sponsors.

Subsequently, and according to the results of this first step, an evaluation of the diagnosis could be envisaged.

For whom is this quality control intended ?

Obviously, internal quality self-assessment should be an integral part of the organisation of every AP laboratory, especially as it does not require any extra investment.

With respect to external national quality assessment, during the initial phase every AP laboratory could be tested for the quality of the technical procedure as well as that of the diagnosis. They could then pride themselves on this control by considering it as a stamp of quality.

Above all, this quality control must be on a **voluntary** basis. It should not be enforced and laboratories should not be subjected to it, for it will fail in its objective.It is not supposed to punish a laboratory or a practitioner. It essentially aims at detecting shortcomings, inadequacies or errors. Its final objective is to advise, to help to find solutions permitting an improvement of the performance of individual pathologists and give a better image to the profession.

Acknowledgements to Lorna Saint Ange for the translation.

Bibliography

1- Howanitz PJ, Howanitz JH. Quality Assurance in Anatomic Pathology. in Laboratory Quality Assurance, New York, McGraw-Hill International Book Co,1987,pp.296-316.

2- Howanitz PJ, Walker K, Bacherer P. Quantification of errors in laboratory reports. A quality improvement study of the college of American Pathologists. Arch Pathol Lab Med 1992;116:694-700.

3- Association of Directors of Anatomic and Surgical pathology. Quality Control in Pathology. Recommendations on Quality Control and Quality Assurance in anatomic pathology. Am J Surg Pathol 1991;15:1007-1009.

4- Association of Directors of Anatomic and Surgical Pathology. Standardization of the Surgical Pathology Report. Am J Surg Pathol 1992;16(1):84-86.

5- Association of Directors of Anatomic and Surgical pathology. Consultations in Surgical Pathology. Am J Surg Pathol 1993;17:743-745.

6- QA/QC Committee : Juan Rosai, chairperson et all. Methods in pathology. Standardization of the Surgical pathology report. Modern Path :197-199

7- Frable WJ. Quality Assurance and Quality Control in Anatomic pathology : Standardization of the Surgical Pathology Report. Modern pathology 1992;5:102a-102b.

8- Cowan DF. Quality Assurance in Anatomic Pathology : An Information System Approach. Arch Pathol Lab Med 1990;114:129-134.

9- Lee FD, Burnett RA. Quality Assurance in Histopathology. Journal of pathology 1987;152:247-251.

10- Lee FD. External quality assessment in histopathology : an overview. J Clin Pathol 1989;42:1009-1011.

11- Macartney JC, Henson DE, Codling BW. Quality Assurance in Anatomic pathology. A J C P 1991;75:467-475

12- Klys HS, Lessells AM. External Quality Assurance in Histopathology. Experience of the East of Scotland Scheme. J Clin Pathol 1992;45:288-291.

13- Weber GF. Current methods in histopathology. Pathol Pol 1992;43:87-91.

14- Cantaboni A, Pezzota MG, Sironi M, Porcellati M. Quality assurance in Pathology, Cytologic and Histologic Correlation. Acta Cytol 1992;36:717-721.

15- Stalsberg H. Quality Assurance in a department of pathology and Anatomy. Tidsskr Nor laegeforen 1992;112:3442-3445.

16- Hutter RVP. The Surgical pathologist as a Diagnostsician and Consultant. A.J.C.P. 1981;75 supp:447-452.

17- Association of Directors of Anatomic and Surgical Pathology. Immediate management of mammographically detected breast lesions. Am J Surg Pathol 1993;17:850-851.

18- Neau JY. Le dépistage du cancer du sein provoque une controverse entre la sécurité sociale et les conseils généraux. Le Monde 1994,04.02.

19- Owings DV, Hann L, Schnitt SJ. How thoroughly should needle localization breast biopsies be sempled for microscopic examination. A prospective mammographic/pathologic correlative study. Am J Surg Pathol 1990;416:578-581.

20- Zafrani B, Contesso G, Eusebi V, Holland R, Millis RR, Peterse JL. Guidlines for the pathological management of mammographiccally detected breast lesions. A paraitre dans The Breast 1994.

21- Friedman S, Bertin F, Mouriesse H, Benchabat A, Genin J, Sarrazin D, Contesso G. Importance of tumor cells in axillary node sinus margins ("clandestine" metastases) discovered by serial sectioning in operable breast carcinoma. Acta Oncologica 1987;27:1-5.

22- Taylor CR. An Exaltation of Experts : Concerted Efforts in the standardization of Immunohistochemistry. Appl Immunohistochem 1993;1:232-243.

23- Beck JS and member of medical research council breast tumour pathology panel associates with United Kingdom trial of early detection of breast cancer. Observer variability in reporting of breast lesions. J Clin Pathol 1985;38:1358-1365.

24- Rosai J. Borderline epithelial lesions of the breast. Am J Surg Pathol 1991;15:209-221.

25- Schnitt SJ, Wang HH, Tavassoli FA and al. Interobserver reproducibility in the diagnosis of ductal proliferative lesions using standardized criteria. Am J Surg Pathol 1992;16:1133-1143.

26- Zuk JA, Kenyon WF, Myskow MW. Audit in histopathology : descriptive scheme with analysis of preliminary results. J Clin Pathol 1991;44:10-16.

27- Ramsay AD, Gallagher PJ. Local Audit of Surgical pathology : 18 month's Experience of Peer Review-based Quality Assessment in an English teaching Hospital. Am J Surg Pathol 1992;16:476-482.

Mastology - Breast Diseases
A.S.S. Figueira Fo et al., editors.

Course on Quality Control in Imaging

Cari Borrás, D.Sc., Pan American Health Organization / World Health Organization Washington, D.C., USA.

Abstract

Quality control in mammography is essential to ensure a diagnostic image with minimum radiation dose. Strict specifications are required for the x-ray generator, the x-ray tube, the exposure geometry, compression devices, grids and phototimers; as well as for the processor and the image receptors. After acceptance-testing, the processor and the following x-ray equipment parameters need to be determined periodically: tube potential, half-value layer, timer accuracy, exposure reproducibility and linearity, source-skin and source-image receptor distances, x-ray beam limitation to the image receptor, congruence between light and radiation fields, spatial resolution and absorbed dose.

Physical Aspects of the Installation

The mammography unit - like any other type of x-ray equipment -needs to be installed following national and/or international radiation safety laws, aimed at protecting the staff and the public from ionizing radiation. Because of the low energy x-ray beams used, the mammography room may not require lead shielding. The operator, however, must remain during the exposure behind a protective barrier, built in such a way that the person can observe and communicate with the patient during the procedure. The integrity and adequacy of such a barrier must be checked before commencing operation. The staff also need to wear personnel dosimeters in order to assess that their occupational exposures are within the dose limits specified by the Regulatory Authority.

Specifications of X-Ray Equipment

Generator[1]. There is a need for an accurate and reproducible tube current and potential supply; a low ripple waveform, obtained with a three-phase or preferably a high frequency generator; sharp rise and fall times, and timers ranging from 0.125 to 4 seconds. The low ripple systems will allow for: 1) shorter exposures times, which will minimize motion blur; 2) greater heat capacity, which will permit the use of smaller focal spots, grid and magnification techniques and longer source-image receptor distances, and 3) lower patient doses.

X-Ray Tube. The x-ray tube is to be constructed with a rotating anode of appropriate backing and adequate angle in a water or air cooled housing in order to increase heat capacity. The window through which the x rays emerge should be made of beryllium.

The target material is very important since it affects the spectra and consequently the contrast. It may be tungsten or molybdenum. For xeroradiography a tungsten target with a 1.5 mm aluminum added filtration operating at tube potentials from 40 to 50 kVp is adequate [2]. For screen-film systems, manufacturers are at present experimenting with different target and filter materials. The best tested combinations are a molybdenum target with a 0.03 mm molybdenum filter and a tungsten target with a 0.05 mm rhodium filter, operating in the range 22-30 kVp. The latter choice is particularly interesting for screening, since at the same image quality than the one afforded by the Mo-Mo combination, it results in lower patient dose. However the Mo-Mo combination still offers overall the best imaging capabilities [3].

The focal spot size needs to be small in order to reduce the penumbra which causes image unsharpness. Since focal spot size affects heating capacity, a compromise is required. Recommended focal spot ranges are: From 0.3 to 0.6 mm for conventional projections without magnification and from 0.1 to 0.3 mm for magnification techniques. [1]

<u>Exposure Geometry.</u> The x-ray tube and collimator assembly are to be constructed in such a way that the center of the x-ray beam does not pass through the center of the collimated field, as in conventional x-ray systems; but close to the edge which is aligned with the thoracic wall. There are several reasons for this "half-field" geometry: 1) It avoids missing the volume which "full-field" systems cannot encompass because of beam divergence and 2) it permits the use of smaller focal spot sizes.

Furthermore the cathode-anode axis of the x-ray tube is to be oriented in such a way that the progressive decrease of tissue from the thoracic wall to the nipple is exposed to the dose gradient caused by the heel effect; i.e. the anode side of the x-ray tube is to be oriented towards the nipple. In that way the density of the resulting film will be more uniform, regardless of the progressive decrease in thickness of tissue exposed.

<u>Scatter Reduction Techniques.</u> There are several methods to reduce scattered radiation which reduces subject contrast and produces image unsharpness. One way would be to lower the tube potential, but this would increase patient dose and patient motion. Another method would be to use air-gap techniques, such as the ones used in magnified views. The best methods are to increase patient compression and to use grids.

Compression reduces 1) geometric and image unsharpness, 2) scattered radiation, and 3) patient dose. Furthermore it increases image contrast by producing a more uniform density throughout the imaged breast and permits the borders of the inside structures to be seen better.

Grids are very effective in reducing scatter, but they should be used judiciously, mainly in patients with large amounts of dense breast parenchyma, since the dose to the patient increases by a factor of 3 or 4. In addition the need for longer exposure times may result in increased patient motion. Grids must be of the moving (bucky) type; the grid lines resulting from stationary grids, which are visible on the film, are not acceptable for high-resolution images [4].

<u>Phototimers.</u> Most mammography units are used today with automatic exposure control, in spite of earlier recommendations to the contrary [2]. Phototimers should be placed in relevant areas of the volume to be imaged and need to be movable to accommodate varying breast sizes. They should yield constant density independent of tube potential and patient thickness and need to compensate for beam hardness [1]. In spite of improved circuits in the new systems, an evaluation of 20 recently manufactured mammography units revealed deficiencies in the density calibration of the automatic exposure control in 15 of them and improper density tracking with tube potential and patient thickness in 8 [5].

Periodic Evaluation of X-Ray Equipment Parameters

Once the right equipment has been selected and accepted, it is essential to set up a quality control program which will periodically check the baseline values established during acceptance testing procedures. The first step is the electromechanical evaluation of the mammographic unit assembly to ensure that all locks, detents, indicators and mechanical support devices for the x-ray tube and image receptor holder assembly are operating properly. To perform these tests a level is needed; the compression may be measured with a bathroom scale.

The following parameters should be determined for all clinical settings: accuracy and reproducibility of the tube potential indication, focal spot size, half value layers, timer accuracy, reproducibility and linearity of the exposure, source-skin distance, source-image receptor distance, limitation of the x-ray beam to the image receptor, congruence between the x-ray and the light fields and spatial resolution. The periodicity of the measurements should depend on the mammography workload; all performance tests on the generator and the x-ray tube should be made at least annually and following any equipment repair and/or servicing. They should be done by a medical physicist proficient in mammography unit evaluations. Collimation tests and image quality assessments should be done more frequently, at least quarterly. They can be performed by a well trained technologist. The methodology and tolerances suggested for each test, which follow, have been adapted from references [1], [6], [7] and [8]. It is important to note that all the instrumentation required to perform the tests need to be calibrated also at periodic intervals, preferably annually.

<u>Tube Potential.</u> Tube potential may be checked with special kVp cassettes or digital kVp meters. The latter are recommended as they speed up the measurement process. The tolerance will depend on manufacturers specifications; recommended values are: $\pm 5\%$ for kVp accuracy and a 0.02 for the kVp coefficient of variation.

<u>Focal Spot Size</u>. Focal spot size may be measured with a pinhole camera, a slit camera or a star pattern. The U.S. National Electrical Manufacturers Association (NEMA) specifies focal spot sizes using a slit camera. Because of the difficulties in aligning the camera with the central x-ray beam and to obtain a high enough density, and the fact that a microdensitometer is required for accurate measurements, the slit camera may only be used during acceptance testing procedures. At that time, star patterns should also be radiographed and their images compared in subsequent quality control tests. Small focal spot sizes require stars with a spoke angle of 0.5°; large focal spots may use a 1° spoke. NEMA tolerance is $+50\%$.

<u>Half Value Layer</u>. The half value layer is a determination of the quality of the beam, needed to assess radiographic contrast and to calculate patient dose. Its measurement requires an ionization chamber and an electrometer, calibrated at mammographic x-ray beam energies, and at least five 0.1 mm thick sheets of 99.9% pure aluminum. The ionization chamber should have a flat energy response in the mammography energy range. At a given tube potential (kVp) below 50 kVp, the measured HVL - in units of mm of aluminum - should be equal or greater than 0.01 kVp.

Timer Accuracy. Timer accuracy is to be tested, for all tube potential and current settings, with an electronic device sometimes incorporated in the dosimetry system. The tolerance will depend on manufacturers specifications; a recommended value is: $\pm 5\%$.

Exposure Reproducibility and Linearity. Exposure reproducibility and linearity in the manual mode are to be tested with an ionization chamber and electrometer for all clinical settings. Tolerances are $\pm 5\%$ for the reproducibility and $\pm 10\%$ for the linearity between adjacent mA stations.

Automatic Exposure Control Reproducibility and Compensation. For mammographic units using automatic exposure control (AEC), the performance of the AEC system is to be checked with regard to short-term reproducibility, tube potential and thickness compensation, and density control selection. For the tests it is required to obtain several radiographs of a phantom of uniform density - preferably made of at least three breast tissue equivalent slabs 2 cm thick - varying phantom thickness and tube potential. For any one phantom thickness, the resulting optical densities and mAs values should have a reproducibility of $\pm 5\%$. As kVp and phantom thickness are increased, the optical density should remain within ± 0.10. Density control selectors, if present, should provide a 0.15 change in film optical density per selector step.

Source-skin and Source-image Receptor Distances. Source-skin (SSD) and source-image receptor (SID) distances are to be measured by triangulation, imaging an object of known dimensions at a known distance. A good method is, during the focal spot size test, to determine the distances from the star to the end of the collimator and to the image receptor and to measure the known dimension of the star imaged on the film. SSD and SID tolerances are $\pm 2\%$ of their nominal value.

Collimator Tests. Accuracy of x-ray field size indicators and congruence between light and radiation field sizes are tested to ensure that the collimator or cone does not allow significant radiation beyond the edges of the image receptor. The test is done by placing opaque markers (such as coins) in the borders of the light field for a nominally specified field size and radiographing their image on a film larger than the image receptor holder. The resulting field should not deviate from the nominal one and/or from the light one by more than $\pm 2\%$ of the SID.

Image Quality. Spatial resolution may be assessed in many ways. Quantitatively it can be done by determining the modulation transfer function of the imaging system. Qualitatively imaging a standard phantom may suffice. For its Accreditation Program the American College of Radiology (ACR) [6] uses a 4.5 cm thick 50% gland / 50% fat equivalent tissue phantom containing fibers, specks and masses. Fiber widths range from 0.40 to 1.56 mm; specks - which simulate microcalcifications - from 0.16 to 0.54 mm; masses -which simulate tumors - from 0.25 to 2.0 mm. Image quality is considered acceptable if one can visualize at least the 0.75 mm fiber, the 0.32 mm speck and the 0.75 mm mass [8].

Periodic Evaluation of Film-Screen Parameters

The evaluation of film-screens as image receptors include periodic testing of the films and screens used and the film processing and viewing conditions. The methodology and tolerances suggested for each test, which follow, have been adapted from references [1], [6], [7] and [8]. Most of the tests can be done by a well trained technologist.

Films and Screens. The choice of the type of film-screens to be used will depend on the contrast vs. latitude and speed vs. detail required by the radiologist. To ensure that these parameters remain constant with time, the film/screen characteristic curve needs to be re-drawn each time the manufacturer sends a new film batch. To do the test it is required to have a sensitometer, which gives precise light exposures to the test film, and a densitometer, which measures the resulting optical densities.

The screen speed uniformity is to be tested radiographing a uniform phantom with all screens in clinical use. The resulting optical densities may not differ by more than 0.30 units. Screens need to be cleaned at least weekly.

Screen/film contact is to be checked by radiographing a copper screen of at least 40 wires per inch placed on top of the image receptor. Good film/screen contact should yield a sharp image on a uniform background. Areas of poor contact greater than 1 cm^2 should not be tolerated.

Darkroom. The darkroom requires to be checked periodically for light-tightness to prevent film fogging. A daily log should be maintained of developer temperature, water temperature, replenishment rate, water flow, cleaning and maintenance. A processor dedicated exclusively to mammography is recommended. To control it, it is necessary to control the transport time, the chemical temperature, the chemical activity and the artifacts. Some manufacturers supply test strips to check the fixer retention on the film. They can be used to know when to change the chemicals. On a daily basis it is necessary to measure and record the solution temperatures and the speed, the contrast and the base and fog on the film.

Illuminators. The high contrast and fine detail in mammograms necessitate special viewing conditions. View boxes need to be uniform in intensity and color and require to have viewing spaces adapted to the height of current mammograms and sliding panels that block extraneous light from the sides. Luminance levels should be of the order of 3,500 nit (candela per m^2). They can be measured with a nit meter. View boxes need also to be cleaned often - at least weekly.

The room ambient illuminance should be 50 lux or less. This can be measured with a photometric system.

Film Repeat Analysis. The ultimate test in film/screen quality control is a periodic -for example quarterly - account of the films that had to be repeated with an analysis of the reason for their repetition: improper patient positioning, patient motion, incomplete view, overexposure, underexposure, fog, processor artifacts, etc. A good quality assurance program should yield repetition rates of less than 5%. Progressive improvements will document financial savings and convince mammography facility administrators of the cost effectiveness of the quality assurance program.

Dosimetry

There appears to be a linear relationship between breast cancer incidence and radiation dose. The data are supported by five major studies: the Japanese A-bomb survivors; women in Massachusetts having received multiple fluoroscopies during pneumothorax treatment; a similar study in Nova Scotia, extended to the rest of Canada; women in New York who were irradiated for postpartum mastitis, and women in Sweden who were treated with radiation for benign breast diseases [2]. The relative risk rate has been estimated as 0.42 per cent per cGy for women 20 to 34 years old, and 0.22 for women beyond age 35 [2].

Thus it is essential that the mammographic examination be conducted with the minimum radiation dose compatible with the diagnostic objective of the examination.

There are many parameters that express radiation dose: Air kerma in air (in-air surface exposure) at the breast entrance surface, surface dose, mid-line dose and mean glandular dose. While the first two magnitudes are easy to measure, they are non-additive for multiple views and they are not representative of relative risk at different beam qualities. On the other hand mid-line dose is difficult to measure and underestimates the risk of softer beams. Mean glandular dose, D_g, is the preferred term to express dose, as it is the most representative of risk for a linear dose-response function [1]. It can be calculated using the relationship:

$$D_g = D_{gN} X_a$$

where D_{gN} is the average glandular dose corresponding to an entrance surface exposure of 2,58 X 10^{-4} C Kg^{-1} and X_a is the entrance surface exposure.

D_{gN} depends on beam quality, tissue composition and breast thickness. Table I, adapted from reference [9]), shows the average glandular dose, D_g, in mGy, as a function of breast thickness for x-ray units of molybdenum target and molybdenum filter and breast composition of 50% breast gland 50% fat. For other target/filter combinations and different breast compositions, data may be found in references [9] and [7].

X_a is measured with an ionization chamber and electrometer or with thermoluminiscent dosimeters (TLDs) placed on the skin of the patient. Either detector has to be calibrated at mammographic x-ray energies. Special care is required when using TLDs as they usually require individual energy calibration factors and fading corrections.

Current ACR recommendations for the average glandular dose to a 4.5 cm compressed breast for screen-film receptors are 1 mGy per view without using the grid and 3 mGy when using it [5]. The 1991 Argentinean legislation on mandatory quality assurance for mammographic facilities - the first such legislation to be enacted [10] - establishes 1 and 4 mGy, regardless of the image receptor used. The U.S. Mammography Quality Standards Act [11], the implementation of which will start in 1994, will follow ACR recommendations.

Table I

Computation of Average Glandular Dose, D_g, in mGy, as a Function of Breast Thickness

X-ray Unit: Molybdenum Target and Molybdenum Filter
Breast Composition: 50% Gland and 50% Fat

(Adapted from [9])

Breast Thickness (cm)	3,0	3,5	4,0	4,5	5,0	5,5	6,0	6,5	7,0
D_{gN}	2,2	1,95	1,75	1,55	1,4	1,25	1,15	1,05	0,95

References

1. American Association of Physicists in Medicine / Radiological Society of North America. The Physics of Radiology; 15: Mammography. (Six cassettes-333 slides). RSNA 1989. Oak Brook, Il.
2. National Council on Radiation Protection and Measurements. Report No. 85, 1986. Mammography -- A User's Guide. Bethesda, MD.
3. Desponds L, Depeursinge C, Grecescu M, Hessler C, Samiri A and Valley JF. Influence of Anode and Filter Material on Image Quality and Glandular Dose for Screen-Film Mammography. Phys. Med. Biol. 1991;36:1165-1182.
4. Eklund GW, Cardenosa G and Parsons W. Assesing Adequacy of Mammographic Image Quality. Radiology 1994;190:297-307.
5. Barnes GT and Hendrick RE. Mammography Accreditation and Equipment Performance. RadioGraphics 1994;14:129-138.
6. American College of Radiology, 1992. Committee on Quality Assurance in Mammography. Mammography Quality Control. Radiologist's Manual; Radiologic Technologists's Manual; Medical Physicist's Manual. American College of Radiology, Merrifield, VA.
7. American Association of Physicists in Medicine, Report No. 29, 1990. Equipment Requirements and Quality Control for Mammography. New York, NY.
8. Farria DM, Bassett LW, Kimme-Smith C and De Bruhl N. Mammography Quality Assurance from A to Z. RadioGraphics 1994;14: 371-385.
9. HHS Publication FDA 85-8239, 1985. Handbook of Glandular Tissue Doses in Mammography. Bethesda, MD.

10. Ministerio de Salud y Acción Social de la República Argentina, 1991. Normas Relativas a la Instalación y Funcionamiento de Equipos Generadores de Rayos X. Buenos Aires, Argentina.
11. U.S.A. Federal Register, 1993. Mammography Quality Standards Act. Washington, DC.

III Breast Cancer

III. 1. Epidemiology and risk factors

Mastology - Breast Diseases
A.S.S. Figueira Fo et al., editors.

Other Risk Factors

Evaldo de Abreu
Coordinator of Cancer Control Programs / National Cancer Institute of Brazil

Emilia Rebelo Lopes
Head of Communitary Education Service

Hormonal and Reproductive Aspects

The reproductive characteristics associated to a major risk of breast cancer include early age at menarche, late age at menopause, first pregnancy after 20 years of age anda nulliparity. The relative risks for each high risk group, when compared to their low risk correspondents, are approximately of 2,0.

Henderson at al reported that women having breast cancer presented regular menstrual first cycles more rapidly than the controls, and that the combination of early age at menarche (age twelve or younger) and the occurrence of regular cycles (within one year after menarche), were associated to an almost 4-fold increased risk when compared to women whith late menarche (age thirteen or older) and long duration of irregular cycles. The rate increase of breast cancer decreases sharply during menopause and the menopause before 45 years of age is associated to a risk of twice, when compared to menopause after 55 years of age. Similarly, the ovariectomy before 40 years of age shows a risk reduction of 50% in comparison to a natural menopause around 50 years of age.

Two of the first reproductive characteristics of the breast cancer epidemiology known were the risk decrease, as a result of parturitions increase, and the risk increase in single women. MacMhon at al made the important advancement towards the understanding of the pregnancy's role in breast cancer, through an analysis of an international joint study of control case: childless single and married women undergone the same increased risk for breast cancer, which was approximately 1,4 times as much than that of married women having kids. Among the married ones, in each country, women with breast cancer had less kids than those of the controls. MacMahon clearly demonstrated, however, that this apparent protecting effect of parturition was in fact due to the protecting effect of the first birth at early age (a complete pregnancy includes the baby's lactation as well). Women whose first gestation occurred before 20 years of age presented half the risk of the childless ones, or of those whose first gestation occurred up to 30 years of age or more. After age control of the first gestation, subsequent gestations had less importance in the development of breast cancer. Women with breast cancer used to have few kids, simply because they had born their first child at a late age. Two other studies in different populations showed a minor residual protecting effect in the number of kid's increase and these suggest that there might be certain circumstances in which the multiparity offers some additional protection. In a recent study performed in Shanghai, it was observed that there was a protecting effect in multiple pregnancies, specially after the fifth child. However, the main protecting effect of pregnancy results from a complete pregnancy at an early age. MacMahon's study shows that a trimester abortion, either spontaneous or induced, before a complete pregnancy, is in fact associated to a risk increase of breast cancer. This observation has been confirmed in a cohort study in women in Connecticut (USA) who had only one gestation with a live child. In this study abortions after the first complete pregnancy did not lead to an increase of breast cancer risk.

The lactation's role has not been clearly defined, neither relating to the risk increase nor to the protection against breast cancer development. If the cumulative number of ovulatory cycles is directly related to the breast cancer risk, a positive effect resulting from a long lactation period would be expected, as cause a substantial delay in ovulation, after a complete pregnancy. Due to a small proportion of mothers with a large cumulative number of lactation months, many previous epidemiological studies have not enabled precise estimates of lactation effects in the risk of breast cancer. Recently, Henderson completed a population-base case control study whose lactation period used to be athe norm. In this study a 30% reduction in the risk of breast was observed for each 5 years of lactation.

Oral contraceptives have been widely used since the early 60's, and today there is a vast literature about its relationship with the risk of breast cancer. Although there are studies evidencing the risk increase, other important studies of case-control and cohort show convincing evidences that when used for long periods, oral contraceptives do not alter the risk of breast cancer. As for their use during adolescence, their role in the alteration of risk is undefined.

Studies with long lasting oral or injectable contraceptives composed only of progestagens depot medroxyprogesterone acetate (DMPA) show little evidence of breast cancer risk increase, although this possibility should not be discarded.

The long use of estrogen replacemente therapy, in moderately high doses, according to reliable data available, increases the risk of breast cancer; as for low doses during long periods of time, studies are insufficient, being less probable that they have substantial effect on risk increase.

Nutritional and Environmental Aspects

Important variations in the incidence rate of breast cancer, at a worldwide level and in studies made with animals - as for example Tannenbaums's pioneer work in 1942, which showed an increase in the number of breast tumours in rats fed with a high-fat diet, raised suspicions on the lipidiums's role in the breast cancer aetiology. However, analytical epidemiology studies performed up to now have not implied any specific factor of the diet. The diet's role on risk increase (from 1,5 to 2 times) for the development of breast cancer has been observed only in postmenopausal women. Willet at al comment that the protecting effect of a high corporal weight in premenopausal women, could be attributed to a great diagnosis facility for breast cancer in the women with low corporal weight, and the risk increase in fat postmenopausal women could be explained through a high conversion of androstenedione to estrone in the adipose tissue, as this is the richest source of endogens oestrogens in these women.

Recent studies indicate that a high-fat diet may be a factor to increase the breast cancer occurrence when fat ingestion is abundant during infancy and adolescence. Some authors attribute a modest increase of breast cancer risk in tall postmenopausal women.

There are indications that Vitamin A and other antiproliferant agents may reduce the risk. Other evidences suggest that a total low-fat diet during the development phase would also be a risk-reducing factor. Alcohol consumption has been presented as a risk factor for breast cancer. However, studies have not consistently demonstrated this association, as well as the necessary quantity of alcohol to cause a risk increase. Additionally, a biologically accepted mechanism to explain this association has not been identified. The smoking habit does not seem to be involved in breast cancer aetiology, although some authors associate tabagism at early ages to a little risk increase. There are evidences on the carcinogenic effect of ionizing radiations over breast, based on studies of survivors of the atomic explosions in Japan, and also of women who have been exposed to high doses of ionizing radiation to treat mastitis and tuberculosis. The risk extension is directly proportional to the radiation dose and indirectly to the women's age when exposure occurred. The effect of low doses, such as those used in clinical diagnosis - mamography and occupational exposures, remain uncertain. Little is known about the breast cancer risk and other types of radiation, for example electromagnetic, however, studies on this subject are under development.

References

01. Bernstein L, Ross RK. Endogenous Hormones and Breast Cancer Risk. Epidemiologic Reviews, 15:48-65,1993.

02. Brinton LA, Schairer C. Estrogen Replacement Therapy and Breast CancerRisk. Epidemiologic Reviews, 15:66-79,1993.

03. Gammon MD, John EM. Recent Etiologic Hypotheses Concerning Breast Cancer. Epidemiologic Reviews, 15:163-168,1993.

04. Hendersen BE, Pike MC, Casagrande JT. Breast Cancer and the oestrogen window hypothesis. Lancet ii:363-364,1981.

05. Hendersen BE, Ross R, Bernstein L. Estrogens as a Cause of Human Cancer:The Richard and Hinda Rosenthal Foundation Award Lecture. Cancer Res., 48:246-253,1988.

06. Howe GR. Epidemiology of radiogenic breast cancer. Prog Cancer Res Ther., 26:119-129,1984.

07. John EM, Kelsey JL. Radiation and Other Environmental Exposures and Breast Cancer. Epidemiologic Reviews, 15:157-162,1993.

08. Kelsey JL, Gammon MD, John EM: Reproductive Factors and Breast Cancer. Epidemiol Reviews, 15:36-47,1993.

09. Lopes ER, Mendonça GA, Mattos IE et al. Câncer e meio ambiente em: Leal MC, Sabroza PC, Rodriguez RH et al. Saúde, Ambiente e Desenvolvimento 1992, Hucitec-Abrasco, Rio de Janeiro.

10. MacMahon B, Cole P, Brown J. Etiology of human breast cancer: a review.

J Natl Cancer Inst., 50:21-42,1973.

11. Malone KE, Daling JR, Weiss N. Oral Contraceptives on Relation to Breast Cancer. Epidemiologic Reviews, 15:80-97,1993.

12. Malone KE. Diethylstilbestrol (DES) and Breast Cancer. Epidemiologic Reviews, 15:108-109,1993.

13. Palmer JR, Rosenberg L. Cigarette Smoking and the Risk of Breast Cancer. Epidemiologic Reviews, 15:145-156,1993.

14. Pike MC, Spicer DV, Dahmoush L et al. Strogens, Progestogens, Normal Breast Cell Proliferation, and Breast Cancer Risk. Epidemiologic Reviews,15: 17-35, 1993.

15. Rosenberg L, Metzger LS, Palmer JR. Alcohol Consumption and Risk of Breast Cancer: a Review of the Epidemiologic Evidence. Epidemiologic Reviews, 15:133-144,1993.

16. Stanford JL, Thomas DB. Exagenous Progestins and Breast Cancer. Epidemiologic Reviews,15:98-107,1993.

17. Trichopolous D, Mac Mahon B, Cole P, et al. The menopause and breast cancer risk. J Natl Cancer Inst.,48:605-613,1972.

18. Willet WC, Browne ML, Bain C. Relative weight and risk of breast cancer among premenopausal women. Am J Epidemiol.,122:731-740,1985.

19. Yang CP, Weiss, NS, Band PR et al. History of Lactation and Breast Cancer Risk. Am J Epidemiol.,138:1050-1056,1993.

Mastology - Breast Diseases
A.S.S. Figueira Fo et al., editors.

Demographics aspect of breast cancer

Au.:Chagas.Carlos Ricardo,MD
Enfermaria 28: Santa Casa de Misericórdia do Rio de Janeiro-Brazil

Summary: Breast cancer is becoming an incresingly important disease in all parts of the world.It is estimated that the annual incidence in the world will be more than 1,000,000 cases by the year 2,000. The recent trends shows a dramatic change in the age-incidence curve. The international differences in the incidence are recognized. Studies in migrant populations suggest that environmental rather genetic factors are responsible for the populational variations. In U.S. differences can be seen among ethinic groups. In Brazil are diagnosed 20,000 cases per year of breast cancer.The highest incidence occur in the places more advanced as Sao Paulo, Rio de Janeiro, and Rio Grande do Sul.

Breast cancer is becoming an incresingly important disease in all parts of the world. It is estimated that the annual incidence of breast cancer in the world will be more than 1,000,000 cases by the year 2000. On basis of current incidence rates, it has been estimated by the American Cancer Society that 1 in 8 women will develop breast cancer at some time during her life (until 85 years old).[1-2]

Although there is considerable circunstantial evidence that environmental factors may be associated with increased risk, it has been more difficult to stablish a tight link between the factors and breast cancer development.

The recent trends in Surveillance,Epidemiology, and End Results (SSER) data shows a dramatic change in the age-incidence curve. In 1973, the incidence rates were typical of those shown earlier, rising steeply, although at low levels, until approximately 40 or 45 years of age, then flattenning out briefly (Clemmensen's hook), and rising again until 85 years of age.By 1987 has found a significantly increase above what had been previously typified. This large increase in disease incidence in women older than 50 years of age within less than 10 years cannot be easily explained.[3]

Some auctors stated that the observed increase in the incidence of breast cancer in the U.S. is consistent with an increase due to early detection by mammography. White et colleagues suggest that this may be true only for women age 45-64.[4] Among older and, possibly, younger women, there may be other factors leading for an increased risk of breast cancer that need further investigations.

In an analysis was undertaken by Gail in situ only and in situ plus invasive are shown, and the patterns are similar.[3]

The probability of a woman will have breast cancer increases throughout her life. Thus, age might be considered the single most important factor for determining breast cancer.[5-6]
In the Japanese data, the climb with increasing age appears almost nil in comparision to western women.[3]
Breast cancer mortality has declined signigicantly from 7,0 per 100,000 women in 1973 to 6,2 per 100,000 in 1988 in women youger than 50 years of age. Probably the advances in adjuvant therapy are responsible of this decline and the increase in early detection also has contributed.[3]
However mortality rates among older women have risen from 88,4 per 100,000 in 1973 to 93,0 per 100,000 in 1988, an increase of 5,2%. This increase in mortality can be explained by the incidence found in the past decade.[3]
The international differences in the incidence of breast cancer are recognized. In general, the incidence is lower in Asia, Africa, and South America than it is in North America and Europe. In recent years, marked rises in breast cancer incidence and mortality rates have been noted in many Asian, Central European, and some South American countries.[6]
Studies in migrant populations suggest that environmental rather genetic factors are responsible for the international variations.[6] For example, the Japanese migrants to the U.S. have breast cancer incidence rates similar to women in Japan, whereas incidence rates in second and third-generation migrants approach those of American-born white women. Buel also noted that Japanese immigrants to the U.S.took longer to exibit a high breast cancer risk than Polish immigrants who had arrived at same time, and suggest that this reflected the rate of cultural assimilation of the two nationalities. In the U.S. differences can be seen among ethnic groups.[6-7] The American white and black women have the highest incidence rates, and the indian women have the lowest incidence.
White women have a higher overall rate of breast cancer than black women. This is not apparent until the age of 40, and the difference is marked only after the age of menopause, and in the working class. While among women under age 40 the rate is higher among black compared whith white women.[6-8]
In U.S., young black women are more likely to undergo an abortion and use contraceptives than are young white women even at same educational level. If either abortion or oral contraceptives use, especially prior to first full term-pregnancy, were linked to increased breast cancer rise, the elevate abortion and the delay of childbearing among black women who try to complete their education, might explain the variation of the incidence between black and white women before age 40 years.[6-8]
Finnaly, we would to talk about the Brazil. Country where this congress are occurring. In Brazil are diagnosed 20,000 new cases per year of breast cancer. The highest incidence occur in the places more advanced and industrialized, as Sao Paulo, Rio de Janeiro, and Rio Grande do Sul. The lowest incidence is found in North Region, Northeast Region, and Central Region.[2]
Breast cancer is the most frequent type of cancer found between women in Rio de Janeiro, Sao Paulo and Rio Grande do Sul. However, uterine cervix cancer is the more frequent in Pará, Goiás, and Pernambuco.[2-9]

References:
1)Kelsey LK,Gammon MD.Epidemiologic Reviews 1990;12:228-240.
2)Rebelo E, Abreu E.Epidemiologia do câncer de mama 1994. Proonco. Ministério da Saúde.Brasil.
3)Kessler LG.Cancer 1992;69(sup):1896-1903.
4)White E, Lee CY, Kristal AR.Journal of the National Cancer Institute 1990;82:1546-1552.
5)Constanza ME.Cancer 1992;69(sup):1925-1929.
6)Henderson UC.Cancer;71:2127-2140.
7)Buell P.Journal of the National Cancer Institute 1973; 51: 1479-1483.
8)Krieger N.American Journal of Epidemiology 1990;131:804-814.
9)Rebelo MS,Abreu E.Câncer no Brasil-Ministério da Saúde.Rio de Janeiro:Proonco.1993.

Mastology - Breast Diseases
A.S.S. Figueira Fo et al., editors.

Clinical management of women at increased risk for breast cancer

Gerardo Hernandez-Muñoz
Unidad de Mastologia Centro Clinico de Maternidad Leopoldo Aguerrevere. Caracas
Address for reprints: P.O. Box 66962, Caracas 1061-A, Venezuela.

A large number of women in the general population are at risk of developing breast cancer. Physicians are being asked, with increasing frequency, to counsel women who might be at increased risk for breast cancer and a number of issues in the management of such women confront the practising clinician.

Risk assessment:

Age

Breast cancer is relatively uncommon before menopause. Most age-incidence curves show a small plateau in the incidence trend observed approximately at 50 years of age when many women are undergoing the menopause and then there is a steeper rise thereafter. The probability that a woman will have breast cancer increases throughout her life, and most breast cancers occur during the postmenopausal years. Thus, age might be considered the single most important factor for determining breast cancer [1].

Family history

Any family history of breast cancer in either maternal or paternal line, increases a woman's risk of having breast cancer but for most relationships, this increased risk is negligible. A more substantial an clinically important increase in risk is associated with breast cancer in a first degree relative: mother, sister or daughter,(or father, brother or son). Breast cancer in mother or sister is associated with an approximately twofold risk increase [2].

A patient without a first or second degree relative having this disease is designated as a sporadic case. The sporadic group comprises the vast majority or about 70% of all breast cancer patients.

Hereditary breast cancer are occurring in patients with a high positive incidence of a family history of breast cancer with a father that is consistent with an autosomal dominant trait. These patients and their affected relatives are usually postmenopausal at the onset of the disease.

The term familial or polygenic breast cancer is then used to include breast cancer in patients who have one or more first or second degree relatives demonstrating breast cancer but who do not fulfil the criteria of hereditary breast cancer. The hereditary or genetic forms make up for 5-9%. The remaining 21-25% are classified as the familial or polygenic type [3].

Endogenous endocrine factors

It has been established and confirmed by many epidemiology studies, that the age at menarche, age at menopause, parity and age at first full term pregnancy are important determinants of risk.

Although age at menarche is by itself an important risk, the time at which a woman establishes a regular ovulatory cycle may be more important [4]. The effects of steroids hormones on the normal breast of women are increasingly well understood; estrogen induces some breast epithelial cell proliferation but estrogen plus progesterone produce greater cell proliferation [5].

The number of pregnancies a woman has is an important determinant of risk, but her age at the time of her full term pregnancy is even more important [6].

Proliferative benign breast disease

Benign breast disease that is serious enough to warrant a biopsy of breast tissue, increases the patient's risk of developing breast cancer subsequent to the biopsy [7]. Non proliferative disease, (fibroadenoma, cysts, duct ectasia, apocrine metaplasia and mild hyperplasia), do not increase the risk of developing breast cancer [8].

Proliferative disease without atypia, (intraductal papilloma, radial scar, sclerosing adenosis, moderate or florid ductal hyperplasia), increase the risk of developing breast cancer by 1.5 to 4 fold. The risk increases in the presence of family history of breast cancer.

Atypical hyperplasia, (ductal or lobular), increases the risk 3 to 4 fold, if atypical hyperplasia is associated with a family history of breast cancer in first degree relatives, the increased risk can be as much as 8 times the baseline rate [8].A diagnosis of lobular carcinoma in situ, (LCIS), increases an individual's risk for breast cancer 10 to 20 fold. The combination of LCIS and a family history of breast cancer further increases the risk [8]. Ductal carcinoma in situ, (DCIS), increases an individual's risk for the subsequent development of invasive malignancy. Any DCIS with a size smaller than 2-3 mm was called atypical ductal hyperplasia even if features of carcinoma in situ were quite well developed [8].

Mammographic parenchymal pattern

The only diagnostic method which has the ability to detect breast cancer at an early stage with high sensitivity is superb quality mammography interpreted by a well trained radiologist.

Wellings and Wolfe attempted to correlate the mammographic appearances with histological findings [9]. Mansel et al [10], and Moskowitz et al [11] were unable to find any association between atypical hyperplasia and P2 or Py. Nonpalpable abnormalities of the breast parenchyma that may be associated with cancer are represented mammographically by microcalcifications, mass densities and architectural alterations.

Management strategies

An effective, prospectively validated management strategy remains to be designed.

Mammographic screening prescriptions

A screening test is not intended to be diagnostic; rather a positive finding will need to be confirmed by special diagnostic procedures. Our main objective in screening is to find patients with the high risk sooner.

Slightly increased risk (RR=1.6 to 2.4)

1- Annual mammography starting at 40 year of age.
2- Biannual clinical examination.
3- Self examination.

Moderately increased risk (RR=2.5 to 7.4)

1- Annual mammography starting at 30 years of age.
2- Clinical examinations 3 times a year.
3- Self examination.
4- Liberal use of fine needle aspiration.

High risk (RR> 7.4)

1- Annual mammography starting at 30 years of age.
2- Clinical examination 3 times a year.
3- Self examination.
4- Liberal use of fine needle aspiration.
5- Option of prophylactic mastectomy.
6- Chemoprevention.

Prophylactic mastectomy

Women who have proliferative changes with or without atypia in the presence of an increased relative risk for breast cancer, are candidates for prophylactic mastectomy. However, the benefits from this procedure is questionable since long term outcome data related to the physical and psychological sequelae from women who have had this procedure is not available. Prophylactic mastectomy is aggressive and even with reconstruction, may be more disfiguring than a lumpectomy for early stage disease. Women at increased risk should be counselled not to undergo breast augmentation procedures because of the difficulty in reading screening mammograms in augmented breasts.

Chemoprevention

After extensive use worldwide in adjuvant treatment trials, Tamoxifen is known to reduce the incidence of contralateral breast cancer by approximately 40% [12], making it a candidate for use in the primary prevention of breast cancer [13]. Tamoxifen also reduces total cholesterol [14] and preserves bone mineral density in postmenopausal women [15].

Postmenopausal estrogen replacement

The potential association between the administration of E.R.T. and the development of breast cancer has been reviewed during the past several decades. All studies suggested that there was a slight increased risk associated with postmenopausal E.R.T., but this increased risk was less than 10% when the analysis was restricted to women whose estrogen exposure exceeded 15 years increasing the relative risk to 1,3. The effects of E.R.T. appeared to be greater in patients with a family history of breast cancer that in those without such a history [16]. The decision to administer E.R.T. to a postmenopausal woman should be carefully individualized.

References

1. Henderson I.C.:Risk Factors for breast cancer development. Cancer 1993,71:2127-2140.
2. Brain C et al. Family history of breast cancer as a risk indicator for the disease. Am J. Epidemiol 1980; 111:301-308.
3. Lynch T.L. et al: Genetic predisposition for breast cancer. Cancer 1984; 53:612-622.
4. Henderson B.E. et al: Breast cancer and the estrogen window hypothesis. Lancet 1981; 2:363-364.
5. Pike M.C. et al: Estrogens, progestogens, normal breast cell proliferation and breast cancer risk.Epidemiol Rev. 1993;15:17-35.
6. MacMahon B et al. Age at first birth and breast cancer risk. Bull World Health Org. 1970;43:209-221.
7. Gail M.H. et al: Projecting individualized probabilities of developing breast cancer for white females who are being examined annually. J Natl Cancer Inst. 1989; 81:1879-1886.
8. Page D.L. et al. Anatomic indicators, (histologic and cytologic) of increased breast cancer risk. Breast cancer research and treatment. 1993;28:157-166.
9. Wellings S.R. et al. Correlative studies of the histological and radiographic appearance of the breast parenchyma. Radiology 1978;129:299-306.
10. Mansel R.E. et al. The interpretation of mammographic ductal enlargement in cancerous breast. Br J Surg 1979;66:701-702.
11. Moskowitz M. et al. Proliferative disorders of the breast as risk factors for breast cancer in a self selected screened population. Radiology 1980; 134"289-291.
12. Early Breast Cancer Trialist's Collaborative Group: Systematic Treatment of early breast cancer by hormonal, cytotoxic or inmmune therapy. Lancet 1992;339:1-15.
13. Love R.R. Prospects for antiestrogen chemoprevention of breast cancer. J Natl Cancer Inst. 1990;82:18-21.
14. Love R.R. et al. Effects of Tamoxifen on cardiovascular risk factors in postmenopausal women. Ann Intern Med 1991;115:860-864.
15. Love R.R. et al Effects of Tamoxifen on bone mineral density in postmenopausal women with breast cancer. N Eng J Med 1992;326:852-856.
16. Steinberg K.K. et al. A meta-analysis of the effect of estrogen replacement therapy. JAMA; 265: 1985-1990.

Mastology - Breast Diseases
A.S.S. Figueira Fo et al., editors.

Genetic perspectives in familial breast cancer

Alberto K. Fuzikawa, M.D. & Sérgio D.J. Pena, M.D., Ph.D.*
Núcleo de Genética Médica de Minas Gerais (GENE), Av. Afonso Pena 3111/9, Belo Horizonte, M.G., Brazil, 30130-909 and Departamento de Bioquímica e Imunologia, Universidade Federal de Minas Gerais, Belo Horizonte, M.G., Brazil.

ABSTRACT
Breast cancer is a disease which affects 5-10% of all women and is responsible for high levels of morbidity and mortality. Although the majority of cases are sporadic, approximately 5% show a pattern compatible with autosomal dominant genetic transmission, mostly due to germinal mutations in BRCA1, a locus that has been mapped to chromosome 17q21. The isolation of BRCA1 by positional cloning is imminent. Once that is achieved, it is hoped that we will achieve a quantum leap in our understanding of the process of tumorigenesis of the mammary epithelium. Moreover, we will have greatly improved genetic counseling of "breast cancer families" and new vistas will be open for the possibility of molecular genetic screening at the population level.

Introduction

In the past decade a major shift occurred in our views about the pathogenesis of malignancy, leading to the new paradigm that cancer is fundamentally a genetic disease. However, cancer differs from conventional Mendelian genetic diseases in two basic aspects: the mutations are predominantly somatic and the process of tumorigenesis is polygenic, depending on the accumulation of several genic or chromosomal mutations involving tumor supressor genes and oncogenes [1]. Nevertheless, it is widely known that cancer often shows familial aggregation generally consistent with Mendelian inheritance, albeit with reduced penetrance [2]. Studies in these families reinforced the genetic paradigm by showing that the germinal mutations segregating in these cancer families also involve tumor supressor genes or, less frequently, oncogenes [2]. Thus, pre-existent germinal mutations accelerate the process of malignant transformation by obviating the need for some of the somatic mutations indispensable in the process.

Familial Breast Cancer

In reference to human breast cancer, it has long been realized that family history is a major clue determining risk, especially when there are cases of breast cancer in first degree relatives. This connection is particularly striking in the presence of premenopausal (early onset) disease and whenever there are also cases of ovary cancer in the family. Women with both a mother and sister affected with breast cancer have as much as a 14 fold increased risk of developing breast cancer themselves [3].

There are two syndromes of familial breast cancer, both segregating in autosomal dominant fashion. Li-Fraumeni syndrome is very rare and is characterized by a very high incidence of premenopausal breast cancer, sarcomas and brain tumors. The greatest importance of this syndrome derives from the demonstration that it is caused by germline mutations in the p53 gene [4], one of the most important tumor supressor genes known [5]. In contrast, the second syndrome, characterized by early onset breast cancer in association with ovarian tumors appears to be very common and will be discussed in detail now.

The BRCA1 gene

In 1990 a locus related to familial breast cancer cases was mapped to chromosome 17q21 and was denominated BRCA1 [6,7]. A recent multicentre study involving 214 breast cancer families, including 57 breast-ovarian cancer families, showed that all families containing at least one case of ovarian cancer were consistent with linkage, whereas only 45% of the families containing exclusively breast cancer cases were linked [8]. This suggests both that BRCA1 also is important in the pathogenesis of ovarian cancer and that more than one gene may be involved in different cases of familial breast cancer.

Lately several groups have attempted to reach BRCA1 by positional cloning. Studies of recombinant events in families demonstrating linkage to BRCA1 have progressively narrowed the region of interest [3,5-11]. Recently, analysis of a single breast-ovarian cancer pedigree with several affected individuals has shown the probable region containing BRCA1 to be 1-1.5 Mb in length, lying between markers D17S857 and D17S183 [11]. These new boundaries have excluded several genes as possible candidates to BRCA1, among them the retinoic acid receptor alpha (RARA1), topoisomerase II (TOPO2), CNP and KRT10. The genes remaining in the minimal region are gastrin and the two 17 SYMBOL 98 \f "Symbol"§-estradiol dehydrogenase genes (EDH17B1 and EDH17B2), the latter two being the most plausible candidates. 17 SYMBOL 98 \f "Symbol"§-estradiol dehydrogenase catalyses the conversion of estrone to the much more potent estrogen, estradiol, the levels of which have been shown to be considerably higher in breast tumors than in normal breast cells. However, sequencing of these genes in genomic DNA from normal and affected individuals in this study did not reveal any germline mutations [11].

Clinical Implications of BRCA1

Although breast cancer attributable to a BRCA1 germline mutation probably accounts for only about 5% of all cases [6], cloning of the gene will likely have very important consequences. First, there are abundant reports of loss of heterozigozity for markers in the BRCA1 critical region in tumors from patients who demonstrate linkage to BRCA1. These losses occur in the wild-type allele at the predisposing locus, reflecting the need for its inactivation, and suggesting that the BRCA1 gene may have tumor-suppressor activity [12]. Thus mutations of BRCA1 are likely to be a relatively uncommon inherited trait but may also be an acquired defect in the majority of sporadic cases. Thus, isolation and cloning of BRCA1 should ultimately lead to a greater understanding of the biology of malignant transformation of the mammary epithelium, leading to major advances in diagnostics and therapeutics benefiting all breast cancer patients [3].

Second, there are specific applications in "breast cancer families". BRCA1 mutation carrier rates have been estimated from 1:200 to 1:700 women. Once identified, genetic alterations in BRCA1 can be assayed in a large number of patients at risk, i.e. daughters and sisters of breast cancer patients. Currently, the dramatic but realistic option for women with more than two affected first degree relatives is bilateral mastectomy in early adulthood. As many as 50% of these women may be at no greater risk than the general population. Unfortunately, at present genetic counseling based on linkage analysis is possible for only very few families (those in which sufficient numbers of affected individuals are available to demonstrate linkage to 17q). Once BRCA1 has been cloned and sequenced and common mutations characterized, it will be possible to identify carriers with certainty, offering prophylactic surgery or intensive surveillance only to those at risk. Non carriers will be spared a disfiguring procedure without fear of compromising their long term survival [3]. If reliable and relatively inexpensive molecular procedures can be developed, it is not too far-fetched to expect that before long, we will be able to offer general population screening for BRCA1 mutations.

ACKNOWLEDGMENTS

We are grateful to Prof. D.T. Bishop from the Imperial Cancer Research Fund and Dr. Francis S. Collins from the National Center for Human Genome Research for access to unpublished information.

REFERENCES

1. Vogelstein B & Kinzler KM. Trends Genet 1993; 9: 138-141.
2. Knudson AG. Nature Genet 1993; 5:103-104.
3. Weber BL, Abel KJ, Brody LL, Flejter WL, Chandrasekharappa SC, Couch FJ, Merajver SD & Collins FS. Cancer 1994 (In Press).
4. Malkin D, Li FP, Strong LC, Fraumeni JF Jr, Nelson CE & Kim DH. Science 1990;250:1233 1238.
5. Harris CC. Science 1993;262:1980-1981.

6. King M-C. Nature Genet 1992; 2:89-90.
7. Hall JM, Lee MK, Morrow J, Newman L, Anderson L, Huey B & King M C. Science 1990; 250:1684-1689.
8. Narod SA, Feunteun J, Lynch HT, Watson P, Conway T, Lynch J & Lenoir GM. Lancet 1991; 338:82-83.
9. Eaton DF, Bishop DT, Ford D, Crockford GP & Breast Cancer Linkage Consortium. Am J Hum Genet 1993; 52:678-701.
10. Bowcock AM, Anderson LA, Friedman LS, Black DM, Osborn Lawrence, Rowell SE, Hall JM, Solomon E & King M C. Am J Hum Genet 1993; 52:718-722.
11. Ketsell DP, Black IM, Bishop DT, & Spurr NK. Hum Molec Genet 1993; 2:1823-1828.
12. Smith SA, Easton DF, Evans DGR, & Ponder BAJ. Nature Genet 1992; 2:128-131.

III. 2. Premalignant lesions

Mastology - Breast Diseases
A.S.S. Figueira Fo et al., editors.

Atypical hyperplasia of the breast

A review of 522 previously diagnosed cases

Prosper Anani MD, Lausanne – Switzerland

Summary

Page and co-workers defined atypical hyperplasia (AH) of the breast as intraductal or lobular proliferative changes that have some but, not all, of the features of carcinoma in situ (1). Histological criteria for the diagnosis of AH have now been standardized and been in use for several years (1,2,3). The diagnosis of AH is a difficult one for pathologists without these criteria, however, the diagnostic outcome is much improved if they are applied. Based upon these criteria, we wished to investigate whether diagnostic ability has changed in our establish- - ment over the last seventeen years. To assess this, we reviewed all slides of benign mammary lesions in which atypical intraductal or lobular hyperplasia (AIH or ALH) was discovered. In the cases from 1974 to 1985, 47% of AIH were confirmed compared to a mere 30% in the cases from 1986 to 1991. For all ALH, these values were 15 and 22% respectively. In contrast the number of cases diagnosed as benign mammary lesions without AH has remained constant over the years. It would appear that AIH have been over-diagnosed during recent years, whereas, statistically, the diagnosis of ALH was not modified.

Materials and methods

All benign breast lesions diagnosed as atypical hyperplasia established by the department of pathology in Lausanne from 1974 to 1991 were recovered from a search strategy in the computer reccords.

Results

A total of 522 cases initially diagnosed as AH (339 AIH and 183 ALH) were reviewed according to the standardized histological criteria by Page and co-workers (1,2,3). Two hundred-nineteen cases of AIH and 148 cases of ALH were excluded as they showed only moderate or florid hyperplasia.

Of the 155 cases retained (from 146 patients), 120 were AIH and 35 ALH. Nine patients demonstrated both types of hyperplasia. Diagnostic reliability was assessed over two periods (Table 1 and 2). a) 1974-1985: three to five pathologists diagnosed 101 cases of AIH and 84 cases of ALH. After reveiwing, only 48 AIH and

Table 1

YEAR	AIH Initialy diagnosed (n)	AIH Corrected cases (n)	% Diag. maintained
1974-1985	101	48	47
1986-1991	238	72	30
total	339	120	35

13 ALH remained valid. b) From 1986 to 1991: seven to eight pathologists diagnosed 238 AIH and 99 ALH. Only 72 AIH and 22 ALH were retained after reveiwing.

Discussion

The object of our study was not to find out whether or not the benign breast lesions contained AH, but to check that, when the diagnosis had been established using the standard histological criteria, that it had been done so correctly (1,2,3). In collaboration with Dr V. Eusebi from Bologna – Italy, in 1990, 1300 consecutive cases of benign breast lesions without AH collected over two years were reviewed in the hope of finding intraductal carcinoma of the clinging sub-type. We did not. Nor did we find AH. However, we did observe moderate or florid hyperplasia.

From 1974 to 1991, 522 cases of AH of which 339 were AIH and 183 were LAH were diagnosed without standardized criteria. When these criteria were applied, only 35% of AIH and 19% of ALH had been correctly diagnosed. For the period from 1986 through 1991, following the publication of Page's paper (1), these values were 35% and 22% respectively for AIH and ALH. On the other hand, from 1974 to 1985 (prior to Page's publication) of the 101 cases of AIH and 84 ALH initially diagnosed, only 47% of AIH and 15% of ALH remained as such after our revision. The difference in the proportion of cases of AIH over-diagnosed between the two afore-mentioned periods is significant ($p<0,01$) but not so for ALH.

Several reasons may possibly explain the over diagnosis of AH in general.

Table 2

YEAR	ALH Initialy diagnosed (n)	ALH Corrected cases (n)	% Diag. maintained
1974-1985	84	13	15
1986-1991	99	22	22
total	183	35	12

Firstly, prior to 1986, no criteria were available, thus each pathologist's interpretation was personal and subjective. Secondly, even when criteria were proposed they were not always applied, either because they were too complex or misunderstood. Finally, and more simply, they were often ignored. One may ask whether their proper use would have tendered correct diagnosis of atypical hyperplasia.

In 1991, Rosai (4) submitted 17 cases of proliferative breast lesions to five pathologists well – experienced in breast pathology. Of these 17 cases, 10 contained intraductal epithelial proliferations and seven lobular epithelial proliferations. Each pathologist was asked to use his own histological criteria. In none of the cases did all five pathologists come to the same diagnosis and in 33% of the cases, the diagnoses differed from hyperplasia without atypia to carcinoma in situ. (4). When a similar test was carried out using standardized criteria (5), diagnostic variability was reduced with a consistancy of 58% for all cases. In this latter test, several conditions should be pointed out: the histological criteria were handed out to the participants, reference slides were available and three of the pathologists had partipated in Rosai's study. From this, we can see that even emminent pathologists needed to refer to criteria in order to diagnose difficult borderline lesions, the diagnoses of which are often prone to personal interpretation and depend largely on experience.

Even if difficult to abide by, criteria do exist to help with borderline lesions of the breast. While it is important that AH not be underdiagnosed , one must keep in mind that therapy may be quite dramatic and when in doubt between AH or carcinoma in situ, it would be wise to consider the more benign diagnosis.

References

1 Page DL. Dupont WP, Rogers LW, Rados MS. Atypical hyperplastic lesions of the female breast: A long-term follow-up study. Cancer 1985; 55: 2698-708.

2 Page DL, Anderson TJ. Diagnostic histopathology of the breast. Edinburgh: Churchill Livingstone. 1987: 120-92.

3 Page DL, Rogers LW. Combined histologic and cytologic criteria for diagnosis of mammary atypical ductal hyperplasia. Hum Pathol 1992; 23: 1095-1097.

4 Rosai J. Boderline epithelial lesions of the breast. Am J Surg Pathol 1991; 15: 209-21.

5 Schnitt SJ, Connolly JL, Tavassoli FA, Fechner RE, Kempson RL, Gelman R, Page DL. Interobserver reproducibility in the diagnosis of ductal proliferative breast lesions using standardized criteria. Am J Surg Pathol 1992; 16: 1133-1143.

III. 3. In-situ carcinoma

Mastology - Breast Diseases
A.S.S. Figueira Fo et al., editors.

The Dilemma of Appropriate Therapy for DCIS The Van Nuys Breast Center Experience

Melvin J. Silverstein, M.D., Medical Director and Senior Surgical Oncologist,
The Breast Center, 14624 Sherman Way, Van Nuys, California 91405, USA

Abstract: During the last decade, the diagnosis of intraductal breast carcinoma (DCIS) has become common. The lesion is generally found by mammography and is often both nonpalpable and non visualizable to both surgeon and pathologist. Because of this, DCIS is difficult to excise completely. Treatment options range from excision only to excision plus breast irradiation to mastectomy. There is an aggressive search for biologic markers that will predict which tumors will recur locally and which will recur in an invasive form.

Text: How do we tell the "bad" DCIS (lesions destined to develop into invasive breast cancer) from the "not-so-bad" DCIS (lesions that will remain *in situ*, never causing significant clinical disease)? How do we choose which patients to treat and which patients to follow? When we treat, how much treatment is required? Is excision with clear margins enough or must the whole breast be treated with either radiation or mastectomy? Which patients are likely to recur after treatment?

Ten years ago, DCIS was a relatively rare lesion and these questions were not asked. All breast cancer, regardless of whether or not invasion was seen, was treated the same way, generally by mastectomy. Today, the incidence of DCIS is increasing rapidly, paralleling the increasing acceptance and use of mammography. DCIS now represents as much as 25% of all newly diagnosed cancers in centers relying on mammography [1] and its treatment is now extremely important.

Mastectomy cures just about all patients with DCIS. With mastectomy there are almost no local recurrences, just about no distant recurrences, and a breast cancer death is a rarity. But what price do we pay to achieve these excellent results? In an era where conservative therapy for small infiltrating tumors is used more frequently than mastectomy, it becomes extremely difficult to justify continued use of mastectomy for noninvasive disease.

When breast conservation therapy is used for DCIS, there will be local recurrences, half of which will be invasive. Some of these will undoubtedly lead to death.

Intraductal breast carcinoma is a biologically and morphologically heterogeneous group of lesions [2]. There are numerous architectural subtypes that can be seen alone or in combination with one another. Nuclear grades vary, some tumors have necrosis, some do not, a high percentage exhibit Her-2 neu (c-erbB-2) over-expression, S-phases vary, some lesions are diploid others are aneuploid [3]. There are many other prognostic factors, most of which have some meaning and prognostic value when evaluated in patients with infiltrating breast carcinoma but have very little meaning for patients with DCIS.

The following is an overview of the patients that make up our study group. From 1979 through 1993, The Van Nuys Breast Center treated 401 patients with DCIS: 50 had evidence of microinvasion (defined as areas of invasive carcinoma less than one mm. in maximum diameter) and 351 patients had DCIS without microinvasion.

DCIS without Microinvasion. The average patient presented with a lesion measuring 24 mm. in maximum diameter. All patients were selectively treated; the least favorable (large tumors with involved biopsy margins) with mastectomy, the most favorable (small tumors with clear margins) with breast preservation. The preservation group was further subdivided into those who received radiation therapy (excision and radiation) and those who did not (excision alone).

In the **mastectomy** group, there were 143 patients (41%) with an average tumor size of 3.4 cm. Fourteen percent (20/143) had multicentric tumors. There have been two local invasive recurrences. Both of these patients have developed distant recurrences, one of whom has died. The 8-year probability of disease-free survival was 99% with mastectomy.

In the **excision and radiation** group, there were 124 patients (35%) with an average tumor size of 1.8 cm. Fifteen patients have had local recurrences (7 invasive and 8 noninvasive), one of whom has died. Two of these patients are currently in remission after inflammatory-type recurrences and are likely to die from breast cancer metastases. The 8-year probability of disease-free survival was 84%, a statistically significant difference when excision and radiation is compared with mastectomy ($P < .001$).

In the **excision alone** group, there were 84 patients (24%) with an average tumor size of 1.7 cm. Eight patients (9%) have had local recurrences, (four of which were invasive) and there have been no deaths. The 4-year probability of disease-free survival was 82%.

Axillary node dissection: 218 axillary node dissections were performed; all were negative.

Conclusions for DCIS without microinvasion: Patients in this series with intraductal carcinoma treated with excision and radiation recurred locally at a statistically higher rate than those treated with mastectomy, in spite of the fact that those chosen for excision and radiation had clinically more favorable tumors. There was, however, no significant difference in overall survival in any subgroup regardless of treatment. However, 52% of the recurrences were invasive. And this is worrisome.

The local recurrence rate for DCIS patients treated with breast irradiation is likely to be approximately 20% at 10 years and higher yet for those treated with excision only. If 50% of recurrences are invasive, I would not be surprised to see a 10-year breast cancer specific mortality rate of approximately 5% for conservatively treated patients. For patients treated with mastectomy, it will be approximately 1% or less.

Conservatively treated patients must be carefully followed until we understand the long-term significance of an invasive local recurrence. Patients with DCIS electing breast conservation must be apprised that theoretically there may be a slightly higher mortality rate. Since DCIS without micro-invasion rarely metastasizes to axillary lymph nodes, routine dissection should not be performed.

DCIS with microinvasion (DCIS-Mi). We have defined microinvasion as up to three foci of invasion all less than one mm. in diameter. These patients could be considered T1a invasive carcinomas with an extensive intraductal component (EIC) [4]. We have 50 patients who meet these criteria. The average DCIS-Mi patient presented with a lesion measuring 38 mm. in maximum diameter. (Statistically larger than our average patient with DCIS without microinvasion $p < 0.01$). Thirty-three patients were treated with mastectomy, two of whom have recurred, one of whom has died; 17 patients were treated conservatively, three of whom have recurred without a death. One patient in this group had a positive node dissection out of a total of 46 dissections. The 8-year probability of disease-free survival and overall survival, while slightly worse for patients with microinvasion than for patients without microinvasion, was not statistically significant.

Conclusions for DCIS with microinvasion: DCIS with microinvasion is not an ominous finding. We are following these patients as a separate subgroup and more time will be required before we can be certain about their outcome. Currently, we are treating them in exactly the same manner as DCIS patients without microinvasion. Over time, they will likely do worse than patients with pure DCIS, but probably not much worse. Axillary node dissection for patients with DCIS-Mi is neither cost effective nor in their best interest.

What factors can we use to predict recurrence? In an attempt to predict recurrence, we have analysed our cases in many different way, using numerous factors like, nuclear size, nuclear grade, the presence of necrosis, differentiation, histologic subtype, P53, c-erbB-2, etc. A classification that interested us was devised by Ian Ellis of the Nottingham Group [5]. It divides DCIS into three groups based upon morphology and cellular necrosis: tumors which showed central lumina with necrotic debris surrounded by large pleomorphic viable cells in solid masses were classified as Predominantly Comedo. Tumors which showed necrotic neoplastic cells of ductal origin within duct lumina, but did not otherwise have a predominantly comedo pattern, were classified as DCIS with necrosis . This group included tumors showing a micropapillary or cribriform architecture with a significant amount of necrotic cellular debris and tumors with a minor but classic comedo component. Tumors that showed no evidence of necrosis were classified as DCIS without necrosis. The following tables show some of our data using this classification. Size, grade, ploidy and S-Phase are mean values.

Type	N	Size (mm)	Grade	Ploidy	S-Phase	c-erbB-2+	ER+
Predominantly Comedo	151	27	2.23	1.37	10.57	32%	65%
DCIS with Necrosis	52	24	2.09	1.29	7.90	42%	73%
DCIS without Necrosis	148	21	1.61	1.20	5.69	8%	79%

Type	**N**	**Recurrences**	**8-Year Disease-Free Survival**
Predominantly Comedo	151	15	(10%) 83%
DCIS with Necrosis	52	5	(10%) 84%
DCIS without Necrosis	148	5	(3%) 92%

If we combine the first two groups (Predominantly Comedo and DCIS with Necrosis), we have sorted the patients by a single pathologic finding: that is, whether or not necrosis is present.

Type	**N**	**Recurrences**	**10-Year Disease-Free Survival**
Necrosis	203	20	77%
No Necrosis	148	5	87%

Can local recurrence be predicted in conservatively treated patients? In our conservatively treated group, there were a total of 23 recurrences; 22 of them (96%) were at or near the initial biopsy. This lead us to believe that the most important cause of local recurrence was probably inadequate resection of the primary. Perhaps local recurrence should be called "local persistence". When we excise a DCIS and the pathologist tells us that the margins are free of disease, what does that mean? Does it really mean that we have excised the entire lesion? Serial subgross microscopic evaluation of excised DCIS specimens reveals that for many patients the lesion is larger than expected, often making complete excision impossible with less than a true quadrantectomy [6]. We have data on 242 patients with DCIS in whom the initial excision was performed using a wide local excision, rather than a true quadrant resection, and who subsequently underwent mastectomy (162 pts) or re-excision (80 pts) of the initial biopsy site, allowing us to histologically evaluate how much DCIS was left behind.

The average size of the initial wide excision was 5.9 cm. All initial specimens were serially sectioned at 2-3 mm. intervals and the margins evaluated microscopically. After 1984, all specimen margins were inked or dyed. Seventy-three patients with microscopically clear margins after initial excision elected re-excision (21 pts) or mastectomy (52 pts) to increase their margin of safety. At mastectomy or re-excision, the previous biopsy cavity was serially sectioned at 4-5 mm. intervals.

Residual DCIS

	at Mastectomy		at Re-excision		TOTAL
Initial Margins	Involved	Clear	Involved	Clear	
Number of Patients	110	52	59	21	242
Residual DCIS	92 (84%)	27 (52%)	42 (71%)	8 (38%)	169 (70%)

Overall, combining mastectomy and re-excision, 79% (134/169) of patients with involved margins had residual DCIS; 48% (35/73) of patients with clear margins had residual DCIS.

DCIS is difficult to excise completely using a wide local excision. If the object is to completely excise DCIS while preserving the breast, a true quadrantectomy may be required in many cases. While we believe that tumor grade and comedo necrosis is important, inadequate excision of the primary lesion is probably the most important cause of local failure after conservative treatment for intraductal breast carcinoma.

References

1. Silverstein MJ, Cohlan B, Gierson ED, et al. Duct carcinoma in situ: 227 cases without microinvasion. Eur J. Cancer 1992;28(2/3):630-634.

2. Lagios MD. Duct Carcinoma *in Situ*: Pathology and Treatment. Surg Clinics N. America 1990;40(4):853-871.

3. Van Dongen JA, Holland R, Peterse JL, et al. Ductal Carcinoma *in situ;* Second EORTC Consensus Meeting. Eur J. Cancer 1992;28(2/3):626-629.

4. Silverstein MJ, Gierson ED, Waisman JR, et al. Axillary Lymph Node Dissection for T1a Breast Carcinoma. Cancer 1994;73:664-667.

5. Poller DN, Ellis I, Galea M. Duct carcinoma in situ of the breast: A proposal of a new simplified histologic classification. In press: Modern Pathology 1994.

6. Holland R, Hendricks JHCL, Verbeek ALM, Mravunac M, and Schuurmans Stekhoven JH.. Extent, distribution, and mammographic/histological correlations of breast ductal carcinoma in situ. Lancet 1990;335:519-522.

Mastology - Breast Diseases
A.S.S. Figueira Fo et al., editors.

Pathology and clinical evaluation of ductal carcinoma in situ (DCIS) of the breast

David L. Page, M.D.[1] and Michael D. Lagois, M.D.
[1] Vanderbilt University Medical Center, Nashville, Tennessee and St. Mary's Hospital, San Francisco, California

Abstract

The therapy of ductal carcinoma in-situ is controversial, but is being more and more decided by the pathologic evidence. What we know of the natural history of ductal carcinoma in-situ is that the comedo and non-comedo examples seem quite different. As detailed in several reviews, the information from studies following patients after biopsy alone indicate a great difference between the small non-comedo examples of ductal carcinoma in-situ and the larger comedo DCIS. The currently available evidence from cases which have been treated by planned surgical excision without radiation therapy would indicate that the non-comedo examples of DCIS may be adequately treated by this modality as indicated in several recent studies.

Introduction

This paper will review the histopathology of DCIS and make the major point that we are currently in a state of transition from a classic posture linked with the premammographic and Halstedian eras. The two postures will be presented and studies supporting the stratification of DCIS by histologic pattern plus cytology and size will be contrasted to the rapidly disappearing classical posture that all DCIS is biologically similar and treatment options need not be stratified by the different subtypes or varieties of DCIS.

Size or extent of ductal carcinoma in-situ

The range of clinical presentations of ductal carcinoma in-situ is immense, extending from large, palpable masses to the tiniest examples which overlap occasionally with atypical ductal hyperplasia [1,2] using current criteria. These smaller lesions should be so recognized as being almost trivial. Size criteria have been helpful at this low end of the DCIS spectrum because lesions that are in the range of 2-5 mm in size are regularly quite circumscribed and obviously usually removed adequately by even the initial biopsy procedures. The natural history of these smaller lesions, when attention is not given to their margins, is detailed in papers published in 1978 [3] and 1982 [4].

The larger examples of DCIS, usually with comedo features are also well-known. They have been assumed to be multicentric in the past but recent studies with careful three dimensional reconstruction [5] make it clear that these lesions are continuous in three dimensions in almost all cases. The biologic event underlying this spread or involvement of much of the breast by a histologically similar process is not yet known. The more extensive examples with higher grade nuclei are often also associated with Paget's disease of the nipple [6].

Histologic type

There is a wide recent acceptance in many countries of the heterogeneity of DCIS [7-9]. Furthermore, many accept that cytology and histologic pattern (see table 1), be used together in order to make assignment into categories more precise, reproducible and clinically useful.

Address for correspondence: David L. Page, M.D., Department of Pathology, Medical Center North, C 3321, Vanderbilt University School of Medicine, Nashville, Tennessee 37232-2561

Table 1: Classification of DCIS

Histology	Cytology	Necrosis	Calcification
Comedo[1]	High grade	Extensive	Linear-branched
Intermediate	Intermediate	Limited	Focal-punctate
Non-Comedo	Low grade	Absent	Micro foci (inconsistent)
Cribriform			
Solid			
Micropapillary[2]			

[1]. Although different terms are used for this high-grade category, the presence of both high grade nuclear atypia and relatively extensive necrosis are necessary criteria

[2]. Some of these are high grade and may be considered comedo. They may be extensive when present in pure form.

Some pathologists have used histologic pattern and cytologic grade as separate determinants, but this approach negates the precise identification of the highest and lowest grade lesions. It is the determination of the highest and lowest grade lesions by the combined approach that is most likely to determine curability by the conservation treatment as indicated by the work of Lagios et al [10]. Initially, separating lesions into four categories with the top two categories having advanced nuclear atypia and necrosis, separated only by the remnants of a micropapillary or cribriform pattern in one of the categories. Later, Lagios [11] felt that these two categories should be combined. Thus, there seems no utility in recognizing minor remnants of cribriform or micropapillary pattern in high grade lesions because a large percentage of these cases recurred after planned wide excision. It is precisely this approach of using patho-anatomic principles in order to identify clinically useful endpoints which distinguishes the modern to histopathology from the historical descriptive approach. It is quite evident that the lower grade, non-comedo lesions are likely to be smaller, and also may be amenable to treatment with very low recurrence rates (table 2).

Table 2. Ductal carcinoma in situ of the breast: Effect of grade on recurrence following excision only

Study	Follow-up (mths)	High grade/Comedo	Low-intermediate grade/ Non-comedo
Lagios [11]	100	30.5% (11/36)	0% (0/32) Low 10% (1/10) Intermediate
Bellamy et al. [12]	60	40% (10/25)	0% (0/6)
Ottesen et al. [16]	63	30.6% (23/76)	5.5% (3/36)
Schwartz et al. [17]	47	47.6% (10/21)	2.0% (1/51)

There is a suggestion, as yet only documented in two studies [7,12] that the pure micropapillary pattern of DCIS (not combined with other patterns) may be associated more frequently with quite extensive disease. This is not true if occasional micropapilli are present intermixed with the solid and cribriform patterns which is frequently the case.

Differential diagnosis

There has been a lack of concordance between different pathologists in determining whether small lesions should be considered atypical hyperplasia or in-situ carcinoma. In general, lesions which involve only a few membrane bound spaces and which measure less than 2-3 mm in greatest dimension should be regarded as hyperplastic lesions (+/- atypia) and not in-situ carcinoma. There is a greater degree of concordance in larger lesions [1]. Even the diagnosis of difficult, smaller, borderline lesions will approach concordance between observers if pathologists agree on criteria [2].

Clinical outcome

After biopsy alone several studies have assessed the risk of subsequent invasive carcinoma in patients where the diagnosis of DCIS was not made at the initial biopsy for small, non-comedo lesions. In these patients approximately one third developed invasive breast cancer in the same region of the same breast within 10-18 years. Attempted wide excision of large, comedo DCIS lesions is notoriously unsuccessful [13, 14].

Developing evidence strongly supports the idea that adequate excision of DCIS lesions without radiotherapy (see table 2) may lead to cure [15]. As noted in other sections of this review, smaller non-comedo examples of DCIS are regularly treated successfully at least with follow-up extending to 7 or 8 years [11,12,16,17]. These surgical protocols have involved careful, planned, wide excision. Most of the cases have been mammographically detected, and a few cases discovered incidentally have been successfully treated also [17].

Role of radiation

What is the role of radiotherapy in reducing local recurrence after wide excision of a localized area of DCIS?

Preliminary data (with follow up of less than 4 years) from a study in the United States [18] suggest that radiotherapy may reduce the rate of disease recurrence within the breast following an adequate excision of a localized area of DCIS. It is not clear from this study whether the benefits of radiotherapy relate to all types of DCIS or whether the benefits will be demonstrable beyond 43 months of follow up. To determine the optimum treatment for screen detected DCIS a number of clinical trials are underway. It is widely accepted that the mammographically-detected DCIS lesion should be considered separately from the regularly larger lesions presenting with palpable masses and nipple discharge [19]. Whether radiation therapy aids in retarding or negating recurrence in some lesions awaits careful subtype analysis of such cases. However, the relevance of stratification by histologic pattern is well also demonstrated in groups of patients treated by radiotherapy after surgical excision [20].

It would appear that small examples of non-comedo ductal carcinoma in-situ are nonobligate precursor lesions, and only 25-30% of them eventuate in invasive carcinomas if left untreated. They may be regarded as increased risk lesions because their relative risk of later invasive cancer development is about 10 x that of the general population. It is obvious that if adequately removed surgically they may be regarded as cured, although it is by no means guaranteed that carcinoma may not develop elsewhere within these breasts in follow-up but that will be rare.

Conclusion

There is strong evidence that small size and low histologic grade interact to produce lesions easily cured by local excision without radiation therapy. This would certainly be true of lesions that are under a centimeter in largest diameter. The greatest extent of a lesion is most easily determined in these smaller lesions with careful pathologic-mammographic correlation, which is mandatory in most instances. It is also abundantly clear that extensive high grade, comedo lesions are not easily cured, and that recurrences are common even after radiation therapy. Precisely which concurrence of histologic grade and size is to be the determinant of therapeutic decision-making is an area under development currently. However, it should be understood that local recurrence in this setting is very unlikely to be a life threatening event and that a woman's desire for breast conservation with a willingness to accept the possibility of local recurrence may be as important with regard to therapeutic decision-making as any other consideration.

References

1. Page DL, Rogers, LW. Hum Pathol 1992;23:1095-1097
2. Schnitt SJ, Connolly JL, Tavassoli FA, Fechner RE, Kempson RL, Gelman R, Page DL. Am J Surg Pathol 1992;16:1133-1143
3. Betsill WL Jr., Rosen PP, Lieberman PH, Robbins GF. J A M A 1978;239:1863-1867
4. Page DL, Dupont WD, Rogers LW, Landenberger M. Cancer 1982;49:751-758
5. Holland R, Hendriks JHCL, Verbeek ALM, Mravunac M, Schuurmans Stekhoven JH. Lancet 1990;335:519-522
6. Chaudary MA, Millis RR, Lane EB, Miller NA. Breast Cancer Res Treat 1986;8:139-146
7. Patchefsky AS, Schwartz GF, Finkelstein SD, Prestipino A, Sohn SE, Singer JS, Feig SA. Cancer 1989;63:731-741
8. Lennington WJ, Jensen RA, Dalton LW, Page DL. Cancer 1994;73:118-124
9. Van Dongen JA, Holland R, Peterse JL, Fentiman IS, Lagios MD, Millis RR, Recht A. Eur J Cancer 1992;28:626-629
10. Lagios MD, Margolin FR, Westdahl PR, Rose MR. Cancer 1989;63:618-624
11. Lagios MD. Surg Clin N A 1990;70:853-871
12. Bellamy COC, McDonald C, Salter DM, Chetty U, Anderson TJ. Hum Pathol 1993;24:16-23
13. Silverstein MJ, Waisman JR, Gamagami P, Gierson ED, Colburn WJ, Rosser RJ, Gordon PS, Lewinsky BS, Fingerhut A. Cancer 1990;66:102-108
14. Dean L, Geschickter CF. Arch Surg 1938;36:225
15. Fechner RE. Am J Clin Pathol 1994;100:654-661
16. Ottesen GL, Graversen HP, Blichert-Toft M, Zedeler K, Andersen JA. Am J Surg Patho 1992;16:1183-1196
17. Schwartz GF, Finkel GC, Garcia JP, Patchefsky AS. Cancer 1992;70:2468-2474
18. Fisher B, Costantino J, Redmond C, Fisher E, Margolese R, Dimitrov N, Wolmark N, Wickerham DL, Deutsch M, Ore L, Mamounas E, Poller W, Kavanah M. N Engl J Med 1993;328:1581-1586
19. Pierce SM, Schnitt SJ, Harris JR. Cancer 1992;70:2576-2578
20. Solin LJ, Yeh I-T, Kurtz J, Fourquet A, Recht A, Kuske R, McCormick B, Cross MA, Schultz DJ, Amalric R, LiVolsi VA, Kowalyshyn MJ, Torhorst J, Jacquemier J, Westermann CD, Mazoujian G, Zafrani B, Rosen PP, Goodman RL, Fowble BL. Cancer 1993;71:2532-2542

Mastology - Breast Diseases
A.S.S. Figueira Fo et al., editors.

Ductal carcinoma in situ
The EORTC experience

E.J.Th. Rutgers, MD, PhD

On behalf of the EORTC Breast Cancer Working Group
Dept. of surgery, The Netherlands Cancer Institute
Plesmanlaan 121
1066 CX AMSTERDAM

Introduction

Ductal carcinoma in situ (DCIS) without invasion is found in 1-3% of the patients with clinically detected breast cancer (1, 2). Improved mammographic techniques, increasing use of mammography for routine use of patients with breast disorders and the introduction of population based screening mammography have resulted in a marked increase in occult, non-palpable breast carcinomas (3). Ductal carcinoma in situ accounts for 10-20% of these tumors (4, 5, 6). Mastectomy has been the standard therapy for clinically detected DCIS. The rationale for this treatment has been the assumed multicentricity of DCIS (7), and the possibility of achieving an almost 100% cure (8). However, the increasing detection of small clinical occult lesions, the doubts on the multicentricity of DCIS (9), the finding that not all DCIS are progressive lesions (10), that only one-third of patients with incompletely excised otherwise untreated DCIS will eventually develop recurrent lesions (11-13), raised the question about the feasibility of breast conservation therapy in DCIS. From retrospective studies, radiotherapy seems to play a role in BCT for DCIS, as after local excision alone a recurrence rate of about 22% in 10 different series was seen (14-23), and after local excision plus radiotherapy 6% recurrences (16, 19, 21, 23-27). To answer the question about the value of radiotherapy in breast conservation after excision of DCIS, several national and international groups started prospective randomized trials (28). Most trials require a complete excision of DCIS. Mastectomy is considered to be the 'Golden Standard' and therefore not taken into account in any trial.

In 1986 the EORTC Breast Cancer Cooperative Group started the trial 10853: "Phase III trial of treatment options for in situ ductal carcinoma of the breast" (29).

DCIS Trial : Annual Entry Rate 86–93
EORTC 10853

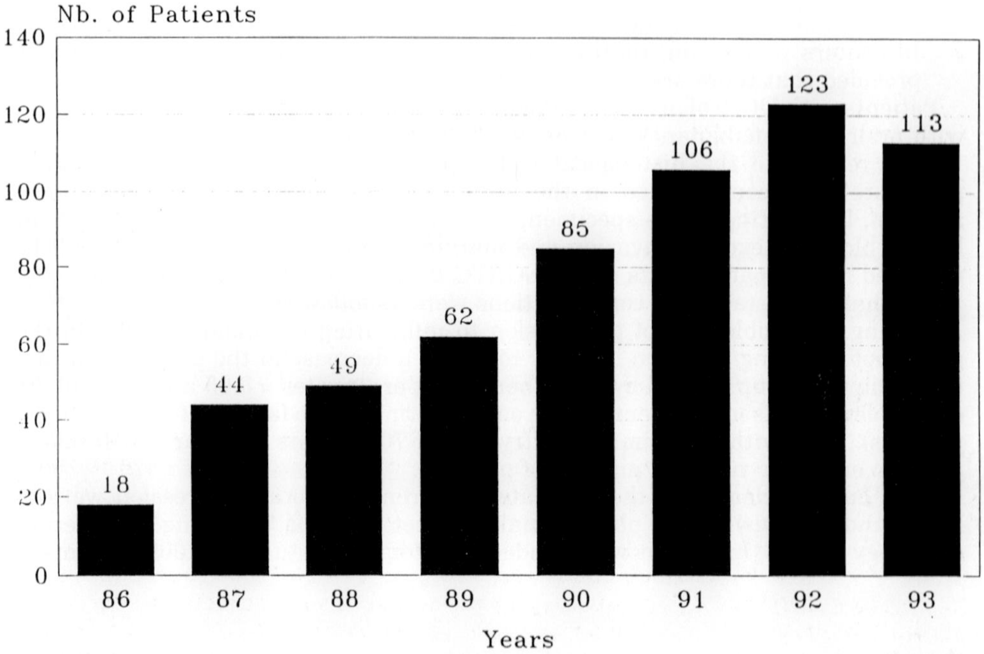

As of October 1993

Trial protocol EORTC 10853

The objectives of this study is to determine as to what proportion of DCIS may be treated by a conservative procedure and whether wide excision in combination with external irradiation provides adequate treatment for DCIS. After wide local excision of DCIS, eligible cases will be randomized between no further therapy and external irradiation of the breast with 50 Gy in 25 fractions in 5 weeks. Ineligible cases will also be registered and followed.
The criteria for eligibility are:

1. Patients will have had a biopsy which confirmed the presence of DCIS (solid, cribriform, papillary, clinging or comedo) without evidence of invasion.
2. Those patients with a lump or an area with microcalcifications less than 5 cm will have had this lump completely excised.
3. Cases between 3 and 5 cm can be excluded if the size of the breast does not allow a conservative surgery.
4. Pathological examination of the wide excision or quadrantectomy specimen

will have confirmed tumor-free margins (in some cases a wide unique excision with clear margins).
5. No evidence of tumor spread after staging investigations.
6. If a patient has a clinically enlarged axillary node suspected to contain tumor, this can be biopsied. If there is histological proof of axillary node metastases the patient will be excluded.
7. In centers performing routine axillary clearance such cases will be eligible provided that there are no axillary metastases.

Patients with DCIS of over 5 cm, Paget's disease of the nipple, who are pregnant, with prior other malignancy, or who are over 70 years of age, are excluded.

With respect to the histological work-up of the resection specimen a strict procedure has been outlined in the protocol, including: inking of the surgical margins, lamellating of the specimen, X-ray of slices in sequence, sampling of at least 8 blocks to exclude invasion and margin involvement. All histology will be reviewed by two pathologists of the EORTC Breast Cancer Working Group.

Originally the statistical considerations were as followed:
Assuming a possible risk of progression to infiltrating carcinoma of 30% in the group not receiving RT, then in order to detect a decrease in the progression rate to 15% in the group treated by radiotherapy (at error rates = 0.05 and = 0.20), 94 evaluable patients must be entered on each treatment arm (a total of 188 evaluable patients). Thus with an estimated entry rate of 70 patients per year it will take 2 years to enter the required number of patients.

As it became clear that the estimated difference in local progression were to large, and the wish to be able to make subset analysis according to different pathology groups, in 1990 it was decided to extend this study to 1.000 patients.

Results

Up to October 1993 600 patients entered this study from 40 different institutes. The great majority (520 pts) was entered by 18 hospitals. Initially the accrual was slow (see figure). In a separate study the reasons for this slow accrual were analyzed in 216 patients with biopsy confirmed DCIS from 6 different participating hospitals (30). Only 77 (36%) were entered and eligible for the trial. The major reason for non-entry was DCIS extending the margin of excision (55%), prior breast cancer (18%), delay in histological diagnosis (6%); only 6 patients (4%) refused to take part in the trial.

As the trial is still open for entry, results are not yet analyzed and can not be disclosed. In October 1993, 48 events in eligible cases were registered: 40 patients with breast relapse (23 DCIS, 16 invasive, 31 same quadrant), 6 contralateral cancers, 1 distant metastases alone and 1 axillary metastases alone.

The final analysis has to be awaited. This trial is of particularly interest with respect to the role of the strict pathology procedure and review, and to the possibility of subset analysis of histological subtypes.

References

1. Smart CR, Meyers MH, Gloecker LA. Implications from SEER data on breast cancer management. Cancer 1978; 40: 787-789.
2. Rosner D, Bedwani RN, Vana J et al. Noninvasive breast carcinoma: results of a national survey by the American College of Surgeons. Ann. Surg. 1980; 192: 139-147.
3. Schnitt SJ, Silen W, Sadowsky NL et al. Ductal carcinoma in situ (intraductal carcinoma) of the breast. N. Engl. J. Med.; 1988; 318: 898-903.
4. Schwartz GF, Feig SA, Patchefsky A. Significance and staging of non palpable carcinomas of the breast. Surg. Gynecol. Obstet.; 1988: 166: 6-10.
5. Peeters PHM, Verbeek ALM, Straatman H et al. Evaluation of overdiagnosis of breast cancer in screening with mammography. Int. J. Epidemiol. 1989; 18: 295-299.
6. Lagios MD, Margolin FR, Westdahl PR, Rose MR. Mammographically detected duct carcinoma in situ. Cancer 1989; 63: 618-624.
7. Lagios MD, Westdahl PR, Margolin FR, Rose MR. Duct carcinoma in situ: relationship of extent of non invasive disease to the frequency of occult invasion, multicentricity, lymph node metastases, and short-term treatment failures. Cancer 1982; 50: 1309-1314.
8. Sunshine JA, Moseley HS, Fletcher WS, Krippaehne WW. Breast carcinoma in situ: a retrospective review of 112 cases with a minimum 10 year follow-up. Am. J. Surg. 1985; 150: 44-51.
9. Holland R, Hendriks JHCL, Verbeek ALM et al. Extent, distribution, and mammographic/histological correlations of breast ductal carcinoma in situ. Lancet 1990; 335: 519-522.
10. Nielsen M, Jensen J, Andersen J. Precancerous and cancerous breast lesions during lifetime and at autopsy. A study of 83 women. Cancer 1984; 54: 612-615.
11. Gelderman WAH, Peterse JL, Van Dongen JA, Cohen P. Het ductale carcinoma in situ van de mamma: een klinisch-pathologisch retrospectief onderzoek. Ned. Tijdschr. Geneesk. 1986; 130: 308-310.
12. Page DL, Dupont WD, Rogers LW, Landenberger M. Intraductal carcinoma of the breast: follow-up after biopsy only. Cancer 1982; 49: 751-758.
13. Eusebi V, Foschini MP, Cook MG et al. Long-term follow-up of in situ carcinoma of the breast with special emphasis on clinging carcinoma. Semin. Diagn. Pathol. 1989; 6: 110-125.
14. Farrow JH. Current concepts in the detection and treatment of the earliest of the early breast cancer. Cancer 1970; 25: 468-477.
15. Ashikari R, Hajdu SI, Robbins G. Intraductal carcinoma of the breast (1960-1969). Cancer 1971; 28: 1182-1187.
16. Millis RR, Thynne GSJ. In situ intraduct carcinoma of the breast; a long-term follow-up study. Br. J. Surg. 1975; 62: 957-962.
17. Temple WJ, Jenkins M, Alexander F et al. Natural history of in situ breast cancer in a defined population. Ann. Surg. 1989; 210: 653-657.
18. Price P, Sinnett HD, Gusterson B et al. Duct carcinoma-in-situ can we predict recurrence after surgery? Lancet 1989; 1: 671-672.
19. Gallagher WJ, Koerner FC, Wood WC. Treatment of intraductal carcinoma with limited surgery: long-term follow-up. J. Clin. Oncol. 1989; 7: 376-380.

20. Ashikari R. Huvos AG, Snyder RE: Prospective study of non-infiltrating carcinoma of the breast. Cancer 1977; 39: 435-439.
21. Fisher ER, Sass R, Fisher B et al. Pathologic findings from the National Surgical Adjuvant Breast Protocol (protocol 6). I. Intraductal carcinoma (DCIS). Cancer 1986; 57: 197-208.
22. Lagios MD, Margolin FR, Westdahl PR, Rose MR. Mammographically detected duct carcinoma in situ. Frequency of local recurrence following tylectomy and prognostic effect of nuclear grade on local recurrence. Cancer 1989; 63: 618-624.
23. Silverstein MJ, Waisman JR, Gamagami P et al. Intraductal carcinoma of the breast (208 cases) Clinical factors influencing treatment choice. Cancer 1990; 66: 102-108.
24. Montague ED. Conservation surgery and radiation therapy in the treatment of operable breast cancer. Cancer 1984; 53: 700-704.
25. Recht A, Danoff BS, Slin LJ et al. Intraductal carcinoma of the breast: results of treatment with excisional biopsy and irradiation. J. Clin. Oncol. 1985; 3: 1339-1343.
26. Zafrani B. Fourquet A, Vilcoq JR et al. Conservative management of intraductal breast carcinoma with tumorectomy and radiation therapy. Cancer 1986; 57: 1299-1301.
27. Findlay P, Goodman R. Radiation therapy for treatment of intraductal carcinoma of the breast. Am. J. Clin. Oncol. 1983; 6: 281-285.
28. Van Dongen JA, Holland R, Peterse JL et al. Ductal carcinoma in situ of the breast: second EORTC Consensus Meeting. Eur J. Cancer 1992; 28: 626-629.
29. Study protocol EORTC 10853. Phase III trial of treatment options for in situ ductal carcinoma of the breast (1982). Study coordinator: Fentiman IS.
30. Fentiman IS, Julien JP, Van Dongen JA, Van Geel B, Chetty U, Coibon M. Reasons for non-entry of patients with DCIS of the breast in situ a randomized trial (EORTC 10853). Eur. J. Cancer 1991; 27: 450-452.

III. 4. Surgical treatment

Mastology - Breast Diseases
A.S.S. Figueira Fo et al., editors.

Controversies in Breast Cancer Surgery

John Hayward, FRCS, Breast Unit, London Bridge Hospital, London, U.K.

The National Surgical Adjuvant Breast Project (NSABP), in the United States, is the largest, and probably the most influential, body which organises clinical trials on breast cancer. In June 1990, as a result of a chance finding by audit clerks at the NSABP headquarters in Pittsburgh, a significant number of errors and falsifications were found in patient data entered by one hospital in Montreal, Canada. Subsequently, similar discrepancies were demonstrated in a number of other contributing centres.

The seriousness of these findings can be judged by the statements made by breast experts enlisted to comment on the implications. They questioned whether any NSABP data were reliable and felt that the integrity of conclusions based on these data could not be assumed. The significance of these developments was compounded by the known effect that the results of NSABP studies have had on current North American, and even worldwide, clinical practice.

The situation was not made public until 1994 when assurances were given that, if patients on whom false data had been recorded, were excluded, the results of the studies were not materially changed. Nevertheless, the basic data were not released and no external review had at this time been undertaken.

The immediate local effects were that the coordinator of these studies was relieved of his post and a subsequent Congressional hearing ordered a complete re-analysis of the database. Moreover, there was understandable unease amongst patients as to whether treatment they had received for breast cancer had been appropriate.

From the scientific point of view, it seems unlikely that the data errors - many of which were trivial - will be found to affect the overall results of previously reported studies. What is more important is the concern that many physicians now feel on the reliability of conclusions which the NSABP drew from their results. Should the interpretation of these conclusions in the management of early breast cancer now be reviewed?

There are two important clinical philosophies, based on the NSABP studies, which have largely been accepted. Firstly is the concept that breast cancer is usually a systemic disease from the start and that variations in loco-regional therapy are unlikely to affect results. Secondly, and as a result of this, that the increased incidence of breast recurrence after many conservative treatments for invasive cancer, or after treatment of DCIS by local surgery and radiation, does not affect the eventual outcome. The inference of these statements is that local control of disease is relatively unimportant and that local recurrence is simply a marker of tumour aggression - not significantly affecting disease-free survival.

Probably the converse view should now be re-examined - that local control of disease is important and that a woman can die of breast cancer if the primary complex is treated ineffectively. There is as convincing evidence to support this thesis as there is to reinforce the NSABP conclusions.

Mastology - Breast Diseases
A.S.S. Figueira Fo et al., editors.

Indications and contraindications to conservative surgery in breast cancer

Paolo Veronesi and Alberto Luini*

Second Division of Surgery and *Division of Senology - European Institute of Oncology - Milan - Italy

Correspondence to: Dr. Paolo Veronesi, Divisione di Chirurgia II, Istituto Europeo di Oncologia, via Ripamonti 435, 20141 Milano, Italy

Abstract

After the drop of the Halstedian theory of demolitive surgery “en bloc”, from the early Eighties on conservative surgery followed by radiotherapy for early breast cancers was applied by all experienced and updated surgeons. Some randomized study showed a high local recurrence rate, due to the limited surgical excision. Extensive intraductal component, high histologic grade, peritumoral lymphatic invasion, young age, lobular histology and margins of resection have been studied as risk factors for local recurrence.

Although many reports on conservative treatment of breast cancer had been available since the beginning of the century, especially those based on X-rays therapy (1-3), the Halstedian theory of demolitive surgery "en bloc" for breast cancer began to be seriously discussed only in the late Sixties. Based on the Halsted theory of lymphatic permeation of cancer cell from the primary tumor, it was decided in 1962 to perform a randomized study on internal mammary node dissection. When, a few years later, it became clear that the dissection of internal mammary nodes did not improve the prognosis in breast cancer patients (4), the need for extensive "en bloc" resection of primary cancer with regional nodes revealed its weakness. In the meantime pathologists showed that the lymphatic spread to regional nodes was "embolic" in nature and the "permeation" process of lymphatic diffusion of cancer cells was thus disproved.

In 1973 a randomized trial started in Milan which compared the traditional Halsted operation with the QU.A.RT. (Quadrantectomy, Axillary dissection, Radiotherapy) technique for Stage 1 breast cancer. The technique which was described in many papers (5-7) involved complete removal of the tumor and the surrounding breast tissue of 2-3 cm, with its portion of skin, down to the fascia of the pectoralis major. Complete axillary dissection (including third level) was performed in continuity or by a separate incision, removing or sparing the pectoralis minor. All patients received postoperative radiotherapy of 50 Gy to the whole breast plus a boost of 10 Gy to the wound area. Adjuvant systemic treatment was given to node positive patients and consisted of chemotherapy: CMF regimen x 12 cycles. There was no difference in the two groups in terms of overall survival (8,9). The cumulative incidence of local recurrences at 18 yr. was 6.9% in the QU.A.RT. group compared with 3.7% in the mastectomy group. The safety of conservative surgical procedures plus radiotherapy was confirmed by several randomized studies (10,11) and from the early Eighties on these procedures were applied by all experienced and updated surgeons, even if the NSABP study experienced a high local recurrence rate due to the limited excision, the so-called "lumpectomy". This procedure consisted in the removal of the tumor with only a small rim of breast tissue. With this kind of surgery, the probability of leaving microscopic foci of neoplastic cells in the breast was high and a radical radiotherapy was necessary to control the disease.

The second generation trials in Milan (Milan II and III) which compared two types of conservative treatment confirmed that when avoiding postoperative radiotherapy or reducing the extent of breast resection, local relapses were higher compared to the QU.A.RT. group. The cumulative incidence of local recurrences at five years shows a risk of 18% for patients treated with quadrantectomy without radiotherapy, and 11.5% for patients treated with tumorectomy plus intensive radiotherapy.

While in the first Italian trial the fear of local relapse limited the indication to quadrantectomy to tumors less than 2 cm in diameter, and to 2.5 cm in the following sudies, many efforts have been made recently to identify patients at high risk of recurrence, and, consequently the type of surgery for any given patient. As a matter of fact, tumor diameter is not the only predictor of local recurrence (LR) and perhaps not even the most important one. Extensive intraductal component (EIC), high tumor grade, peritumoral lymphatic invasion (PLI), young age, infiltrating lobular histology and positivity on margin resection were studied as risk factors for LR.

EIC

Moderate or marked intraductal cancer in the primary tumor and intraductal cancer involving the surrounding breast tissue are both predictors of LR and were combined together and labeled EIC by Schnitt et al. in 1984 (12). From then on, many reports stressed the importance of EIC as (the most important) predictor of LR (13-16), even if some investigators failed to find a significant correlation between EIC and breast relapse (17,18). The most important study describing the growth pattern of breast cancer was recently reported by Holland et al. (19) who performed a radiologic-pathologic mapping study on 217 specimens from mastectomies. They found 33% of prominent residual disease more than 2 cm from the primary tumor in the EIC (+) group, compared with only 2% in the EIC (-) one. These percentages drop to 14% and 1% at 3 cm from the primary tumor. These findings underline the importance of extensive resection in patients with EIC (+) cancer.

Histologic grade

Fisher (17), Clarke (18) and Kurtz (20) found a significant difference in local recurrence rate between patients with G3 tumors (12% to 17%) compared with patients with G1 and G2 tumors (2% to 4%). As most of the breast failures occurred in the original tumor bed, it seems reasonable to administer a higher tumor-bed boost to patients with high-grade cancers.

Peritumoral lymphatic invasion

The correlation between PLI and LR has been shown by Fisher et al. (17), especially in patients treated with conservative surgery without radiotherapy. Similar conclusions have been reported by Fourquet et al. (14).

Young age

There is significant controversy regarding the importance of young age as a risk factor for LR. Many reports showed an increased incidence of local failures in young patients (14, 21, 22) even if others failed to demonstrate a correlation between young age and LR (18, 23). Data published by Recht et al. (21), Fourquet et al. (14) and Kurtz et al. (15) showed that young age appears to be correlated with EIC positive, high grade and incomplete gross excision. In absence of these findings, young age does not affect the risk of LR.

Lobular carcinoma

Although invasive lobular carcinoma represents only 6 to 10% of breast cancers, literature supports the view that this subtype has a slightly higher risk of local failure after breast conservative surgery (24,25). In these series the higher incidence of local failure was probably due to limited excision (lumpectomy). In a review of 2,233 breast cancer patients operated on at the National Cancer Institute in Milan between 1973 and 1987 with a median follow-up of 10.5 years according to the QUART technique, no difference in recurrence rate was observed between 1,633 infiltrating ductal carcinomas and 258 infiltrating lobular carcinomas (5.3% and 5.0% respectively)(26).

Margin of resection

In the Milan II trial, 46 out of 345 T.A.RT. (Tumorectomy, Axillary dissection, Radiotherapy) patients showed positive margins of resection. In this group of patients radiotherapy was performed according to the protocol. In these cases, the LR rate was 20% (50% in EIC. positive patients). Moreover, the cases with negative margins showed a LR rate of 8% (20% in EIC. positive patients). These results suggest that the methods to define positivity of margins are inadeguate, as they detect only one fourth of cases with residual cancer cells. Consequently, in patients with negative margins, postoperative radiotherapy is necessary also because of the high rate of false negatives.

It is difficult to describe a treatment plan for each breast cancer patient based only on the tumor diameter. The real problem is to perform a breast excision which is wide enough to obtain a 2-3 cm margin of normal tissue all around the tumor. Therefore the ratio between tumor diameter and breast size is of great importance. In large breasts it is possible to perform a safe quadrantectomy or wide resection even for tumors up to 3 cm in diameter, while in very small breasts it could be difficult to obtain a safe margin even for small cancers.

Preoperative mammography is necessary to plan the extension of the resection. The presence of microcalcifications suggests an extensive intraductal component, thus requiring a wider excision. Moreover, mammography could detect occult multicentric lesions, thereby suggesting total mastectomy. In selected cases, when multifocality is limited to a breast quadrant, conservative treatment may be considered provided the resection is sufficiently extensive.

For patients who do not fulfill the requirements for a conservative procedure, primary chemotherapy could be considered. Three cycles of full-dose primary chemotherapy can safely induce prompt tumor shrinkage and allows for conservative surgery. Our experience indicates that several drug regimens as primary chemotherapy can down-stage a large, but resectable, breast cancer to less than 3 cm in most patients (initial tumor size 3-5 cm, 91%; larger than 5 cm., 73%).(27).

REFERENCES

1. Finzi NS. X-Rays and radium in the treatment of carcinoma of the breast. Br Med J 1908; 2: 728-733.

2. Hirsch J. Radiumchirurgia des Brust Krebses. Dtsch Med Wochenschr 1927; 53: 1419-1421.

3. Baclesse F. Roentgen therapy as the sole method of treatment of cancer of the breast. Am J Roent Radium Ther Nucl Med 1949; 62: 311-313.

4. Veronesi U and Valagussa P. Inefficacy of internal mammary nodes dissection in breast cancer surgery. Cancer 1981; 47: 170-175.

5. Veronesi U. New trends in the treatment of breast cancer at the Cancer Institute of Milan. Am J Roentgenology 1977; 128: 287-289.

6. Veronesi U, Banfi A, Saccozzi R et al. Conservative treatment of breast cancer. A trial in progress at the Cancer Institute of Milan. Cancer 1977; 39: 2822-2826.

7. Veronesi U. Value of limited surgery for breast cancer. Seminars in Oncology 1978; 5: 395-402.

8. Veronesi U, Saccozzi R, Del Vecchio M et al. Comparing radical mastectomy with quadrantectomy, axillary dissection, and radiotherapy in patients with small cancer of the breast. New England J Med 1981; 305: 6-11.

9. Veronesi U, Banfi A, Del Vecchio M et al. Comparison of Halsted mastectomy with quadrantectomy, axillary dissection, and radiotherapy in early breast cancer: long-term results. Eur J Cancer Clin Oncol 1986; 22: 1085-1089.

10. Sarrazin D, Lè MG, Fontaine MF and Arriagada R. Conservative treatment versus mastectomy in T1 or small T2 breast cancer. A randomized clinical trial. In: Harris JR, Hellman S and Silen W (eds.) Conservative Management of Breast Cancer. Philadelphia: Lippincot, 1983; 101-112.

11. Fisher B, Bauer M, Margolese R et al. Five-year results of a randomized clinical trial comparing total mastectomy and segmental mastectomy with or without radiation in the treatment of breast cancer. New England J Med 1985; 312: 665-673.

12. Schnitt SJ, Connolly JL, Harris JR et al. Pathologic predictors of early local recurrence in stage I and II breast cancer treated by primary radiation therapy. Cancer 1984; 53: 1049-1057.

13. Bartelink H, Borger JH, van Dongen JA, Peterse JL. The impact of tumor size and histology on local control after breast conserving therapy. Radiotherapy and Oncology 1988; 11: 297-303.

14. Fourquet A, Campana F, Zafrani B et al. Prognostic factors of breast recurrence in the conservative management of early breast cancer: a 25 years follow-up. Int J Radiat Oncol Biol Phys 1989; 17: 719-725.

15. Kurtz J, Jacquemier J, Almaric R. Risk factors for breast recurrence in premenopausal and postmenopausal patients with ductal cancers treated by conservation therapy. Cancer 1990; 65: 1867-1878.

16. Lindley R, Bulman A, Parson P. Histologic feature predictive of an increased risk of early local recurrence after treatment of breast cancer by local tumor excision and radical radiotherapy. Surgery 1989; 105: 13-20.

17. Fisher ER, Sass R, Fisher B et al. Pathologic findings from the National Surgical Adjuvant Breast Project (protocol 6): II. Relation of local breast recurrence to multicentricity. Cancer 1986; 57: 1717-1724.

18. Clarke DH, Le MG, Sarrazin D et al. Analysis of local-regional relapses in patients with early breast cancers treated with excision and radiotherapy: Experience of the Institut Gustave-Roussy. Int J Radiat Oncol Biol Phys 1985; 11: 137-145.

19. Holland R, Connolly JL, Gelman R et al. The presence of an extensive intraductal component following a limited excision correlates with prominent residual disease in the remainder of the breast. J Clin Oncol 1990; 8: 113-118.

20. Kurtz JM, Jacquemier J, Amalric R et al. Risk factors for mammary recurrence in pre- and post-menopausal women with infiltrating ductal cancers. Proceedings of the 7th Annual Meeting of the European Society of Therapeutic Radiology and Oncology 1988, 216.

21. Recht A, Connolly JL, Schnitt SJ et al. The effect of young age on tumor recurrence in the treated breast after conservative surgery and radiotherapy. Int J Radiat Oncol Biol Phys 1988; 14: 3-10.

22. Kurtz JM, Spitalier JM, Amalric R et al. Mammary recurrences in women younger than forty. Int J Radiat Oncol Biol Phys 1988; 15: 271-276, 1988.

23. Solin LJ, Fowble B, Schultz DJ et al. Age as a prognostic factor for patients treated with definitive irradiation for early stage breast cancer. Int J Radiat Oncol Biol Phys 1989; 16: 373-381.

24. Kurtz JM, Jacquemier J, Torhorst J et al. Conservation therapy for breast cancers other than infiltrating ductal carcinoma. Cancer 1989; 63: 1630-1635.

25. Schnitt SJ, Connolly JL, Recht A et al. Influence of infiltrating lobular histology on local tumor control in breast cancer patients treated with conservative surgery and radiotherapy. Cancer 1989; 64: 448-454.

26. Veronesi P, Zurrida S, Greco M, Del Vecchio M. Infiltrating lobular histology is not a contraindication to conservative surgery in the management of breast cancer patients. Br J Surg (in press).

27. Bonadonna G, Veronesi U, Brambilla C et al. Primary chemotherapy to avoid mastectomy in tumors with diameters of three centimeters or more. J Natl Cancer Inst 1990; 82: 1539.

Mastology - Breast Diseases
A.S.S. Figueira Fo et al., editors.

SURGICAL TREATMENT OF BREAST CANCER: TOTAL MASTECTOMY OR LIMITED RESECTION

JOHN G. GOGAS, M.D.

Second Department of Propaedeutic Surgery,

University of Athens, Athens-Greece

Breast cancer is a major public health problem of great interest. The epidemiologic increase of this cancer is of grave concern to the international health care community. In this short paper the surgical management of Stage I and II breast cancer is discussed.

Local treatment of infiltrating breast cancer is directed to the breast and the adjacent lymph nodes. The principal objective of local treatment is the eradication of local disease. In patients without metastasis this treatment can cure the disease.

Surgical treatment for local and regional breast cancer has changed considerably during the past decade. Modified radical mastectomy and breast concerving surgery with axillary dissection followed by radiation offer alternative approaches of comparable efficacy.

Until the early 1980´s the standard treatment was mastectomy. Then reports of several trials were published showing that breast conserving surgery followed by radiotherapy was a valid alternative for many women. Retrospective reviews of the clinical outcome of breast conserving treatments, some with very long periods of follow-up have shown low rates of local recurrence, high rates of satisfactory cosmetic results and a very low rate of complications [1,2,3].

The frequency with which modified radical mastectomy and breast conserving treatment are used has changed during the recent years. The incidence of modified radical mastectomy from 55.6% in 1977 increased to 72%

whereas the use of partial mastectomy from 2.8% to 7.2% in the United States of America [4]. In a recent survey in England 64% of breast cancer cases were treated by conservative surgery and 22% by mastectomy [5].

Although the concept of breast conservation is not a new one utilization of this therapy has been somewhat slow . In a recent article it was demonstrated that there were remarkable geographic regional differences in the United States of America in the utilization of such therapy for early breast cancer. The proportion of women with localized breast cancer who underwent brast conserving surgery ranged from 19.6 percent (Iowa) to 41.5 percent (Seatle) in 1985-1986 [6]. At Memorial Hospital the utilization of breast conservation almost equals that of modified radical mastectomy in the treatment of 950+ annual primary operable breast cancers [3]. At a consensus conference in 1985 there was an attempt to define the proper conserving procedure [7]. Most faculty members advocated a wide excision. A simple excision without regard to margins was thought to carry high risk of local recurrence and quadrantectomy was considered to be too deforming to permit an acceptable cosmetic result. Microscopic assessment of the margins of resection has been used by some to determine whether further resection is necessary. If the margins are involved by tumor a reexcision of the primary site is performed as involved margins in fact lead to an increased risk of local recurrence.

Patient selection criteria for conservation surgery versus mastectomy

The actual selection of therapy for an individual patient is complex confusing and controversial. The patient selection plays a pivotal role in obtaining excellent local regional control. There are few absolute or relative contraindications to breast preservation. The commonly accepted contraindications in Stage I and II breast cancer involve multicentricity and tumor size. Steroid dependent collagen-vascular disease remains an absolute contraindication because of the poor cosmetic results after radiotherapy [3].

Multicentricity is a very common characteristic of breast cancer [8]. In a prospective study of 366 specimens of modified radical mastectomy multicentricity was found in 49.1 per cent samples. It was found factors related to multicentricity were the young age of the patient, the size and histologic type of the tumor levels of progesterone receptors more than 50f mol/mg of protein and the amount of solid tissue in the breasts. It was more common in young and premenopausal women and in large tumors. Multicentricity is associated with increased risk of local recurrence (40 percent in patients with multiple lesions versus 11 percent in patients with a single lesion [9].

Extensive intraductal component: The patients who are extensive intraductal component positive have a higher rate of local failure rate (18%-25%) than patients who are extensive intraductal component negative (5%-10%) [2,10,11]. Histologic type and grade of the lesion.Lobular infiltrating carcinoma as well tumors with high grade of malignancy have an increased rate of local recurrence compared to those with infiltrating ductal carcinoma and of low grade of malignancy [3].

Young age and extensive intraductal component are the most significant risk factors for local recurrence after conservation surgery [2].

Although no patient or tumor characteristics have been identified that preclude the use of conservation procedures and radiation therapy [1]. It seems that patient selection plays a pivotal role in obtaining excellent local-regional control and there are certain early stage breast cancers who are better served with mastectomy [3].

REFERENCES

1. Fisher B, Anderson S. World J Surg 1994; 18: 63-69.
2. Veronesi M, Luini A, Galimberti V, Zurrida S. World J Surg 1994; 18: 70-75.
3. Moore MP, Kinne DW. World J Surg 1994; 18: 58-62.
4. Wilson RE, Donegan WL, Mettlin C, et al. Surg Gyn Obst 1984; 159: 309-314.
5. Morris J, Royle GT, Taylor I. J R Soc Med 1989; 290: 12-14.
6. Farrow D, Hunt WC, Samet JM. N Engl J Med 1992; 326: 1097-1101.
7. Harris JR, Hellman S, Kinne DW. N Engl J Med 1985; 313: 1365-1370.
8. Anastassiades O, Iakovou E, Stavridou N, Gogas J, Karameris A. Am J Clin Path 1993; 99: 238-243.
9. Leopold KA, Recht A, Schnitt SJ et al. Int J Radiat Oncol Biol Phys 1989; 16: 11.
10. Recht A, Silen W, Schnitt SJ, et al. Int J Radiat Oncol Biol Phys 1988; 15: 255.
11. Lindle R, Bulman A, Parsons P, Phillips R, Henry K, Ellis H. Surgery 1989; 105: 13-20.

Mastology - Breast Diseases
A.S.S. Figueira Fo et al., editors.

Surgical implications of preoperative chemotherapy in large-size breast cancer.

M. Greco*, S. Zurrida, V. Galimberti, R. Agresti.

Istituto Nazionale Tumori, Via Venezian 1, 20133 Milano, Italy

*To whom correspondence should be addressed.

Abstract

Preoperative chemotherapy in 226 women with large breast cancers reduced tumour size sufficiently for breast conservation surgery, according to our criteria, in 203 (90%). After 50 months' mean follow-up there were 13/203 local relapses (5.3%). This approach is therefore valid but only if the breast can be conserved with good aesthetic result, otherwise mastectomy plus reconstruction is preferable. What surgery to perform must be decided during the operation after careful assessment of tumour regression, resection margins, tumour size in relation to breast size and extent of microcalcifications.

Cytoreductive chemotherapy is routinely applied preoperatively in advanced tumours (a) to help achieve surgical radicality, (b) to permit conservative surgery when the local situation indicates a demolitive approach, and (c) to combat micrometastases at an early stage. The literature on these applications is abundant [1]. Primary chemotherapy was first used against locally advanced breast cancer (T3b, T4): to rapidly reduce tumour size and allow safe surgery or radiotherapy [2]. Numerous studies have shown that overall survival in breast cancer mainly depends on the number and invasion level of involved axillary lymph nodes and the initial size of the tumour; the type of local surgery having little influence on prognosis [3]. Taking this as our starting point, we sought to explore the problems that the surgeon faces in attempting to conserve the breast when operating on large breast cancers pre-operatively treated by chemotherapy.

Patients and methods

From January 1988 to October 1990, 226 consenting patients, less than 65 years of age, with cytologically or histologically confirmed breast malignancy >3 cm on mammogram, were studied to evaluate the efficacy of different chemotherapy regimens in reducing the initial size of the primary and allow quadrantectomy as described by Veronesi [4,5]. In 220 patients the treatment was completed as scheduled. The location and size of the tumour mass was tattooed on the skin surface before beginning chemotherapy. Three weeks after the last cycle each patient was clinically and mammographically re-evaluated, and if the tumour was sufficiently reduced, conservative surgery planned. The proportion of patients whose breasts were conserved was the same for all chemotherapy regimens. During the operation the removed tissue was carefully examined for multifocality and to assess residual tumour size and resection margins. If the margins were positive another resection was performed and the new margins examined. If the new margins were still positive, the macroscopic dimension of the lesion too large to allow a secure procedure, or the neoplasm was multifocal, the breast was removed completely. In all cases total axillary dissection was performed. Conservatively treated patients were always given complementary radiotherapy (breast only). All patients were checked clinically and instrumentally every four months. Mean follow-up to date is 50 months (range 38 – 76).

Results

Of the 226 patients operated on, 203 (90%) received conservative, and 23 (10%) received demolitive treatment. Table 1 shows the type of surgery in relation to initial tumour size. The larger the initial size the less likely the tumour would

Table 1
Treatment according to initial tumor size

Initial size of tumour (cm)	No of patients	QUART*	Mastectomy
3.0 – 4,0	141	138	3
4.1 – 5.0	56	46	11
>5	29	20	9
Totals	226	203	23

shrink to a size compatible with conservative treatment, but: where the initial diameter was <5 cm conservation was usually possible. At surgical inspection it was impossible to find any trace of lesion in 26 instances, eight of which also showed no microscopic evidence of cancer. Histology revealed multifocality of the primary in 37 patients (16.3%); in 22 of which (60%) mammography showed carcinoma associated with microcalcifications. Multifocality was slightly more frequent in larger tumours, probably because they had not been uniformly destroyed by the chemotherapy. Local recurrences were more frequent in node positive (13/136) than node negative patients (4/90), and were also more frequent in mastectomy (22%) than quadrantectomy (5%) patients. Metastases occurred in 10/23 mastectomy patients (44%) and 56/203 quadrantectomy patients (27%). Mastectomy patients had larger initial lesions (mean 5.5 cm vs 4 cm) and were more frequently axillary node positive (19/23 vs 117/203) than quadrantectomy patients.

Discussion

We are the first to consider the surgical problems raised by preoperative chemotherapy in breast cancer. Our study shows that preoperative chemotherapy reduces the size of the primary in a high percentage of cases, often consenting conservative surgery. Accurate estimation of tumour size in the operating room is crucial for deciding the type and extent of operation to be performed. The tumour may become soft to palpation following destruction of much of the tumour mass; so that tattoo marks are essential for locating the part to be completely removed. When microcalcifications are observed in the initial mammogram, intraoperative x-ray of the specimen helps to ensure that the whole lesion is removed. Obviously, dispersed calcifications contraindicate preoperative chemotherapy. Of 23 mastectomies, 9 involved primaries of diameter <3 cm but with multiple foci in the surrounding tissue as revealed by examination in the operating room. Conversely, 21/203 conservative treatments (10.3%) were carried out when the tumour was >3 cm; here the favourable ratio between tumour size and breast volume assured a good cosmetic result while fulfilling our radicality criteria. After a mean follow-up 50 months there have been 13 local relapses (5.3%) in 203 quadrantectomies. In all these cases the original tumours were >3 cm and sometimes >6 cm, so this relapse rate appears acceptable. Contrastingly a high rate of local recurrences occurred in the mastectomied patients (5/23; 21.7%); showing that in this subgroup carcinoma was resistant to chemotherapy and aggressive, and indicating that additional treatments, such as postoperative chest-wall radiotherapy, should be considered in the future. We conclude that conservative breast surgery always followed by radiotherapy (QUART) is a valid treatment for large tumours if preoperative chemotherapy reduces tumour size to <3 cm. We emphasise, however, that the final decision on which surgery to perform should be taken in the operating room after careful assessment of tumour regression, resection margins, tumour size in relation to breast size, and extent of microcalcifications. A further fundamental point is that the aim of preoperative chemotherapy is aesthetically acceptable breast conservation. If this is not reasonably achievable, then mastectomy followed by one of the newer and highly effective breast reconstruction approaches should be applied.

References

1. Harris DT, Mastrangelo MJ. Theory and application of early systemic therapy. Semin Oncol 1991; 18: 493-503.
2. Valagussa P, Zambetti M, Bonadonna G, et al. Prognosis factors in locally advanced non-inflammatory breast cancer. Long term results following primary chemotherapy. Breast Cancer Res Treat 1990; 15: 137-147.
3. Veronesi U, Galimberti V, Zurrida S, et al. Prognostic significance of number and level of axillary node metastases in breast cancer. The Breast 1993, 2: 224-228.
4. Veronesi U, Costa A, Saccozzi R, et al. Surgical technique of breast quadrantectomy and axillary dissection. In: Strombeck JO, Rosato FE (eds) Surgery of the

breast. Diagnosis and treatment of breast disease. Thieme Verlag, Stuttgart 1986; 127-131.
5. Veronesi U, Salvadori B, Luini A, et al. Conservative treatment of early breast cancer. Ann Surg 1990; 211(3): 250-259.

Mastology - Breast Diseases
A.S.S. Figueira Fo et al., editors.

CONSERVATIVE X RADICAL TREATMENT OF BREAST CANCER SELECTION OF PATIENTS FOR CONSERVATIVE TREATMENT

MAURÍCIO MAGALHÃES COSTA, M.D., M.S.
CENTRO MÉDICO SOROCABA
RUA SOROCABA 464 / 401
BOTAFOGO - RIO DE JANEIRO - BRAZIL
22271-100

Major changes have occurred in the last century, mainly in the last decade, in the overall management of the patient with malignant lesion of the breast.

The comprehension of the natural history and tumor biology guided toward less disfiguring surgery combined to other therapeutic modalities.

The primary procedure used in the treatment of breast cancer was the radical mastectomy. In 1894, Halsted published a classical research with the results of radical mastectomy and a local recurrence of 6% [1] that was markedly lower than the previously described for this disease.

Although the radical mastectomy was an important advance in the treatment of patients with breast cancer, it resulted in significant functional and cosmetic deformities. The modified radical mastectomy was developed as an attempt to avoid these problems by sparing the pectoral musculature and at the same time achieving the same ultimate results. Retrospective studies, such as Handley e Patey [2,3] attest to equivalent results attainable with a modified radical mastectomy as compared with the classical radical mastectomy.

The knowledges about tumor biology demonstrating that the neoplasia can be systemic, even in early stages, have introduced the concepts of multimodality therapeutic, combining chemotherapy, surgery and radiotherapy in order to treat the micrometastases.

Based on the success obtained with the modified radical mastectomy, and in an attempt to further limit the extent of resection, there has been a great deal of interest in examining the results that can be obtained without a mastectomy in the treatment of breast cancer [table 1].

Based on these data, the recent NIH Consensus Development conference on the treatment of early breast cancer made the following statement [7]:

" *Breast conservation treatment is an appropriate method of primary therapy for the majority of women with Stage I and II breast cancer and is preferable because it provides survival equivalent to total mastectomy and axillary dissection while preserving the breast*"

The final decision in the management of a patient is determined by multiple factors and some patients are not candidates for breast conservation. There are two broad categories of patients who might be better treated with mastectomy than with breast conservation: 1) those patients in whom the cosmetic appearance of the breast would be unacceptable despite optimal attempts at breast conservation; and 2) those patients who are at high risk for local failure after breast conservation.

Although there is not an absolute size cutoff for breast preservation, patients who have tumors that are relative large compared with the size of the breast may have an unacceptable cosmetic result with conservative surgery. Patients with underlying collagen vascular disease tend to have a poor cosmetic result with radiation therapy.

Controversy exists about the contraindication to breast conservation based on the likehood of a particular tumor to develop local recurrence in the breast. It is reasonable to examine risk factors for local failure; for those patients at high risk for local recurrence, considerations should be given to a mastectomy.

Patients with multifocal disease or those with diffuse microcalcifications on mammography are at high risk for local recurrence, consideration should be given to a mastectomy. Of some controversy is the role of specific pathologic and patient features, including: extensive intraductal component, extensive lymphatic vascular invasion, comedonecrosis, histologic grade, axillary node metastases, presence of inflamatory infiltrate, tumor size and young patients(< 35 years).[8,9]

Reviews from the Joint Center for Radiation Therapy have shown that the primary predictor for local failure after breast conserving therapy in the presence of an extensive intraductal component, defined as intraductal cancer making up > 25% of the tumor mass and intraductal cancer extending beyond the margins of the tumor mass. Patients with EIC-positive tumors had an acturial local recurrence rate of 25% at five years, compared with 5% for patients with EIC-negative tumors.[10]

Size restriction is based on several factors. There is a correlation between local recurrence and increasing tumor size [table 2] and large tumors are more likely to involve pectoral muscle or skin invasion.

Patients with two nonadjacent primary tumors in the same breast, determined either clinically or mammographically, are generally considered poor candidates for breast-conserving treatment. The cosmetic result of multiple wide excisions is likely to be poor and patients with multicentric primary tumors are more likely to have local recurrence elsewhere within the breast[11].

There is an increased local recurrence rate in patients with less than 35 years old. Matthews [15] showed an incidence of 13% in patients < 35 and 8% > 35 years.

There are some contraindications for the conservative treatment of breast cancer: tumor size > 5 cm, multicentric tumors, bad prognosis factors, breast cancer and pregnancy, breast cancer in man and previous conservative treatment

The current accepted criteria for selecting candidates for conservative surgery and radiation therapy are:

- Tumor size < 4 or 5 cm
- Single tumor within the breast
- Discrete microcalcifications only
- Absence of certain systemic diseases as collagen vascular diseases or scleroderm
- Good prognosis tumor

We concluded that primary breast cancer treatment is becoming increasingly complex, with rapid changes in management policy based on maturing clinical

Table 1 . Randomized prospective trials of stage I and II breast cancer: Conservative vs. mastectomy

Institute Reference	% local recurrence	% DFS	% OS
Stage I			
NCI-Milan	1/2	84/86	90/92
Institute Gustave-Roussy	10/6	72/84	92/92
Stage I and II			
NSABP B-06	- / 7.7	66/72	76/85

Table 2 Relationship between tumor size and % breast recurrence

Author	T1	T2
Fisher	7	10
Clarke	5	9
Delouche	7	14
Solin	5	8

trials, new data and the exploration of cellular prognostic indicators that may enable better treatment selection in more specific ways in the future. Because of this complexity, patient involvement in decision making is fundamental.

References

1-Halsted WS. The results of operations for the cure of cancer of the breast performed at Johns Hopkins Hospital from June 1889 to January 1894. Ann Surg 1894;20:497-555.

2-Handley RS. The conservative radical mastectomy of Patey: 10 year results in 425 patients' breasts. Dis Breast 1976; 2:16-19.

3-Patey DH, Dyson WH. The prognosis of carcinoma of the breast in relation to the type of operation performed. Br J Cancer 1948;2:7-13.

4-Veronesi U, Saccozzi R, Del Vecchio M, et al. Comparing radical mastectomy with quadrantectomy, axillary dissection and radiotherapy in patients with small cancers of the breast. N Engl J Med 1981;305:6-11.
5-Sarrazin D, Le MG, Arrigada R, et al. Ten year results of a randomized trial comparing a conservative treatment to mastectomy in early breast cancer. Radiother Oncol 1989;14:177-184
6-Fisher B, Bauer M, Margolese R, et al. Five-year results of a randomized clinical trial comparing total mastectomy and segmental mastectomy with and without radiation in the treatment of breast cancer. N Engl J Med 1989;312:665-673.
7-National Institutes of Health Consensus Development Conference Statement on the Treatment of Early Breast Cancer. J Am Med Assoc 1991,265:391-395.
8-Lindley R. Bulmam A, Parsons P, et al. Histologic features of an increased risk of local recurrence after treatment of breast cancer by local tumor excision and radiotherapy. Surgery 1989;105:13-20.
9-Osteen RT, Connolly JL, Recht A, et al. Identification of patients at high risk for local recurrence after conservative surgery and radiation therapy for stage I or II breast cancer. Arch Surg 1987,122:1248-1252
10-Holland R, Connolly JL, Gelman R, et al. The presence of an extensive intraductal component following a limited excision correlates with proeminent residual disease in the remainder of the breast. J Clin Oncol 1990;8:113-118.
11- Fisher ER, Sass R, Fisher B, et al. Pathologic findings from the National Surgical Adjuvant Breast Project (Protocol 6).II. Relation of local breast recurrence to multicentricity. Cancer 1986;57:1717-1724.
12- Clarke DH, Le MG, Sarrazin D, et al. Analysis of local-regional relapses in patients with early breast cancers treated in patients with early breast cancers treated by excision and radiotherapy: experiences of the Institute Gustave-Roussy. Int J Radiat Oncol Biol Phys 1985;11:137145.
13- Delouche G, Bachelot F, Premont M, Kurtz JM. Conservation treatment of early breast cancer: long term results and complications. Int J Radiat Oncol Biol Phys 1987;13:29-34.
14- Solin LJ, Fowble B, Matz KL, Goodman RL. Definitive irradiation for early stage breast cancer: the University of Pennsylvania experience. Int J Radiat Oncol Biol Phys 1988;15:271-276.
15- Matthews RH, McNeese MD, Montague ED, Oswald MJ. Prognostic implications of age in breast cancer patients treated with tumorectomy and irradiation or with mastectomy. Int J Radiat Oncol Biol Phys 1988;14:659-663.

Mastology - Breast Diseases
A.S.S. Figueira Fo et al., editors.

Conservative versus radical treatment of breast cancer The management of the axilla

E.J.Th. Rutgers, MD, PhD

Surgical Oncologist, Dept. of surgery, Netherlands Cancer Institute Amsterdam, Plesmanlaan 121, 1066 CX Amsterdam

Introduction

The axilla contains the major lymph drainage basin of the breast and is therefore the principal site of regional metastases from invasive breast cancer. The chance of lymph node metastases is determined by the metastatic potential of the primary tumor, which is, to a large extend, simply a function of tumor size (1). About 40 – 50% of patients with clinically operable breast cancer have nodal metastases at presentation. The prediction of the existence of lymph node metastases is difficult, either by physical means or by primary tumor parameters. The accuracy of physical examination in predicting histological involvement of axillary nodes is low with a false positive rate of about 25% and a false negative rate of 40% (3). Only a meticulous histological examination of a complete axillary dissection specimen will reveal the presence and number of lymph node metastases.

The existence of lymph node metastases is the most important marker for the prediction of haematogenic spread and thus the chance of dying from disseminated disease. This chance increases with the number of affected lymph nodes: not any other prognostic factor discriminates better the chance of surviving breast cancer. The nodal status is therefore successfully used for the identification of patients at high risk for eventual dissemination: the benefit of adjuvant systemic treatment is most obvious in node positive patients (2).

The early treatment of regional lymph node metastases inevitably leads to a better regional tumor control, which aim probably is equally set by surgery as by radiotherapy (3), at a comparable complication rate. Whether early regional treatment adds to overall survival is still a matter of debate (4, 5), albeit that persistent loco-regional tumor growth has to be detrimental to some individual patients. It is clear that axillary treatment can be avoided in patients with histological proven non invasive – in situ- breast cancers.

This paper discussed the pro's and con's of complete axillary dissection. The discussion concerning 'radical' versus 'conservative' treatment of the axilla is focused on 3 statements:

1. Staging: complete axillary dissection and histological examination provides the best prognostic information and is therefore the optimal staging procedure.
2. Regional therapy: immediate axillary treatment is mandatory for an optimal loco-regional control.
3. Survival benefit: immediate treatment of regional lymph nodes will result in a survival benefit.

Arguments pro complete axillary dissection

1. The axillary status is the best way to determine prognosis in patients with primary breast cancer and thus to identify patients at increased risk for dissemination (18). For the purpose of staging, the axillary nodal status has to be determined completely: the surgeon should perform a complete axillary clearance, at least including the so called levels I and II, and the pathologist should examine the specimen thoroughly. According to an interesting Danish study by Axelson et al (6) in over 7.000 low risk node negative patients, it is advised that at least 10 lymph nodes should be examined to exclude misclassification of node positive patients. Patients in whom 10 or more negative lymph nodes were examined histologically -and thus removed- had significantly better recurrence free, distant disease free, and overall survival. The better survival of patients with 10 or more negative lymph nodes compared to the patients with less negative lymph nodes is most probably due to understaging and consequently the denial of misclassified node positive patients from proper adjuvant systemic therapy. Furthermore, one might speculate that the worse survival is partly due to a less optimal loco-regional treatment. Also other studies showed that so called node sampling will predict insufficiently nodal status (7, 8, 9).

   With the emancipation of the patient and their legal rights on information, the wish to be informed about their prognosis is expressed more and more, which obviates the need of the knowledge of her axillary nodal status.
2. A complete axillary dissection provides the patient with an excellent regional control. In a series of 691 patients who underwent a modified radical mastectomy at the Netherlands Cancer Institute from 1979 – 1988 and 1.026 patients who underwent breast conserving treatment in the same period, only 0.6 respectively 1.0% had axillary recurrence; post operative irradiation on the axilla was only rarely applied (8 and 3% of all patients), and the node positive rate was respectively 44% and 28%. Many other studies conform this experience. Lesser axillary procedures give way to the risk of leaving involved lymph nodes, varying in different studies from 21 – 82% (1, 10), even if no lymph node metastases are encountered in the sampling specimen (17). To achieve optimal regional control, patients with incomplete axillary dissection and positive nodes are subjected to post operative irradiation. The combination of radiotherapy and, even lesser, axillary surgery increases markedly the risk of lymph oedema and shoulder function disturbances. In fact, for this reason a combination of surgery and radiotherapy should be avoided as much as possible. Recurrent axillary metastases after insufficient surgery are sometimes difficult to manage because of the extend of the disease. Salvage surgery of the axilla is difficult and might cause more complications. Furthermore, the re-occurrence of breast cancer, also loco-regionally, is a major psychological burden and drawback to the patient.
3. A better initial regional control by complete axillary dissection leads to a better overall survival. This statement is most controversial but supported by a number of randomized studies. In a prospective phase III trial by the Institut Curie 658 patients were randomized between lumpectomy alone versus lumpectomy plus axillary dissection (11). Both groups received radiotherapy to the breast. After a median follow-up of 54 months, the 5 years survival rates were 92.6% for the lumpectomy group and 96.6% for the plus axillary dissection group, with a significant difference between the two survival curves (p. 0.014).

As adjuvant chemotherapy was only given to very few patients in the axillary dissection group, the survival benefit in this group can hardly be accounted only to the adjuvant treatment. Also other randomized trials suggested a survival benefit of immediate axillary dissection (12, 13). So, immediate axillary treatment might lead to a better survival. However, the difference is probably rather small and thus very difficult to prove with statical significance in randomized trials (15).

Arguments contra radical axillary treatment

1. Staging. Many other factors have been studied with respect to prognosis: tumor size, hormone receptor content, tumor grade, vascular invasion, proliferative index, C-erb B2 oncogene expression, cathepsin-D, tumor aneuploidy, lymphocytic infiltration, mitotic index and so on. In multifactorial analysis all these factors are less predictive comparing to the nodal status. Furthermore, it is unclear and unproven whether patients with unfavourable prognostic factors as above mentioned are the ones who will respond to systemic therapy (except for hormone receptors and adjuvant hormonal therapy). If one is prepared to give every breast cancer patient adjuvant systemic treatment, a discriminatory tool is not necessary. But, it is hardly to justify to give every low risk premenopausal women a potentially toxic course of adjuvant chemotherapy. As the far less tamoxifen improves survival as well as in node positive as node negative post menopausal women (3), it is defensible to treat all these women with tamoxifen, thus making axillary staging in this group less important.
2. Regional therapy. Axillary irradiation of at least over 50 Gy in 2 Gy fractions appears to be an as effective means to control axillary disease as axillary dissection (3, 5, 14, 15). However, one can doubt about the long term effect on clinically obvious positive nodes and the long term serious sequelae of radiotherapy to the axilla, particularly with respect to the nerval plexus. The complication rate of radiotherapy of the axilla appears to be comparable to that of axillary dissection (3). Leaving a clinically unsuspected axilla untreated has some advocates but opens the way to uncontrollable regional disease when neglected and will lead to a substantional number of patients who needs a secondary treatment.

   As a result of increasing breast cancer screening activities, more women with very low risk invasive breast cancers are diagnosed. The risk of axillary involvement of post menopausal (over 50 years) patients with well differentiated (grade I) small (<1 cm, usual clinically occult) breast cancers is about 5% (16). Since 95% unnecessary axillary clearances is overdone, this patients group could be offered a wait and see policy concerning the axilla. However, this implies an initial careful examination of the primary tumor to identify this low risk group.
3. Survival benefit. The NSABP B-04 trial comparing radical mastectomy versus total mastectomy with or without irradiation (4) is the most important trial that appears to prove that delayed treatment of the axilla does not influence overall survival. However, some critics on this trial are made (5), the most important being that the number of patients in this trial might be too small to show any difference in survival concerning the axillary treatment.

Conclusion

Since the effectiveness of adjuvant chemotherapy in node positive premenopausal women is proven and the lack of a better predictor to response of chemotherapy, complete axillary dissection and its careful microscopic evaluation is mandatory in premonopausal patients with invasive breast cancer. In very low risk postmenopausal patients, usually with screen detected clinically occult breast cancers, one might advocate to leave the axillary untreated, since the chance of axillary metastases in these patients is small. All other postmenopausal women two treatment options could be offered: breast conserving therapy including radiotherapy of the breast and axilla followed by tamoxifen (20 mg at least 2 years) for all patients, or the classical breast conserving therapy consisting of lumpectomy, axillary dissection and radiotherapy to the breast, and consequently in increased risk -node positive- patients adjuvant systemic treatment, usually being tamoxifen. Patients for whom mastectomy is indicated an en bloc axillary dissection is the easiest way to control the axilla with only a slight increasing morbidity and thus appears to be the treatment of choice and with the advantage of having prognostic information (of which the patient may wish to know). For patients with proven non invasive breast cancer axillary treatment is not necessary.

References

1. Veronesi U, Luini A, Galimberti V, Marchini S, Sacchini V, Rilke F Extent of metastatic axillary involvement in 1446 cases of breast cancer. Eur. J. Surg. Oncol. 1990; 16: 127-133.
2. Early Breast Cancer Trialists Collaborative Group. Systemic treatment of early breast cancer by hormonal, cytotoxic or immuno therapy. Lancet 1992; 339: 1-5, 71-85.
3. Sacks MPM, Barr LC, Allan SM, Baum M. The role of axillary dissection in operable breast cancer. The Breast 1992; 1: 41-49.
4. Fisher B, Redmond C, Fisher ER. Ten years result of a randomized clinical trial comparing radical mastectomy and total mastectomy with or without irradiation. New. Eng. J. Med. 1985; 312: 674-881.
5. Harris JR, Osteen RT. Patients with early breast cancer benefit from axillary treatment. Breast Cancer Res. Treat. 1985; 5: 17-21.
6. Axelsson CK, Mouridsen HT, Zedeler K et al. Axillary dissection of level I and II lymph nodes is important in breast cancer classification. Eur. J. Cancer 1992; 28A: 1415-1418.
7. Kissin MW, Thompson EM, Price AB et al. The inadequacy of axillary sampling in breast cancer. Lancet 1982; 1: 1210-1212.
8. Cant ELM, Shivas AA, Forrest APM. Lymph node biopsy during simple mastectomy. Lancet 1975; 1: 995-997.
9. Kjaergaard J, Blichert-Toft M, Anderson JA et al. Probability of false negative nodal staging in conjunction with partial axillary dissection in breast cancer. Br. J. Surg. 1985; 72: 365-367.

10. Danforth DN, Findlay PA, McDonald HD et al. Complete axillary lymph node dissection for stage I-II carcinoma of the breast. J. Clin. Oncol. 1986; 4: 655-62.
11. Cabanes PA, Salmon RJ, Vilcoq JR et al. Value of axillary dissection in addition to lumpectomy and radiotherapy in early breast cancer. Lancet 1992; 339: 1245-1248.
12. Langlands AO. Prescott RJ, Hamilton TA. Clinical trial in the management of operable breast cancer. Lancet 1980; 2: 55-60.
13. Hayward JL. The Guy's trial of treatments of 'early' breast cancer. World J. Surg. 1977; 1: 314-316.
14. Amalric R, Santamaria F, Robert F et al. Radiation therapy with or without primary limited surgery for operable breast cancer. Cancer 1982; 49: 30-34.
15. Mazeron JJ, Otmezguine Y, Huart J, Pierquin B. Conservative treatment of breast cancer: results of management of axillary lymph node area in 3353 patients (letter). Lancet 1985; 1: 1387.
16. Walls J, Boggis, CRM, Wilson M et al. Treatment of the axilla in patients with screen-detected breast cancer. Br. J. Surgery 1993; 80: 434-438.
17. Graverson HP, Blichert-Toft M, Anderson JA, Zedeler K. Breast cancer: risk of axillary recurrence in node negative patients following partial dissection of the axilla. Eur. J. Surg. Oncol. 1988; 14: 407-412.
18. Fisher B, Bauer M, Wickerham DL et al. Relation of number of positive axillary nodes to the prognosis of patients with primary breast cancer: A NSABP update. Cancer 1983; 52: 1551-1557.

Mastology - Breast Diseases
A.S.S. Figueira Fo et al., editors.

Axillary Lymph Node Dissection for Small Invasive Breast Carcinomas: Is It Indicated?

Melvin J. Silverstein, M.D., Eugene.D.Gierson , M.D., James.R.Waisman, M.D.
Parvis Gamagami,M.D., Melinda Epstein, B.S., and William. J. Colburn, M.D.
The Breast Center, 14624 Sherman Way, Van Nuys, California 91405, USA

Abstract: Axillary node positivity is the single most important prognostic variable in patients with breast cancer. We used a combination of tumor size (T category) and method of diagnosis (whether or not the tumor was palpable) to predict patients with a low likelihood of nodal positivity in whom node dissection could be eliminated.

Palpability was a poor prognostic sign. Breast cancer specific survival decreased for T1b, T1c, and T2 lesions when they become palpable. There was a statistically significant increase in nodal positivity when palpable T1b, T1c, and T2 lesions were compared with similar sized nonpalpable lesions. Palpable T1b lesions had a higher risk of nodal positivity than larger nonpalpable T1c lesions ($p = 0.05$). It may now be time to consider eliminating axillary node dissection for invasive cancers with a low probability of axillary lymph node positivity; this includes all T1a lesions and nonpalpable T1b lesions.

Background: Axillary lymph node dissection has been a routine part of breast cancer treatment for more than 100 years. The status of axillary nodes continues to be the single most important prognostic variable regarding invasive breast cancer survival [1-3]. Axillary node positivity increases as the size of the invasive component increases and it is an excellent predictor of both disease-free and breast cancer specific survival [4,6,7]. With cost-containment a high priority and with the development of numerous new immunochemical prognostic indicators, it now may be time to consider eliminating routine node dissection for selected patients with infiltrating breast cancers [4,5].

We question whether a combination of tumor size and method of diagnosis (palpable versus mammographic) can be used to select a group of patients with invasive breast carcinomas, in whom the probability of nodal positivity is so low, that axillary dissection can be safely omitted?

Patients and Methods: From 1979 through 1993, 1192 axillary node dissections were performed for patients with invasive cancer. Nodal positivity and breast cancer specific survival were analyzed by T category and whether or not the lesion was palpable. A combination of tumor size and the method of tumor detection was used to predict patients with a low probability of nodal positivity who were unlikely to benefit from node dissection.

Results: Overall, 411 of 1192 (34%) node dissections contained metastases. Table 1 presents axillary node positivity by both T category and whether or not the lesions were palpable.

ble 1: Nodal Positivity by T Category and Palpability

	NONPALPABLE	PALPABLE	
ategory	No. Pos/Total	No. Pos/Total	P Value
a (1-5 mm)	2/56 (4%)	2/42 (5%)	NS
b (6-10 mm)	5/82 (6%)	25/100 (25%)	0.0006
c (11-20 mm)	12/88 (14%)	113/330 (34%)	0.0002
(21-50 mm)	10/45 (22%)	157/325 (48%)	0.001
(51 mm or more)	2/5 (40%)	58/96 (60%)	NS
(Locally Advanced))	None	22/23 (96%)	NS
TAL 34/276 (12%)	377/916 (41%)	0.0001	

le 2 presents breast cancer specific survival by both T category and whether or not the lesions were pable.

ble 2: 7-Year Breast Cancer Specific Survival by T Category and Palpability

ategory	NONPALPABLE	PALPABLE	P Value
	98%	100%	NS
)	100%	90%	0.05
	91%	87%	0.015
	80%	75%	0.08
	60%	62%	NS
	None	50%	NS

Discussion: During the last 20 years, the surgical approach to the breast has become less ressive. This is evidenced by a decrease in the percentage of mastectomies being performed with a comitant increase in the percentage of breast conservation procedures. During the same time period, lary dissections have become less radical but, nevertheless, continue to be a routine part of breast cer treatment. Current medical dogma suggest that axillary dissection is only prognostic [8,9]. But some ors [10,11] feel that axillary dissection may also be therapeutic, curing a small percentage of patients. If agement decisions regarding adjuvant therapy can be made regardless of axillary node status (based umor size, nuclear grade, ER, PR, c-erbB-2, etc.), the rational for axillary node removal will ntially be eliminated for physicians who believe that the procedure is only prognostic.

In this series, palpability was a poor prognostic sign. Breast cancer specific survival decreased T1b, T1c, and T2 lesions when they became palpable. There was a statistically significant increase in nodal positivity when palpable T1b, T1c, and T2 lesions were compared with similar sized nonpalpabl lesions. A palpable T1b lesion had a higher risk of nodal positivity than a larger nonpalpable T1c lesion ($p = 0.05$).

It is interesting that equally sized tumors had differing outcomes depending on whether or not they were clinically palpable. It is possible that palpable tumors have a much greater tumor burden than nonpalpable tumors of equal size and hence their poorer prognosis. There may also be other biochemic and genetic factors, currently not understood, that worsen the prognosis for palpable lesions.

It may now time to consider eliminating axillary node dissection for invasive cancers with a lo probability of axillary lymph node positivity; this includes all T1a lesions and nonpalpable T1b lesions

References:

1. Valagussa P, Bonadonna G, Veronesi U. Patterns of relapse and survival following radical mastectomy. Cancer 1978;41:1170-1178.
2. Nemoto T, Vana J, Bedwani RN, Baker HW, McGregor FH, Murphy GP. Management and surviv of female breast cancer: Results of a national survey by The American College of Surgeons. Cancer 1980;45:2917-2924.
3. Fisher B, Slack N, Katrych D, Wolmark N. Ten-year follow-up results of patients with carcinoma the breast in a cooperative clinical trial evaluating surgical adjuvant chemotherapy. Surg Gynecol Obste 1975;140:528-534.
4. Silverstein MJ, Gierson ED, Waisman JR, et al. Axillary lymph node dissection for T1a breast carcinoma: It it indicated? Cancer 1994;73:664-667.
5. Cady B. The need to reexamine axillary lymph node dissection in invasive breast cancer. Cancer 1994;73:505-508.
6. Ciatto S, Cecchini S, Lossa A, et al. T category and operable breast cancer prognosis. Tumori 1989;75:18-22.
7. Ciatto S, Rosselli Del Turco M, Bonardi R, et al. Nonpalpable lesions of the breast detected by mammography - Review of 1182 consecutive histologically confirmed cases. Eur J Cancer 1994 30A(1):40-44.
8. Fisher B. The surgical dilemma in the primary therapy of invasive breast cancer: A critical appraisal Current Problems in Surgery. October 1970:1-53.
9. Fisher B, Redmond C, Fisher ER, Bauer M, Wolmark N, Wickerham L, et al. Ten-year results of randomized clinical trial comparing radical mastectomy and total mastectomy with or without radiation Engl J Med 1985;312:674-681.
10. Harris JR, Osteen RT. Patients with early breast cancer benefit from effective axillary treatment. Breast Cancer Res and Treatment 1985;5:17-21
11. Hellman S, Harris JR. The appropriate breast cancer paradigm. Cancer Res. 1987;2:339-342.

Mastology - Breast Diseases
A.S.S. Figueira Fo et al., editors.

Breast-conserving surgery after induction chemotherapy

George N. Peters, M.D.

Baylor-Charles A. Sammons Cancer Center, Baylor University Medical Center, Dallas, Texas

Correspondence: George N. Peters, M.D., 300 Sammons, 3409 Worth Street, Dallas, Texas 75246, USA

Since the early 1980s, standard treatment for nonmetastatic stage IIIa and IIIb breast cancer in the United States has centered on induction chemotherapy. After confirmation of breast cancer by needle biopsy, chemotherapy is given for at least four cycles and is followed by surgery, which in the past primarily has been modified radical mastectomy. Postoperative chemotherapy is then given with radiation therapy. Several authors have reported on breast conservation in patients who have undergone induction chemotherapy for locally advanced breast cancer. At the M.D. Anderson Cancer Center in Houston, Texas, a retrospective study revealed that 23% of patients undergoing induction chemotherapy are potential candidates for breast conservation at the completion of their treatment. Criteria for breast conservation after induction chemotherapy include 1) solitary primary tumors that are 4 cm or less in size or two primary tumors within a sphere of less than 4 cm; 2) no involvement or fixation to chest wall; 3) tumor-to-breast-size ratio small enough for a good cosmetic result, 4) no palpable or small, low, or axillary lymph nodes; 5) absence of collagen vascular disease or other contraindications for radiation therapy; and 6) no extensive lymphatic involvement in the breast. This study concluded that induction chemotherapy at the M.D. Anderson Cancer Center is an effective treatment for locally advanced breast cancer and that it provides some patients with the option of breast conservation for locoregional control.

A prospective study by Dr. Bonadonna in Milan estimated that 81% of patients undergoing induction chemotherapy can have objective responses to allow more breast conservation with no adverse survival effects. Eighty-six percent of patients with tumors 3.0 to 5.0 cm and 59% of patients with initial tumors 5.1 to >7.0 cm responded with reduction of their tumors to less than 3.0 cm. A multicenter report on patients with tumors 4.0 to 12 cm showed an overall 76% survival with locoregional occurrence of 8.5% at a follow-up of 46 months.

Dr. Gordon Schwartz, in a review of his data from 1979 to 1991 in 189 patients, noted an 85% response to induction chemotherapy in patients with stage IIb and III breast cancer. Overall, 34% of his patients underwent breast conservation, but 75% since 1990 have been candidates for breast conservation. The projected 2-year, 5-year, and 10-year disease-free survival is 81%, 61%, and 55%, respectively. At surgery, 10% of the patients had no tumor, and 7% had only ductal carcinoma in situ. Dr. Claude Jacquillat of France evaluated 250 breast cancer patients entered in a protocol combining neoadjuvant chemotherapy and radiation therapy as the exclusive treatment for locoregional control. After a five-year follow-up, breast preservation was approximately 94% in the overall series, with disease-free survival in stage IIIa of 46% and stage IIIb of 52%. In our series of stage IIb to stage III tumors, over 60% of the patients treated with induction chemotherapy did undergo pathologic downstaging to stage IIa or better. It is therefore concluded that induction chemotherapy is an effective treatment for locally advanced breast cancer. Induction chemotherapy can provide some patients with the option of breast conservation for locoregional control with no adverse effects on survival.

References

1. Khanna MM, Mark RJ, Silverstein MJ, Juillard G, Lewinsky B, Giuliano AE. Arch Surg 1992;127:1038-1043.
2. Bonadonna G, Veronesi U, Brambilla C, Ferrari L, Luini A, Greco M, Bartoli C, de Yoldi GC, Zucali R, Rilke F, Andreola S, Silvestrini R, Di Fronzo G, Valagussa P. Journal of the National Cancer Institute 1990;82:1539-1545.
3. Schwartz GF, Birchansky CA, Komarnicky LT, Mansfield CM, Cantor RI, Biermann WA, Fellin FM, McFarlane J. Cancer 1994;73:362-369.
4. Singletary SE, McNeese MD, Hortobagyi GN. Cancer 1992;69:2849-2852.
5. Jacquillat C, Weil M, Baillet F, Borel C, Auclerc G, de Maublanc MA, Housset M, Forget G, Thill L, Soubrane C, Khayat D. Cancer July 1, 1990:119-129.

III. 5. Advanced diseases

Mastology - Breast Diseases
A.S.S. Figueira Fo et al., editors.

Locally advanced breast cancer diagnostics aspects

Dr Carlos Vazquez Albaladejo and Dra Josefina Camps Roig

Instituto Valenciano de Oncologia, Valencia, España

Introduction

The mechanism working step by step up to the regional lymphonodulus, which was gathered in the technique of radical mastectomy published by Halsted in 1894, expressed the fact that for this author there was a locoregional evolution of the tumour in a direction that could be qualified of lineal, with subsequent haematogenic dissemination, after the overflowing of the ganglionic stations (1).

But the disseminative and mechanic lymphophilo pattern of Halsted loses ground because a number of patients with undamaged regional adenopathies evolve toward the metastatic dissemination (2). It is confirmed that a bigger local action is not followed by better results at long term, and it changes the reason of the chirurgical perfomance, and so to be defined as the practice of an exeresis at the proper time and in due manner.

Definition of the clam tumours

The locally advanced carcinoma of mamma (CLAM) is the way in which appears the cancer of mamma, being characterized by a significant enlargement of the mammary glands, with a tumour of variable size, which infiltrates the skin and the regional lymphatic ganglia, and with an evolution not necessarily fatal, as the survivals after five years are up to the 30%.

It has to do with a local or regional ample range of the neoplasia, sometimes as a consequence of a quick development of the same with ganglionic dissemination (N1-2), or on the contrary of a great local progression of the mammary tumour by a long and slow evolution since its diagnostic (T4).

Historically, and although this type of tumours were technically able to be dried, the patients were lost due to the dissemination at a distance and many times being the tumour present. With the result that the therapeutic planning nowadays includes usually the systemic attack as from the beginning, mostly when, after the examination of the patient and of the biopsy specimen, it has been determined the possibility of response to such treatments.

Its definition is subject to various particularities. For some doctors it is a question of patients not susceptible of a conservative treatment, for others they are the non-tributary ones of surgical resection at the beginnig, and for most of them they correspond to stadium III, if excluded the inflammatory carcinoma.

The concretion of this stadium has had several variations since the UICC has published the TNM classification. Previously Haagensen and Stout described the serious signs of mammary cancer by elucidating some judgments of inoperability which are still in force, such as the oedema of the mamma skin, the ulceration, the fixation of the tumour to the thoracic wall, and the massive affectation of axillary ganglia, with fixation of the same to the superlying skin or to other axillary structures. With the above data the classification of the university of Columbia has been prepared, where they labelled the CLAM in stadium C (4,5).

The UICC has redefined Stadium III in 1987, by introducing several variations, which had already been proposed in some publications (6). The big tumour (T3), without affected ganglia, has been segregated and included in stadium II, in view of its better prognostic, and also to contrast it with those tumours which, having a smaller size, had already disseminated the armpit. It had also been estimated that the N3 had to be assigned to the lymphonodulus of the inner mammary, and the old N3, which was the ganglionic supraclavicular affectation is classified as metastasic. So, nowadays, they consider as CLAM tumours any Carcinoma that infiltrates the skin and or the thoracic wall, with ganglionic invasion in any degree, either being axillary or pertaining to the group of the inner mammary (7). (Table 1)

The CLAM is composed of a heterogeneous group of tumours. Some of them are of a large size, with local infiltration and scarce sytemic aggressiveness, with no ganglionic affectation, and others are smaller tumours that grow quickly and have little local affectation, but with a serious dissemination towards the ganglia. This variety makes the studies of its evolutional process to be complex, as a great number of publications effect the global analysis of all the tumours in this stadium, and even in some cases they include the inflammatory carcinoma. (T4d).

This kind of tumourous presentation, the inflammatory carcinoma, which are also CLAM, must be segregated due to its special characteristics. It has to do with non-concret tumours from the exploratory and radiological point of view, which grow quickly, with flush, skin oedema, local heat, with anatomopathological affectation of the dermic lymphatics, and very bad prognostic. (3,7,8).

This very histological fact is basic for the appointment to the group, and it must be differentiated from the lymphatic peritumourous infiltrations of the tumours that ulcerate the skin or from the so called inflammatory hidden carcinoma. These also of very bad prognostic are the kind of cancer which, having the lymphangitical infiltration of the skin, lack of the clinical inflammatory signs (10).

Putting aside these clinico-pathological variantes, one gradation for a better interpretation of the results is the division in substadiums like III A-B, which for some authors is also an indicative of the surgical dessication at start (11).

Table 1
TNM. Classification. Breast tumours

III A	III B	
T0 N2	T4	N0
T1 N2	T4	N1
T2 N2	T4	N2
T3 N1-2	T0-1-2-3-4	N3

The prevailing of the CLAM is very changeable, but in our medium it presupposes between 15-20% of the tumours. However, these figures are different according to the place the patients come from; in fact, the percentage is smaller if they come from a centre with precocious diagnosis or from a social welfare ambit (Table 2). Also the type of hospital, if public or private, shows important differences in the sick people being studied, having in mind their cultural and social levels. In our experience 48% of the presentations CLAM happens in women over 60 years old. In this subgroup of patients we have detected tumours of slow evolution, of moderated biological agressiveness, and low fractions of growth, which give place to a scarce local response to the medical treatments.

Tumourous size

An important fact to be considered is the valuation of the tumour size (T). When it is a matter of lesions bigger than 5 cm its evaluation is not difficult at all, but there exists some difficulty in identifying the T4.

It is really a tumour that, by affecting the skin from a conceptual point of view, individualized, can embrace a range going from a small nodule, which produces a scarce coutaneous retraction , up to the big neoplastic ulcer, sometimes with the metastasis in the very skin of the mamma (T4 b). There are also included the ones infiltrating the thoracic wall (T4 a), and the combination of the two forms (T4c)

The diversity of the presentations gives place to the different variations in the initial local treatment and they have also repercussion on the SG, which after 5 years is of 54% in the whole of the series, in front of the 85% of the ones which could be denominated as false T4. (12).

Lymphonodal affectation

The corresponding axillary invasion is significant (N2-3), and this fact conditions absolutely the survival, which is actually of 20-30% after 5 years. In view of the histological report it is difficult the adscription to a definite group (N1-N2).

The capsular infiltration, overflowing it, (pN1biii), with more than 50% of the ganglia being affected, is not easily differentiated from the N2, mostly if this is not very evident surgically speaking. In fact some groups consider the capsular infiltration as N2.

The difficulty is much bigger if the capsular incision occurs only in one ganglion. On the other side, these gradations in the intensity of the affectation of the lymphatic ganglia, still seem to drag along mechanized concepts with regard to the dissemination of the tumourous cells. Really, under the protection of the biological concepts with immunological support about the meaning of the ganglionic tumourous infiltration, the size of the metastasis of the affected ganglion does not seem important, if the tumour infiltrates the capsule at only one point, or if it infiltrates it totally, or if it breaks it, or if it gets in contact with other ganglia; in any case, if the surgical axillary resection was complete. The complexity of the

Table 2
Results of diagnosis cancer center. 1993. Dr. R. maraña. Valencia. Spanish cancer association

Size	No	%
Invasive	15	5.7
T <2CMS(T1)	92	35.3
T 2-5CMS(T2)	115	44.1
T 3-4	39	14.9
Total	261	100

adscription of the female patients for its ganglionic stratification gives occasion for interpretations by the working groups, that have a repercussion on the results being published. At all events, these data, which have on one side a value of prognostication and on the other side a therapeutic repercussion, and consisting of the necessity of systemic treatment (13).

Valuation of the N3

Ganglionic stages being considered as N3, such as the supraclaviculars, are nowadays classified as metastatic, and the internal mammaries are valued as N3. The ganglia of this chain are placed by the intercostal cartilages and muscles. Their size is from 2 to 5 cm and their number varies betwem 3 and 9, and they are more freguent in the first intercostal spaces.

The lymphatic current they receive is above all the one coming from the internal quadrants of the mamma, although some studies effected by lymphoscintigraphy indicate that qualitatively as well as quantitatively any quadrant can send lymphatic flux to the same. By the way, there are few possibilities for the lymph to cross the midline in spite of the frequent existence of anastomotic vias between the lymphatic nets on both sides of the body (14). But these descriptions of lymphatic kinetic are not in harmony with the frequency the said chain is affected in the totality of the mammary carcinomas, having in mind even the cases in which the axillary ganglia are infiltrated and the tumour is medial.

The imagenological identification of the same is very difficult, as there is not any diagnostic procedure reliable enough for its identification. Several publications have been made for its detection by means of lymphoscintigraphy, echography, computerized tomography and magnetic resonance. According to some authors, with the first technique, a high specificity is obtained, but other studies indicate for the echography a positivism of 84 % after the biopsia of the suspicious noduls, which are those of more than 6 mm of size.(15)

We have studied with magnetic resonance a group of 19 patients between 38 and 77 years, all of them with tumours with internal quadrants, T 1-2-3, and with axillary infiltration in 9 cases. It has been imposible in any case to detect in the

Table 3
Results of regional lymphonide. Valoracion with magnetic resonance tomography on 19 patients with internal quadrants breast cancer.

	PTNM			
Size	No	N1	N2	N3
T1	6	2	1	0
T2	4	1	1	0
T3	0	2	2	0

spectrum the presence of adenopathies in the internal mammary, although the affected axilaries were made evident, in 8 out of the 9 cases in which they were mestastatized. (Table III)

In any case, with the exception of the scintigraphy which evaluates eventual possitiveness to tumourous infiltration as per the repletion defects, the rest of the techniques consider an eventual macroscopic affectation of the lymphonodules due to their size, mostly the ones situated on the second, third and fourth intercostal spaces, although not being able to determinate with accuracy whether there is or not a tumourous infiltration (16,17,18,19,20)

There are difficulties in obtaining a ganglionic sample, as a surgical routine, to confirm its infiltration. For this reason, its understanding as far as the stadium is concerned, still motivates studies to determine which non-invasive technique is the best for its identification.

References

1. Halsted WS. The results for operations for the cure of cancer of the breast performed at the Jhon Hopkins Hospital from June to January 1894. Ann Surg 1894; 20: 497-555
2. Fisher B. The revolution in breast cancer: science or anecdotalism?. Wolrd J Surg 1985; 9: 655-666.
3. Hortobadgyi GN, Blumenschein GR, Spanos W, et al. Multimodal treatment of locorregionally advanced breast cancer. Cancer 1983; 51: 763-768.
4. Haaegensen CD. Enfermedad de la mama. Edit. Beta SRL. Buenos Aires. 1972;685-691
5. Manual for Satging of Cancer. Third Edition. American Joint Commitee on Cancer. J.B. Lippincott. Co. 1988.
6. Garcia Vilanova A. Sistema TNM 1978 en cáncer de mama: propuesta de su modificación. Rev Esp Oncología 1985; 32:95-108
7. UICC. TNM atlas Illustrated Guide for the TNM/pTNM classification of malignant tumours. Third Edition. Springer-Verlag. 1989.
8. Ellis DL, Teitelbaum SL. Inflammatory carcinoma of the breast: A pathologic definition. Cancer 1974; 33:1045-1047.

9. Lucas FV, Perez- Mesa C. Inflammatory carcinoma of the breast. Cancer 1978;41:1595-1605.
10. Salzstein SI. Clinically occult inflammatory of the breast. Cancer 1974; 34:382-388
11. De Lena M, Zuccali R, Vimagoti G el al. Combined chemoterapy-radiotherapy approach in locally advanced (T3b-4) breast cancer. Cancer Chemother. Pharmacol. 1978; 1:53-59.
12. Vazquez Albaladejo C. Conservacion o reconstruccion en el cancer de mama en estadios iniciales. En: Cancer de mama. Avances en diagnostico y tratamiento. Diaz Faes (ed).Leon.1990;183-202.
13. Bonadonna G, Valagussa P, Rossi A, et al. Ten-years experience with CMF-based adjuvant chemotherapy in resectable breast cancer. Breast Cancer Res. Treat.1985.5:95-115.
14. Vendrell E. Linfogammagrafía de la mama. Tesis Doctoral. Universidad de Barcelona. Secretariado de Publicaciones. Romagraf. pp 1-33.1971.
15. Scataridge JC, Hamper Um, Stheth S et al. Paraesternal sonography of the internal mammary vessels: Technique, normal anatomy and lymphoadenopathy. Radiology 1989; 172: 453-457.
16. Noguchi M, Michigishi T, Nakajima K, et al. The diagnosis of internal mammary node metastases of breast cancer. Int Surg 1993; 7:171-175.
17. Toruglu HT, Janjan NA, Thorsen MK, et al. Imaging of regional spread of breast cancer by internal mammary. Clin Nucl Med 1992; 17:482-484.
18. Taylor JL,Taylor DN, Lowry C, el al. Radioinmunoescintigraphy of metastasis breast carcinoma. Eur J Surg Oncol 1992; 18-57-63.
19. Linden A, Reusch K, Smolarz K. Retroesternal lymph node metastases in breast cancer: Lymphoescintigraphy and magnetic resonance tomography. Nuclearmedizin 1991; 30:279-282.
20. Scott WW, Fishman EK. Detection of internal mammary limph node enlargement: comparison of CT and conventional roentgenograms. Clin Imagin 1991;15:268-272.

Mastology - Breast Diseases
A.S.S. Figueira Fo et al., editors.

Locally advanced breast cancer

Sérgio Bruno B. Hastschbach, José Clemente Linhares, Nils Skare, Rosane Johnsson, Andrea Hilgenberg, Sônia Bozko, Andreia Andraus

Erasto Gaertner Hospital, Ovande do Amaral street, N 201, Cep: 81520.060

Locally advanced breast cancer

Locally advanced breast cancer includes huge removable tumors and tumors considered inoperable but without distant metastasis.

We notice there is a lot of different opinions in literature whether patients with locally advanced breast cancer should be classified in stagement EC IIIa and/or EC IIIb according to with UICC 1983/1987.

A clear definition about the results published is neccessary, for a patient T3 No Mo will have absolutely different resuls from a patient T3 N2 Mo.

Breast cancer is a malignant disease that presents many peculiar caracteristics. While incipient cases correctly conduced may progress unfavourably, others locally advanced cases, at the same time, reach surprising good answers to the treatment.

Nevertheless the knowledg that the majority of the cases present subclinic disseminated disease at the time of diagnosis, it is very important that the physician guides carefully the patients to obtain the local control of that disease. At the same time a sistemic therapy (chemotherapy)* started aiming to destroy the circulating neoplasic cells in the subclinic disease.

Technologycal, social and cultural evolution have reduced greatly the locally advanced breast cancer in countries of the first world. Despite of this fact, our experience shows that in our ambiency these cases are still expressive in numbers. While in USA, ECIII represents 19%, in our service (Erasto Gaertner Hospital) ECIII is of 25,2%.

The local control of breast cancer is important not only because it offers a better survival curve for the patients, but also because it offers better quality of life. The evolution and quality of life is different when comparing a patient with locally controlled disease to another with a huge tumor, observing her own bad progression.

The prognostic of locally advanced cancers may be variable especially if we regard the subjects SIZE (T) and axilary metastasis, that certainly worsen prognosis.

Arnold and Leesmick presented results of 77 to 78% for tumors T3 No Mo and 58% for T3 N1 Mo.

The relationship with tumor size and axilary metastasis is clear.

Fisher presented that tumors with more than 6 cm showed 63% of axilary metastasis in about 2000 cases. Whereas, tumors with 1,0 to 1,9 cm presented 38% of axilary metastasis.

In this way, Fisher prooved that tumors bigger than 6 cm and with axilary metastasis in more than 4 linfonodes presented 94% of recurrence. And tumors with 6 cm or more with negative axila presented 24% of recurrence.

Stewart and cols have analised another prognostic factor in ECIII, the estrogenic receptors. They concluded that in operable cases (T3 N0/N1) with negative and positive estrogenic receptors, patients have had benefits with estatistic relevance. For patients with inoperable tumors and estrogenics receptors + or-, there have been no prognostic value or influence.

Others factors may be important to the prognosis, for example, the cellular proliferating factor, the hystological types and so on.

Surgical treatment

It is important to identify the operable locally advanced tumors from those considered inoperables, that present signs of advanced disease, that are: ulcerated tumors, lesions fixed to the toraxic chest wall, axilary metastasis with more than 2,5 cm and fixed axilary linfonodes (Haagensen).

Obviously that surgycal treatment of locally advanced breast cancer must be added with post operative radiotherapy and with hormone and chemotherapy.

Haagensen and Stout observed that in cases that presented inoperability criteria the survival results in 5 years were of 0%. Fracchia published results of 27% in 10 years of survival of patients with operable ECIII treated only with surgery. According to this author a local recurrence index of 25% for patients with + axila is comprooved. Considering these uncertain results, the majority of especiallized services agree that it is necessary to treat patients with chemo and radioterapy and also eventual surgery to obtain better results.

Primary radiotherapy

The uncertain and poor results obtained with surgycal treatment in locally advanced breast cancer compelled the services to use radiotherapy as another way of local treatment for these cases.

Exclusive radiotherapy may be used when it is associated with surgery, but local recidive index is higher than in cases treated with exclusive surgery.

Local recidive index in exclusive RXT is about 50%, while in exclusive surgery is abou 25%.

In 1975, Buckmann and cols reduced the local recidive with higher irradiation doses adding interstitial irradiation. An important work reported in literature as from Zucali and cols comprooves that in a group of patients treated with radiotherapy and surgery 62 to 100% remained with residual tumor in irradiated breast.

An important point observed was that in huge tumors, radiotherapy was not effective. So, we conclude that surgery associated with radiotherapy are the best procedings features for local control.

Radiotherapy may be pre operative or post operative.

Pre operative radiotherapy followed by surgery have worse results, with index of local controll varying form 11 to 45% developing distant metastasis in 65 to 89%.

Surgery followed by radiotherapy results in a local controll of 70 to 86% of tu mors and survival index for 5 years of 30 to 45%. The ideal moment and sequence for the therapeutic introduction is still unknown. More effective and intensive approaches are requered to obtain lower rates in local recidive. Hormone and chemotherapy previous to or after local treatment are the approaches being used in cases of locally advanced breast cancer.

Related to this subject many works were reported since 1978. For example, Caceres in 1980, Schaake Koning in 1985 and Wong in 1986. CMF, FAC, Tamoxifen and occasionally surgycal or actinic ooforectomy are the most used schemes for systemic chemo therapy.

Works reported by EORTC for treatin, patients ECIII used many combinations as exclusive RXT, RXT and endocrinotherapy, or RXT + QT without surgery.

The conclusion of this attempt was that systemic treatment produces an effective local controll but not in the global survival in patients with worse prognosis and advanced disease.

Another important study from Delena that used neo adjuvant chemotherapy is what follows:

There were 2 groups:

1) Patients with previous surgery.
2) Patients with previous radiotherapy.

The conclusion was that the local recidive index was exactly the same in both.

So, the kind of local treatment does not interfer neither in survival rate nor in local controll of the disease.

In 1988, Dr. Anderson published results obtained from patients with ECIIIa and ECIIIb. In there he were considered 3 cicles of chemotherapy (FAC) followed by surgery, radiotherapy or both. Afterwards chemotherapy was hold for 9 months.

The work conclusion is that the treatment of choice for disease ECIIIa and ECIIIb must be multidisciplinar.

Local E systemic therapeutic association

The work is about a retrospective study of 186 cases of locally advanced breast cancer treated at Hospital Erasto Gaertner in the period of january 1986 to december of 1989.

For the patients to be included in the project, there were requested the following criterias:

1) Patients with malignant breast neoplasia hystologically confirmed.
2) Locally advanced breast cancer based on T N M classification: T3 N0, T3 N+, T4 N0 or +, without distant or local metastases at the time of diagnose.
3) Treatment exclusively done at the referred institution (Erasto Gaertner Hospital).

There have been excluded cases with impossible staging as those who have had parcial or total treatment in other institution, cases of bilateral breast cancer, patients not submitted to surgycal treatment or without hystological comprooving. Patients who did not complete the programmed treatment or who abandonned the follow up were also out.

Staging had been done according to the results of UICC of 1987, and the group of patients T3 N0 M0, T3 N+M0, T4 N0 M0 and T4N+M0 have been considered in the analysis.

Follow up was done with periodic clinical examination every 3 months in the first year, and every 4 months during 2nd year. Then, twice a year (each 6 months) during two years and finally once a year.

The annual routine comprised the requirement of contralateral mamography, RX of torax and hepatic ecography.

Treatment

Patients have been gathered into one of the four clinical stagements. It was observed the index of assyntomatic patients, patients with local recidive or with distant metastasis during the period of follow up, and also the survival rate and lifetime free of disease. These criterias were adopted in order to choose the kind of treatment.

The four groups are the following:

1) Patients submitted only to surgery without other systemic treatment. It was done simple mastectomy with or without axilary dissection, radical or modified mastectomy and conservative treatment.
2) Patients submitted to associated surgery and radiotheraphy (per or post operative) without systemic treatment at all.
3) Patients submitted to associated surgery and systemic treatment (chemotherapy per or post operative) and hormone therapy, separetedly studied)
4) Patients submited to associated surgery, radiotherapy (pre or post operative) and chemotherapy (adjuvant or neoadjuvant).

Cases that presented recidive were separetedly studied in order to investigate what could have interferred in the evolution of that group.

Results

186 patients were studied and 100% were female. The age varied between 28 to 83 years.

The subject 'T'analysed showed 102 (54,8%) patients T3 and 84 (45,2%) patients T4 according to UICC.

Considering the axilary condition, 52 (27,9%) of patients were free of linfonodes involvement by the disease.

The predominant hystological type was invasive ductal carcinoma with 181 (97,3%) of cases. Medullary carcinoma, lobular carcinoma and Paget disease comprised about 0,5%.

The minimal follow up time was of 5 years.

In general, cases as T3 N0 M0 (EC IIIby UICC, 1983) were in number of 26, and the majority of them remained free of disease (66,2%). The local recidive index was of 11,5%.

Patients T3 N+ M0 corresponded to 40,3% of cases and had a local recidive index of 6,6% and 28,6% of them developed distant metastases.

Analysing T3/T4 we noticed that T4 N0 M0 comprised 12,9% and there dind happen local recidive at all. (Fig 2)

The group T4 N+ M0 presented a local recidive index of 13,1%. The axilary involvement was the most important factor responsable for the worsening of the patients, independently of them being T3 and T4.

In our material we studied the results according to the adopted kind of treatment. There was four different groups of treatment types: (Fig. 4)

1) Exclusive surgery (8,6%)
2) Surgery + Chemotherapy (neoadjuvante or adjuvant) (36,4%)
3) Surgery + Radiotherapy (15,4%)
4) Surgery + Chemotherapy + Radiotherapy (39,5%)

In this way, the analysis of the different types of treatment revealed that in cases treated only with surgery there was any case of local recidive. On the other hand, 85,7% of patients had distant metastases.

Is the group submitted to surgery and chemotherapy we had an index of local recidive of 8,4% and 22 (37,2%) of cases with distant metastases.

The group treated surgically associated with radiotherapy reached 70% of cases with distant metastases and 4% of local recidive.

Patients treated with surgery, radio and chemotherapy showed 10,9% of local recidive and 46,8% of distant metastases.

Conclusions

Actual indication for patients with locally advanced breast tumors is the treatment with higher doses of systemic chemotherapy, intending to destroy micrometastasis before local proceedings.

Radiotherapy and surgery may be necessary to reduce the local recidive index. Nevertheless the use of surgery and radiotherapy do not change survival rates.

Patients with negative axila presented the best prognosis.

Figure 1:

Therapeutics Modalities X Results

Group	No. Cases	Recurrence	Metastases	Disease free
Surgery	14	0 —	12 (85,7 %)	2 (14,2 %)
Surgery + Qt	59	5 (8,4%)	22 (37,2%)	32 (54,2%)
Surgery + XRT	25	1 (4%)	17 (70,8%)	5 (20%)
Surgery + Qt + XRT	64	7 (10,9%)	30 (46,8%)	24 (37,5%)

* E.G.H.

Future

In fact, chemotherapic effect not only reduces the local recidive index but also brings important benefits for the survival rates.

According to this, we should include the use of chemotherapy in higher doses and a rescue with own's bone marrow grafting.

These results are not so effective perhaps because this proceeding is being indicated in bad prognostic cases.

World literature starts now to show works related to growing factores and monoclonal antibodies, etc...

Figure 2:

Clinical Stage X Results

Group	No. Cases	Recurrence	Metastases	Disease free
T3 N0 M0	26	3 (11,5%)	6 (23%)	18 (68,2 %)
T3 N+ M0	75	5 (6,6%)	29 (38,6%)	37 (49,3%)
T4 N0 M0	24	0 —	7 (29,1%)	15 (62,5%)
T4 N+ M0	61	8 (13,1%)	23 (37,7%)	29 (14,7%)

* E.G.H.

Bibliography

1) Davila E, Vogel CL. Management of locally advanced breast cancer (ECIII) Review. Intl. Adv. Surg. oncol F: 297-327-1984.
2) Hortobagyi GN, Ames PC, Buzdar AV, et al. Management of stage III primary breast Cancer with Primary chemotherapy surgery and radiation therapy (Can 62 2507 2516, 1988)
3) Arnold DJ, Lesnick GJ. Survival Following mastectomy for stage III breast cancer: Am J surg 137 362-366 1979.
4) Bruckman JE, Harris Jr, Levine MB. Results of treating stage III carcinoma of the breast by Primary radiation Therapy. Cancer 43-985-993, 1979.
5) Donegan WL. Cancer of the Breast, ed 2, Philadelfia, W.B Saunders, 1979 pg. 263
6) Sheldon T, Hayes DF, Candy B, et al. Primary radiation therapy for locally advanced breast cancer. Cancer 60-1219-1225-1987.

Mastology - Breast Diseases
A.S.S. Figueira Fo et al., editors.

Locally advanced breast carcinoma: present surgical treatment modalities

Ruben Orda, MD MS FACS

Professor and Chairman, Sackler Faculty of Medicine, Tel Aviv University, Assaf Harofeh Medical Center, Israel.

Address for correspondence: Professor Ruben Orda, Chairman of Surgery, Department of Surgery "A", Assaf Harofeh Medical Center, Zerifin 70300, Israel.

Abstract: The surgical treatment for locally advanced breast cancer is reviewed and discussed. A multimodality approach - intensive neoadjuvant systemic chemotherapy, followed by local control - is the recommended strategy. The need for further evaluation by well controlled studies, is stressed.

The management of patients with locally advanced breast carcinoma presents a formidable therapeutic challenge. Optimal treatment still remains controversial.

Haagensen and Stout [1] classified these patients in the Columbia as clinical class D, or inoperable cases. After reviewing 1135 breast cancer patients treated with radical mastectomy at the Columbia Presbyterian Hospital in New York, from 1915 to 1942, they identified a condition that was beyond cure, even by radical surgery. It was associated with a zero percent, 5-year cure rate, and a more than 50 percent probability of local recurrence.

Unimodality experiences demonstrated that good, local control rates by surgery or radiotherapy alone [2,3] were associated with poor prognosis. Systemic micrometastases could not be controlled with either surgery or radiotherapy alone [4]. Nevertheless, the value of surgery can now be reconsidered on the basis of new, more effective, multimodality treatments.

Multimodality trials from the Milan National Cancer Institute [5,6] and from the University of Texas, M.D. Anderson Cancer Center [7], reported encouraging results after using primary induction or neoadjuvant systemic chemotherapy as an integral part of the primary management of locally advanced breast cancer. The treatment strategies included the combined use of three modalities: chemotherapy, surgery and radiotherapy. Most patients achieved substantial tumor reductions. Downstaging of primary tumors renders many inoperable tumors operable. Patients who would previously have required radical surgery, can now be treated with modified radical mastectomy, or in some cases breast conservation procedures.

The M.D. Anderson Cancer Center proposed an alogarithm for the treatment of stage III breast carcinoma. Three courses of FAC (5-Fluorouracil, Adriamycin and Cyclophosphamide) are used for induction chemotherapy, and patients are assessed for clinical response and classified accordingly. If the patient responds to induction chemotherapy, surgical resection is then attempted. Otherwise, radiotherapy is given followed by surgical resection.

The surgical procedure is a total mastectomy with level I/II axillary dissection for pathological node assessment. The resection is performed

3 weeks following the last chemotherapy cycle. Surgery is performed before radiotherapy because better radiotherapeutic local control can be achieved after having debulked the tumor surgically. After the surgical procedure, six courses of adjuvant chemotherapy are given. At the completion of chemotherapy, radiotherapy is given. Many authors have shown that aggressive induction chemotherapy, followed by local surgical treatment, can result in good local control, with improved survival and relapse-free survival rates [9-15].

Frank et al. [16], reported a 5-year overall survival rate of 54% in a series of patients with locally advanced breast cancer who were treated with neoadjuvant systemic therapy prior to surgery.

Canavese et al. [17] reported better results in a randomized study of patients treated with a combined modality approach, when compared to an historical non-randomized control. He reported an actuarial survival of 71.5%. The disease-free survival rate was 43%.

On the other hand, Rainer [18] reported the results of a randomized clinical trial on locally advanced breast cancer, comparing perioperative chemotherapy with perioperative radiotherapy. A group of 19 patients having undergone chemotherapy or radiotherapy before scheduled surgery, refused operation. These patients, despite not being operated upon, had a relapse-free survival that was at least as good as that in those operated by modified radical mastectomy.

Although in most cases local control can be achieved with a standard mastectomy, sometimes skin invasion or chest wall fixation may demand more radical procedures which should be followed by reconstructive techniques. If the defect involves skin and subcutaneous tissue only, it can sometimes be handled by skin graft. Most larger defects are best reconstructed with myocutaneous flaps [19,20].

The latissimus dorsi flap has two main advantages: its lack of donor site morbidity and its reliable blood supply. Its main disadvantage is its limited size.

The rectus abdominis myocutaneous flaps are larger. There are three types of flap: the vertical flap, the single pedicle transverse rectus abdominis myocutaneous (TRAM) flap, and the double pedicle TRAM flap. The single pedicle TRAM flap is widely used in non smoking and non diabetic patients who have an adequate blood supply and an intact chest wall; based upon the single pedicle TRAM, the double pedicle TRAM flap doubles the blood supply by basing the flap on both rectus abdominis muscles.

When the chest wall is not intact, the flap reliability becomes more critical. The latissimus dorsi mycocutaneous flap is a good choice for small defects located within the arc of rotation. For defects lower on the chest wall, the vertical rectus abdominis flap and the double pedicle TRAM flap are good options.

Although the surgical procedure classically used for locally advanced breast cancer is a radical or modified radical mastectomy, breast conservation surgery after induction chemotherapy was also proposed.

In 1990, Bonadonna et al. [21] reported that the delivery of relatively short-term primary chemotherapy in large breast tumors, can induce down staging of the primary lesion to less than 3cm in most patients, thus allowing breast conservation. Tumor shrinkage was documented in 81% of 157 women subjected to surgery, thus allowing a breast-saving procedure, rather than mastectomy. In all patients, postoperative irradiation was performed. The approach of primary chemotherapy and conservative treatment with limited surgery and radiotherapy, was also supported by others [22,23]. The role of breast conservation therapy is now the subject of ongoing trials. The purpose of these studies is to evaluate whether or not this treatment strategy is a safe alternative for women with locally advanced breast carcinomas who are responders to an induction chemotherapy.

Inflammatory breast carcinoma is a special condition. This is a T4 tumor, according to the TNM classification, and is considered to be a stage III B breast carcinoma. It accounts for 1-4% of all cases of breast cancer and is the most aggressive form of primary breast cancer. Neither surgical treatment nor radiotherapy alone, has little impact on survival. Even the combination of both has little effect.

Inflammatory breast carcinoma is a systemic disease at diagnosis and local therapy alone is inadequate for treatment. The classical contraindication of surgery has been challenged. An intensive combination therapy regimen should be used prior to local therapy. This multimodal treatment (preoperative chemotherapy and mastectomy) may improve survival.

In 1989, Thoms et al. [24] reported that a prospective study of patients with inflammatory breast cancer, revealed that the locoregional control rate and the 5-year disease-free rates were not improved by the addition of mastectomy. Nevertheless, he concluded that mastectomy can be justified in those patients with the highest probability of prolonged disease-free survival on the basis of reduced late sequelae of irradiation. Multimodality treatment of inflammatory breast carcinoma, has resulted in 27% of patients attaining 5-year disease-free survival. The incidence of failure is low if clinical or pathological response is obtained following initial chemotherapy. Zylberberg et al. [25] reported that lesions cooled by chemotherapy could evolve following a pattern very similar to that of non-inflammatory lesions.

In conclusion, we can say that at the present time, an intensive combination chemotherapy regimen should be used prior to local therapy for the treatment of locally advanced breast carcinoma. This will reduce local tumor burden and thereby optimize local control, eradicate systemic micrometastases, and may increase the probability of survival. The long-term benefit of this strategy must be evaluated in well designed controlled studies.

REFERENCES

1. Haagensen CD, Stout AP. Ann Surg 1943;118:1032-1051.
2. Fletcher GH, Montague ED. AJR 1965;93:573-584.
3. Zucali R, Uslenghi C, Kenda R, Bonadonna G. Cancer 1976;37:1422-1431.
4. Davila E, Vogel CL. Int Adv Surg Oncol 1984;7:297-327.
5. Lena MD, Zucali R, Viganotti G, Valagussa P, Bonadonna G. Cancer Chemother Pharmacol 1978;1:53-59.
6. Valagussa P, Zambetti M, Bignami P, Lena MD, Varini M, Zucali R, Rovini D, Bonadonna G. Clin Exp Metastasis 1983;1:191-202.

7. Hortobagyi GN, Ames FC, Buzdar AU, Kav SW, McNeese MD, Paulus D, Hug V, Holmes FA, Romsdahl MD, Fraschini G, McBride CM, Martin RG, Montague E. Cancer 1988;62:2507-2516.

8. Morrow M, Braverman A, Thelmo W, Sohn CK, Sand J, Mora M, Forlenza T, Marti J. Arch Surg 1986;121:1291-1296.

9. Swain SM, Sorace RA, Bagley CS, Danforth DN Jr, Bader J, Wesley MN, Steinberg SM, Lippman ME. Cancer Res 1987;47:3889-3894.

10. Schwartz GF, Cantor RI, Biermann WA. Arch Surg 1987;122:1430-1434.

11. Piccart MJ, De Valeriola D, Paridanes R, Balidjian D, Mattheiem WH, Loriaux C, Arrigo RN, Contraine F, Heuson JC. Cancer 1988;62:2501-2506.

12. Broadwater JR, Edwards MJ, Kuglen C, Hortobagy GN, Ames FC, Balch CM. Ann Surg 1991;213:126-129.

13. Danforth DN Jr, Lippman ME, McDonald H, Bader J, Egan E, Lampert M, Steinberg SM, Swain SM. Am Surgeon 1990;56:6-11.

14. Rodger A, Jack WJL, Hardman PDJ, Kerr GR, Chetty U, Leonard RCF. Br J Cancer 1992;65:761-765.

15. Sauter ER, Eisenberg BL, Hoffman JP, Ottery FD, Boraas Mc, Goldstein LJ, Solin LJ. World J Surg 1993;17:237-242.

16. Frank JL, McClish DK, Dawson KS, Bear HD. J Surg Oncol 1992;49:220-225.

17. Canavese G, Catturich A, Battistini G, Caroti C, Pronzato P, Gardin G, Amoroso D, Bertelli G, Conte PF, Tomao S. Oncology 1989;46:353-356.

18. Rainer H. Lancet 1988;1(8580):295.

19. Bostwick J, Vasconez LO, Jurkiewicz MD. Plast Reconstr Surg 1978;61:682.

20. Pollock RE, Kroll SS, Balch CM. In: Bland KI, Copeland III EM (eds.) The Breast. WB Saunders Company, 1991;948-956.

21. Bonadonna G, Veronesi U, Brambilla C, Ferrari L, Luini A, Greco M, Bartoli C, Coopmans de Yoldi G, Zucali R, Rilke F, Andreola S, Silvestrini R, Di Fronzo G, Valagussa P. J Natl Cancer Inst 1990;82:1539-1545.

22. Singletary SE, McNeese MD, Hortobagyi GN. Cancer 1992;69:2849-2852.

23. Calais G, Descamps P, Chapet S, Turgeon V, Reynaud-Bougnoux A, Lemarie E, Fignon A, Body G, Bougnoux P, Lansac J, Le Floch O. Int J Radiat Oncol Biol Phys 1993;26:37-42.

24. Thoms WW, McNeese MD, Gletcher GH. Int J Radiat Oncol Biol Phys 1989;17:739-745.

25. Zylberberg B, Salat-Baroux J, Ravina JH, Dormont D, Amiel JP, Diebold P, Izrael V. Cancer 1982;49:1537-1543.

III. 6. Recurrences

Mastology - Breast Diseases
A.S.S. Figueira Fo et al., editors.

Detection of Recurrences in Breast Cancer Following Primary Therapy

M. Seifert, L. Auerbach , S. Vogl, E. Kubista, Department of Obstetrics and Gynecology, Spitalgasse 23 University of Vienna, A-1090 Vienna.

In a total of 677 computer documented and primarily operated breast carcinomas at the First Department of Obstetrics and Gynecology, University of Vienna between 1980 and 1989, we diagnosed 178 recurrences of tumor (distant metastases as well as local recurrences), this amounted to 26.4%.

The aim of this study was to evaluate the importance of examinations in quarterly intervals between 1 and 3 years, in half-yearly intervals between 3 and 5 years, and in yearly intervals, including routine determination of blood parameters, mammography and clinical examinations as well as routine bone scans, chest x-rays and sonography of the liver with regard to their clinical relevance in the demonstration of distant metastases.

After complete primary treatment, oncological postoperative care in its exact sense involves regular follow-up examinations for the diagnosis of the tumor recurrences and metastases. Further, psychological and human contact with patients and their rehabilitation are also the aim of this postoperative care [1]. Today there are extreme opinions regarding the significance of postoperative care. On the one hand there is the view that the time when metastases are exposed is irrelevant for the survival time of the patients. On other hand it is believed that earliest possible recognition and therapy are of prime importance and the entire spectrum of diagnostic procedures should be used for this purpose at regular intervals.

Material and Methods

At the First Department of Obstetrics and Gynecology, University of Vienna the patients were examined according to a certain model. During the first three years this consisted to the following: Calling the patient to the Aftercare Outpatient Department, preparation of an intermediary case history and a physical examination as well as half-yearly blood tests for determination of tumor markers, determining blood count and blood chemistry values including liver parameters. Further, mammography of the contralateral side, chest x-ray, sonography of the liver and bone scans were done in yearly intervals. From the third to the fifth year following primary therapy half-yearly follow-up examinations were done and from the fifth to the tenth year following primary therapy a thorough examination was carried out yearly; this included mammography, bone scan, liver sonogram, chest x-ray, tumor marker and blood chemistry.

Screening recommendations for follow- up after primary treated breast cancer are based on the likelihood of recurrence in general and the clinical utility of early detection of any recurrence.

This model proved the fact that 60 to 80% of tumor recurrences and metastases occur within the first three years following primary therapy.

Regular use of the various diagnostic procedures is based on two rational assumptions. First, it is assumed that their application helps to locate the metastases or the local recurrence earlier and the second is that metastases which are discovered early can be treated more effectively.

Results

Of 677 patients with primary mammary carcinoma who were primary operated between 1980 and 1989 at our clinic, there were 178 recurrences of metastases; 89 of these cases (49 metastases, 34 local tumor recurrences) could be analyzed retrospectively.

Of 20 bone metastases (43%) as first site of recurrence 14 patients showed symptoms of pain, one patient had a pathological fracture. Only 6 patients showed no symptoms at all. In 5 of 20 cases there was obvious evidence of metastatic spread although the bone scan was negative.

Liver metastases as first localisation of relapse appeared in 7 cases (15%), 4 patients were symptomatic and 3 were symptomless; 3 of 7 had increased transaminases, one patient had a heightened tumor marker.

Lung metastases as first site of recurrence were found in 7 cases (15%); 6 of 7 patients showed marked clinical symptoms with irritating cough or dyspnoea; only in one patient the routine chest x-ray revealed the metastatic changes already in progress.

In symptomless patients the interval during which they were free of tumor recurrence (lead time) was three weeks to three months less than in patients presenting with symptoms.

Discussion

Several retrospective studies have shown, that well over 50%, approximately 70% of all patients who relapse bring attention to the physician with more or less specific symptoms [2-9].

As per our present state of knowledge metastases of a breast carcinoma represent an incurable state of disease, regardless of the tumor mass at the time of detection [1,2,4,9,10].

Although the responsiveness of tumors depends partly on their volume one doesn't expect cures even in tumors of smaller volume [11-13]. Thus all forms of therapy are purely palliative measures. The question which arises in the context of exploding health costs is whether patients without symptoms should be subjected to a large number of diagnostic procedures for earliest possible diagnosis of distant metastases.

Though the advances of diagnosis may allow detection of some recurrences earlier, the question remains, whether or not such detection is clinically and for the patients relevant [14]. More effective treatment implies that the patients can be cured, or at least their survival prolonged combined with an improvement of quality of life [15-17].

Metastases represent an incurable stage of the disease, only local recurrences after breast conserving therapy and breast carcinomas of the contralateral side can be possibly cured [18-24].

Patients with prior breast cancer have a fourfold risk to develop a new contralateral primary breast cancer when compared with a normal age- matched control population [4].

Ipsilateral recurrences after breast conserving therapy seems to have the same prognosis as primary breast cancer. Accordingly the diagnosis and treatment of these ipsilateral recurrences and primary breast carcinomas of the contralateral breast at an early stage is important [25-28].

In contrast, the survival benefits of treatment of metastases remain unproven [12,13,29]. Even if early treatment does result in a delay to onset of symptoms - this issue has not been addressed in any major trial- whether such an outcome would justify the toxicity related to systemic therapy of asymptomatic patients is unclear.

In summary general treatment of asymptomatic metastases cannot be justified.

Since the usefullness of early diagnosis of metastases for improving palliative care is not proven, the physician has to asses whether early treatment of asymptomatic recurrences may lead to an improvement by palliation, weighting the toxicity and quality of life versus the benefits of delaying or preventing future symptoms.

Our present status of medical knowledge regards the metastatic stage of breast cancer as incurable. Hence it becomes even more important to give attention to the living quality of the patient [30].

Patients with breast cancer may never be free of fear to relapse even after a long period and if their basic prognostic factors are favourable.

This involves special emphasis on their psyche, oncological patients rarely miss follow-up examinations, nevertheless each examination recalls the memory of cancer and the fear associated with the outcome of the examination. On the other hand the patients regard the examination as rather natural event, this is partly due to the easy applicability and availability of the various diagnostic procedures.

Finally this raises another problem: the obligation of the doctor to inform the patient and explain her condition. If the doctor is faced with a symptomless patient in whom routine examination has indicated metastases, should he inform the patient of the examination result?

Further, false-positive tumor markers lead to follow-ups which involve calling the patient to the hospital; this increases the anxiety of the patient, who, is already sensitive on the subject.

Summary

In most cases symptoms, anamnesis and physical examination lead to the detection of metastases. Special attention should be paid to the psyche and the living quality of the patients. The knowledge of asymptomatic metastases may substantially reduce the patients quality of life.

Determination of the status of patients for analyzing the results of primary therapy or adjuvant therapy is mostly possible after exact investigation of case history and physical examination.

References

1. Schmidt-Matthiesen H: Allgemeine Prinzipien der Nachsorge. Arch Gynec 232:218, 1981.
2. Stierer M, Rosen HR: Influence of early diagnosis on prognosis of recurrent breast cancer. Cancer 64:1128 1989.
3. Tomin R, Donegan WL: Screening for recurrent breast cancer- its effectiveness and prognostic value. J Clin. Oncol 5:62, 1987.
4. Rutgers EJ, Van SEA, Kluck HM: Follow -up after treatment of primary breast cancer. BR J Surg 76:187, 1989.
5. Pedrazzini A, Gelber R, Isley M, et al: First repeated bone scan in the observation of patients with operable breast cancer. J Clin Oncol 4:389, 1986.
6. Winchester DP, Sener SF, Khandekar JD, et al: Symptomatology as an indicator of recurrentor metastatic breast cancer. Cancer 43:956, 1979.
7. Pandya KJ, Mcfadden ET, Kalish LA, et al: A retrospectiv study of earliest indicators of recurrence in patients on Eastern Cooperative Group adjuvant chemotherapy trials for breast cancer: A preliminary report. Cancer 55:202, 1985.
8. Scanlon EF, Oviedo MA, Cunningham MP, et al: Preoperative and follow-up procedures on patients

with breast cancer. Cancer 46:977, 1980.

9. Zwaveling a, Albers GHR, Felthuis W, Hermans J: An evaluation of routine follow-up for detection of breast cancer recurrences. J Clin Oncol 34:194, 1987.
10. Broyn T, Froyen J: Evaluation of routine follow-up after surgery of primary breast carcinoma. Acta Chir Scand 148:401, 1982.
11. Harris J, Hellman S: Observations on survival analysis with particular reference to breast cancer treatment. Cancer 57:925, 1986.
12. Rosen P, Groshen W, Siago P, et al: A long-term follow-up study of survival of stage I (T1 N0 M0) and stage II (T1 N1 M0) breast carcinoma. J Clin Oncol 7:355, 1989.
13. Langlands A, Pocock S, Kerr G, Gore S: Long-term survival of patients with breast cancer: A study of curability of the disease. Br Med J 2:1247, 1979.
14. Paterson AHG, Szafran O, Cornish F, et al: Effect of chemotherapy on survival in metastatic breast cancer. Breast Cancer Res Treat 1:357-363, 1981.
15. Paterson AHG, Szafran O, Hanson J, et al: Response on treatment and its influence on survival in metastatic breast cancer. Am J Clin Oncol 8:283-292, 1985.
16. Powles TJ, Smith IE, Ford HT, et al: Failure of chemotherapy to prolong survival in a group of patients with metastatic breast cancer. Lancet 1:580-582, 1980.
17. Kaufman RJ: Advanced breast cancer - Additive hormonal therapy. Cancer 47:2398-2403, 1981.
18. Recht A, Schnitt SJ, Connolly JL, et al: Prognosis following local or regional recurrence of conservative surgery and radiotherapy for early stage breast carcinoma. Int J Radiat Oncol Biol Phys 16:33-9, 1989.
19. Kurtz JM, Amalric R, Brandone H, et al: Local recurrence after breast- conserving surgery and radiotherapy: Frequency, time course, and prognosis. Cancer 63:1912-1917, 1989.
20. Stotter AT, McNeese MD, Ames FC, et al: Predicting the rate and extent of locoregional failure after breast conservation therapy for early breast cancer. Cancer 64:2217-2225, 1989.
21. Harris JR, Recht A, Amalric R, et al: Time course and prognosis of local recurrence following primary radiation therapy for early breast cancer. J Clin Oncol 2:37-41, 1984.
22. Fisher ER, Fisher B, Sass R, et al: Pathologic finding of the NSABP (protocol no.4). Bilateral breast cancer. Cancer 54:3002-3011, 1984.
23. Finney GC, Finney GG, Montague AC, et al: Bilateral breast cancer, clinical and pathological review. Ann Surg 175:635-646, 1972.
24. Slack NH, Nemoto T, Fisher B: Experience with bilateral breast primary carcinoma of the breast. Surg Gynecol Obstet 136:433, 1973.
25. Egan RL: Bilateral breast carcinomas: Role of mammography. Cancer 38:931-938, 1976.
26. Sears HF, Janus C, Mc Dermott A, et al: Bilateral breast carcinoma: Prospective evaluation of factors assisting diagnosis. J Surg Oncol 32:203-207,1986.
27. Holmberg L, Adamo HO, Ekbom A, et al: Prognosis in bilateral breast cancer. Effect of time interval between first and second primary tumors. Br J Cancer 58:191-194, 1988.
28. Senofsky GM, Wanebo HJ, Wilhelm MC, et al: Has monitoring of the contralateral breast improved the prognosis in patients treated for primary breast cancer? Cancer 57:592-602, 1986.
29. Rutqvist LE: Increasing incidenceand constant mortality rates of breast cance: Time trends in Stockholm County 1961-1973. Breast Cancer Res Treat 4:233, 1984.
30. Mueller CB: Asymptomatic metastases: To treat or not to treat? Surgery 93:328, 1983.

Mastology - Breast Diseases
A.S.S. Figueira Fo et al., editors.

Management of locally recurrent breast cancer after mastectomy.

Riccardo Masetti, M.D., Daniela Terribile, M.D., Armando Antinori, M.D., Alessandro Marra, M.D., Miriam Valentini, M.D., Claudio Breccia, M.D., Paolo Magistrelli, M.D. and Aurelio Picciocchi, M.D.

Department of General Surgery I, Catholic University, Largo A. Gemelli, 8 - 00168 Rome - Italy

Summary

Although locoregional recurrences following mastectomy have a poor prognosis, many patients will live for years after recurrence. Uncertainties remain about the therapeutic approaches. Fourty-eight patients with chest wall recurrence of breast cancer after mastectomy were retrospectively reviewed in this study.

Mean interval to recurrence was 31 months (range 3-166). Actuarial 5-year overall and disease-free survival were respectively 37% and 24%. Univariate analysis showed a significant correlation between survival and time interval to recurrence, axillary node status and number of recurrent nodules. Patients with time interval shorter than two years, positive axillary node status and multiple recurrences manifested a poorer prognosis.

Text

Locoregional recurrence is commonly the first and most distressing indication of therapeutic failure for women with breast cancer.

The incidence of local recurrence after definitive surgery varies from 4 to 30% in reported series [1-4]. It depends on many of the same factors that predict the likelyhood of developing distant metastases, among which the most important is the pathological status of the axillary limph nodes [5]. The chance of a local recurrence following radical mastectomy with pathologically negative nodes varies from 4% to 6%, while it increases up to 28% when the axillary nodes are positive [1-5].

Most local relapses occur relatively rapidly after mastectomy. The median time is less than two years in 60-80% of cases, with almost all remaining recurrences appearing before the end of 10 years [6]. However, local recurrences occurring 15 to 50 years after initial surgery have been occasionally reported [7-8].

Clinical presentation, etiology and prognostic factors

Chest wall recurrence most commonly appears as single or multiple, tiny (1-2 cm) asymptomatic nodules, usually located in or near the scar of mastectomy. The number of separate nodules initially found on the chest wall is usually small. The nodules may ulcerate or the skin of the chest wall may become indurated. Occasionally, inflammatory skin changes may progress to a "carcinoma en cuirasse", with diffuse infiltration of the skin and subcutaneous tissue and spread of tumor on the chest wall beyond the limits of standard surgical or radiation therapy boundaries.

The exact mechanism of local recurrence remains uncertain. Proposed etiologies include tumor cells left by inadequate initial resection of the primary tumor, surgical transection of disease-containing lymphatic channels or hematogenous spread to the surgical wound [6-7].

The overall prognosis of local recurrence after mastectomy is poor. Despite aggressive local treatment, as many as two-thirds of patients will go on to develop distant metastases [9].

Several factors have been shown to correlate with distant relapse and survival. One of the most potent indicators for rapid progress is the initial disease-free interval (DFI). In a review of 128 patients with local recurrence, Bedwinek et al. [10] demonstrated a 5-year disease-free survival rate of 21% for patients with DFI greater than 2 years as compared to 8% for patients with shorter intervals. Similar findings concerning overall survival were reported by Aberzik et al. [11] (58% versus 33%) and Schwaibold et al. [12] (67% versus 30%). Other prognostic indicators have been evaluated. Multiple rather than single relapses, increasing size of lesion or axillary nodal involvement by the primary tumor all are associated with poor prognosis [9,13].

Treatment

The rationale for treatment of local recurrence after mastectomy is that local control of patients with no evidence of systemic disease is associated with a better rate of freedom from distant metastases and better survival. On the contrary, uncontrolled local disease is often painful, may present problems of hygiene and infection and is psychologically disabling as an evidence of previous treatment failures.

The many differences in presentation and the variable courses of patients with local recurrence have made it difficult to evaluate the benefits of available treatments; so little agreement exists on which patients should be treated, with which modalities, and when.

Radiation therapy is the mainstay of management if the initial treatment did not include irradiation [9,12]. Complete response rates and 5-year overall survival rates varying between 63-67% and 10-39% respectively, have been reported [7-14].

Optimal technique should include treatment to the entire chest wall and probably to the supraclavicular fossa. Elective treatment of other uninvolved sites, as the axilla and the internal mammary region, does not appear necessary and may increase complication [12]. The dose of radiation required is dependent on the volume of the disease. Doses of 4500 cGy are adequate for electively treated sites. For excised regions a minimum dose of 5000 cGy is required. For gross disease higher doses are required. Lesions < 4 cm require a minimum dose of 6000 cGy. No dose response is evident for larger lesions with up to a 50% failure rate despite doses of 7000 cGy [12,14].

Despite adequate dose and technique, a disappointingly large number of patients suffer further recurrences, while only a few may expect to have an extended period of disease-free survival. Efforts to improve locoregional control with the use of hyperthermia are in progress [15].

The benefits of systemic therapy, either alone or in combination with radiotherapy or surgery, remain controversial [1,6]. Candidates for systemic therapy should include patients at higher risk of developing distant metastases (brief disease-free interval and multifocal or bulky relapses).

Complete excision of the local recurrence should be performed whenever possible as it allows lighter schedules of radiation and adjuvant therapies and enhances the probability of local control and occasionally of cure. Complete excision may not always be technically feasible, mainly due to local spread of the recurrent tumor. In these cases a biopsy should always be performed for histological diagnosis and for estrogen and progesterone receptor assay.

When complete excision requires an extended surgical procedure (wide excision of soft tissues with flap reconstruction or chest wall resection with or without prosthetic reconstruction), indications to surgery should be modulated considering the patient's overall condition, the likelyhood of effective local control, the morbidity of salvage treatment and the prediction of survival [16].

Chest wall resection can be achieved with low morbidity and mortality if performed only by surgeons with expertise on thoracic surgery.

If used in selected patients, extended radical procedures can offer significant palliation of pain and other sequelae of tumor ulcerative (local control rates: 75% - 97%) and improved survival (5-year overall survival rates: 31% - 70%) [17-19].

Personal experience

Between 1967 and 1989, 769 patients underwent radical surgery for breast cancer at the Department of General Surgery I of the Catholic University of Rome.

With a median follow up period of 149 months, 48 patients (6.2%) developed an isolated local recurrence. The median age of these 48 patients was 53 years (range 23-77 years). Initial surgery consisted of radical mastectomy in 24 cases and modified radical mastectomy in 24 cases. Pathological axillary nodal involvement was assessed in 37 patients. Eleven patients had negative nodes initially.

The median time to recurrence was 23 months (range 3 - 78 months), with the latest failure occurring at 14 years.

Complete excision of the local recurrence was achieved in 67% of patients, followed by radiation treatment in 36% of cases. Complete excision required a chest wall resection with prosthetic reconstruction in 4 cases.

In the remaining 33% of patients an incisional biopsy was performed, followed by radiotherapy (23% of cases) or chemo-hormonal therapy (10%).

Mean follow up after recurrence was 38 months (range 2- 86 months). Actuarial 5-year overall and relapse-free survival were respectively 37% and 24%.

Univariate analysis of survival showed a significant correlation with the time interval to recurrence, the axillary node status and the number of nodules. Actuarial overall 5-year survival was significantly worst for patients that developed recurrence within the first two years after mastectomy, had axillary nodal involvement by the primary tumor or had multiple recurrences as compared to patients with longer disease-free intervals after mastectomy, uninvolved axilla and single recurrences on the chest wall (respectively 18%, 25% and 25% versus 75%, 76% and 56%).

Conclusions

The overall prognosis of local recurrence after mastectomy is poor, but many patients will live for years after recurrence.

Analysis of prognostic factors indicates that survival seems to be related to the tumor biology more than to the single treatment modalities. Uncertainties persist concerning therapeutic approaches. Efforts should be made to achieve locoregional control in the hope of occasional cure.

A multimodal therapeutic approach is warranted and an accurate selection of patients is mandatory to optimize the choice of treatment and enhance the chances of cure.

References

1) Kennedy MJ and Abeloff MD. Cancer 1993; 71: 2395-409.

2) Rosenmann J, Bernard S. et al. Cancer 1986; 57: 1421-5.

3) Valagussa P, Bonadonna G. et al. Cancer 1978; 41: 1170-8.

4) Fowble B, Gray R. et al. J Clin Oncol 1988; 6: 1107-17.

5) Clark GM, Dressler LG et al. N England J Med 1989; 320: 627-33.

6) Gilliand MD, Barton RM et al. Ann Surg 1983; 197: 284-7.

7) Chen KKY, Montague E. et al. Cancer 1985; 56: 1269-73.

8) Chu FCH, Lin FJ et al. Cancer 1976; 37: 2677-81.

9) Magno L, Bignardi M et al. Cancer 1987; 60: 240-5.

10) Bedwinek JM, Fineberg B. et al Int J Radiat Oncol Biol Phys 1981; 7: 581-5.

11) Aberzik WJ, Silver B. et al. Cancer 1986; 58: 1214-8.

12) Schwaibold F, Fowble BL. Int J Radiat Oncol Biol Phys 1991: 21:299-310

13) Ames FC, Balch CL et al. Surg Clin North Am 1990; 70: 1115-24.

14) Halverson KJ, Perez CA et al. Int J Radiat Oncol Biol Phys1991; 19: 851-8.

15) Dragovic J, Seydel H et al. J Clin Oncol 1989; 7: 30-5.

16) McCormak PM, Bains M. et al. Arch Surg 1989; 124: 158-61.

17) Miyauchi K, Koyama H et al. Eur J Cancer 1992; 28: 1059-62.

18) Kluiber R, Bines S et al. Am Surg 1991; 57:523-30.

19) Zoetmulder FAN, Van Dongen JA. Eur J Surg Oncol 1988; 14: 127-32.

III. 7. Special forms

Mastology - Breast Diseases
A.S.S. Figueira Fo et al., editors.

Breast cancer in elderly patients: issues related to the surgical management.

F. Badellino, G. Canavese, A. Catturich, C. Vecchio, D. Tomei.
Divisione di Oncologia Chirurgica - Istituto Nazionale Ricerca sul Cancro - Genova (Italia).

There is no consensus on the optimum local treatment for breast cancer in elderly women. In fact, elderly patients with the same stage of disease may be treated in different centres by mastectomy, by local excision or by tamoxifen alone. From 1980 to 1991 out of 1157 patients with stage I-II breast cancer operated at our Division 269 were aged over 70 years. Eight years overall survival rate was 59% and progression free survival rate was 39%. Elderly patients should receive standard therapy that control disease long term.

There is not a clear agreement on how the elderly have to be defined; generally they have been considered as being aged from 65 years to over 85 years.

The patient aged over 70 years up to now have been excluded from the clinical trials; so by default this can be described as "the oncological definition of old age".

Although the elderly women have been often excluded from the clinical trials, women aged 70 have a live expectancy of 14 years.

Several studies have suggested that cancer is less likely to be diagnosed at a local stage in elderly compared to younger patients (1, 2) and that older subjects are less likely to receive a standard treatment than are younger after the diagnosis of cancer.

A part from the comorbidity, other factors that might affect the treatment choice in the elderly include decreased social support, low economic status, lack of information on efficacy and toxicity of cancer therapies, and physician, patient, or family bias against treating the elderly (3).

The data derived from the NCI' Surveillence Epidemiology and End Result (SEER) showed that surgery was less likely to be performed in those patients aged over 85 and in this group was less likely to be extensive. When divided into stages and after adjusting for non-cancer deaths was no difference in survival of those with localized disease, irrispective of age (4).

In 1980, uncontrolled studies with a short follow-up suggested that Tamoxifen as the sole treatment was effective for elderly cancer patient.

Horobin achieved long-term control in 37% of 113 patients aged 70 years treated by Tamoxifen only (minimum follow-up: 5 years) (5).

The result of two prospective trials comparing Tamoxifen vs surgery in elderly patients are controversial. Gazet et al. reported no difference in time to disease progression between the two group (6).

These data have been criticised either because of its small number and large proportion of inoperable cancer and because the surgery was sub-optimal.

In the randomized study of Robertson (wedge mastectomy vs Tamoxifen) the patients receiving Tamoxifen alone showed a significative increased risk of local recurrence (7).

The CRC trial compared Tamoxifen vs Tamoxifen plus optimal surgery (8).

In most patients the surgical treatment was wide local excision: one in four had a mastectomy. At a follow-up of 34 months local recurrence rates were more than five higher in the patients treated by conservative surgery.

Kantorowitz and others have reported that in Rochester, NY, of women over 60 who underwent segmental mastectomy by community surgeon, only 40% were referred for postoperative RT. Local or regional recurrence developed in 39,1% of the women who had no radiation therapy and in only 4% of those who received both modality of treatment (9).

Consequently these data suggest that wide local excision without postoperative RT is not a satisfactory local treatment for elderly with breast cancer.

The EORTC trials n° 10850 (tumorectomy plus Tamoxifen vs modified radical mastectomy and modified radical mastectomy vs Tamoxifen only) will be analyzed. Then the surgical approach is mandatory in elderly patients with stage I-II breast cancer. What is the best surgical choice?

Simple mastectomy seems to be associated with an unacceptable rate of axillary relapse when compared with a modified radical mastectomy (10).

The segmental mastectomy or lumpectomy could be performed in a small subset of patients with lesions less than 1 cm. and in absence of palpable axillary nodes. The segmental mastectomy and axillary dissection plus RT or modified radical mastectomy are the standard treatment options with proven safety efficacy. The average mortality in elderly patients undergoing mastectomy is less than 1%; this is comparate to minor surgical procedure (11, 12). Conservative treatment plus RT is an important advance in the management of "young" and "middle age"women with breast cancer; this does not be the same for the "older" women. A study performed at a Maidstone Hospital (U.K.) conclude that, when a choice is available, 90% of elderly women prefer breast conservation (13). An elderly women who is already faced with the decline in physical appearance associated with aging, can find the loss of a breast a severy injury. Also, women with large breasts have sometimes difficult to use a external prosthesis.

From 1980 to 1991 out of 1157 patients with stage I-II breast cancer operated at our Division 269 (23.2%) were aged over 70 years.

Out of these cases 25 underwent conservative surgery plus RT, 173 radical or modified radical mastectomy and 71 total mastectomy with or without axillary nodes sampling.

Axillary nodes metastases were found in 115 (47%) of pts. The estrogen receptors assays was positive in 147 cases (54.6%) and unknown in 74 (27%). Seven (12%) patients received chemotherapy, 61 hormonal therapy and 2 both treatments.

Eight years overall survival rate was 59% and progression free survival rate was 39%. Clearly, elderly patients should receive standard therapy that control disease long term (conservative surgery plus RT or radical modified mastectomy). They should receive adjuvant therapy. Only in case of comorbid disease a less intensive treatment could be choosed.

More of elderly patients who did not receive a standard treatment developed a local recurrence. This event required further therapy and unpaired the quality of life.

REFERENCES

1) Goodwin JS, Samet JM, Key CR, Humble C, Kutvirt D, Hunt C
Stage of diagnosis of cancer varies with the age of the patient.
Am Geriat Soc 1986; 34: 20-26.

2) Holmes FF, Heanne E
Cancer stage to stage relationship in the elderly.
Am Geriat Soc 1981; 29: 55-58.

3) Godwin JS, Hunt WC, Samet JM
Determinants of cancer therapy in elderly patients.
Cancer 1993; 72: 594-600.

4) Yancik R, Riess LG and Yates JW
Breast cancer in aging women.
Cancer 1989; 63: 976.

5) Horobin JM, Preece PE, Dewar JA, Wood Rab, Cuschieri A
Long-term follow-up of elderly patient with loco-regionale breast cancer with Tamoxifen only.
Br J Surg 1991; 78: 213-217.

6) Gazet JC, Markopoulos CH, Ford HT, Coombers RC, Bland JM, Dixon RC
Prospective randomized trial of Tamoxifen versus surgery in elderly patients with breast cancer.
Lancet 1988; 679-81.

7) Robertson JFR, Todd JH, Ellis O, Elston CW, Blamey RW
Comparison of mastectomy with Tamoxifen for treating elderly patients with operable breast cancer.
Brit Med J 1988; 297: 511-514.

8) Bates T, Riley DL, Houghton J, Fallowfield L, Baum M
Breast cancer in elderly women: a Cancer Research Campaign trial comparing treatment with Tamoxifen and optimal surgery with Tamoxifen alone.
Br J Surg 1991; 78: 591-594.

9) Kantorowitz D, Poulter CA, Sischy B
Treatment of breast cancer among elderly women with segmental mastectomy or segmental mastectomy plus postoperative radiotherapy.
Int J Radiat Oncol Biol Phys 1988; 15: 263.

10) Fentiman IS
Breast cancer in the elderly. In: Detection and treatment of early breast cancer.
London: Martin Dunitz, 1991: 193-206.

11) Amsterdam E, Birkenfeld S, Gilad A, Krispin M
Surgery for carcinoma of the breast in women over 70 years of age.
J Surg Oncol 1987; 35: 180-183.

12) Svastics E, Sulyok Z, Besznyk I
Treatment of breast cancer in women older than 70 years.
J Surg Oncol 1989; 41: 19-21.

13) Jones PA, Philiphs RM and Wright P
Breast conservation or mastectomy; choice of women over seventy.
European Journal of Surgical Oncology 1993; 19: 491.

Mastology - Breast Diseases
A.S.S. Figueira Fo et al., editors.

Biology of breast cancer in elderly women

Rosella Silvestrini, Elvira Benini, Antonella Luisi, Silvia Veneroni, Barbara Valentinis, Maria Grazia Daidone

Oncologia Sperimentale C, Istituto Nazionale Tumori, Via Venezian 1, 20133 Milan, Italy

Abstract

The biology of breast cancers in elderly patients has been scarcely investigated up to now. A basic analysis carried out on a large series of patients recruited over a 20-year period showed that breast cancers from elderly women were characterized by the highest positivity for estrogen receptors (ER) and the lowest proliferative rate compared to tumors from younger patients. Conversely, DNA ploidy and progesterone receptors (PgR) were only marginally affected by the increase in patient age. As already observed for younger patients, even in cancers from elderly patients biologic markers were independent of tumor size and nodal involvement, except for a high incidence of lack of hormone receptors within large tumors. In elderly patients with node-positive tumors treated with adjuvant hormonal therapy, besides lymph nodal involvement cell proliferation, hormone receptors and the expression of P53 were significantly discriminant of 4-year relapse-free survival. The combined consideration of biologic and pathologic variables allowed us to identify patients markedly differing in the risk of relapse on the basis of tumor features. These findings could represent the biologic basis of a tailored therapy to improve clinical results.

In the last few decades, studies on breast cancer biology have been progressively intensified and biologic information has substantially contributed to improve knowledge on the natural history of the disease, to define the clinical role of biologic markers such as hormone receptors, cell proliferation and ploidy (i.e., nuclear DNA content) and to give clinicians information for treatment-decision making [1]. However, these studies have been generally performed on tumors from relatively younger patients who entered therapeutic clinical protocols. Conversely, tumors from elderly patients have been marginally investigated until now, so that little information is available to establish whether these cancers are biologically different from cancers of younger women and whether clinical outcome could be improved by planning therapeutic protocols according to the biologic characteristics [2].

On a series of more than 1000 primary breast cancers from patients over 70 years of age, we determined biologic features, including cell proliferation, (expressed as the ^{3}H-thymidine labeling index, ^{3}H-dT LI), ER and PgR (evaluated by using the dextran coated-charcoal absorption technique), and DNA ploidy (evaluated by flow cytometry). The relations among these biologic variables and among these and conventional pathologic factors were comparatively analyzed for the different decade age classes.

From this basic analysis we observed a slight decrease in the frequency of aneuploid tumors (i.e., tumors with gross DNA abnormalities) with increasing age, with the highest frequency (80%) in patients younger than 30 years and the lowest value (70%) in patients older than 80 years. The age-related behavior of PgR was rather discontinuous, with a peak of 75%

positive tumors and the highest levels of PgR in tumors from patients aged 30-50 years, and with a decrease to 50% positive tumors for older patients. Conversely, a marked and direct age-related pattern was observed for ER, in terms of presence of the receptor and in terms of concentration. In fact, a progressive and relatively constant increase in ER positivity was observed from 65%, in the youngest patients, to more than 80% in patients over 70 years of age. Such an increase was paralleled by a similar increase in ER content, whose median value was around 40 fmol in premenopausal patients and 3 and more then 4 times higher in patients older than 70 and 80 years, respectively. As expected, the opposite finding was observed for cell proliferation, which progressively and consistently decreased with increasing of patient age. In fact, in a series of about 10,000 cases recruited since 1973, the median ^{3}H-dT LI of 5.5%, reported for the youngest patients, decreased as age increased and plateaued around 3% in tumors from patients over 70 years of age. In conclusion, breast cancers from elderly patients were characterized by the highest positivity for ER and the lowest proliferative rate.

The pattern of association between biologic and pathologic variables was unaffected by patient age. It showed a general independence of biologic markers from nodal involvement at time of diagnosis, and a trend of an association of tumor size with hormone receptors (with larger tumors more frequently hormone-receptor negative) but not with cell proliferation and ploidy. Anyway, the presence or lack of an association was consistent regardless of patient age [3].

According to the guidelines proposed by McGuire [4], the assessment of the clinical relevance of biologic markers should be carried out on substantial series of patients with an adequate follow-up and homogeneous for tumor stage and clinical treatment. Within the subset of elderly patients, such requirements were fulfilled by node-positive tumors treated with tamoxifen for at least 1 year and with a median follow-up of 4 years. In this case series of about 100 patients, the probability to relapse was unaffected by tumor size, whereas it was significantly related to the number of involved axillary lymph nodes, ER, PgR and ^{3}H-dT LI, although with a different discriminating power, In fact, the relapse rate in patients with tumors without hormone receptors or rapidly proliferating was about twofold that of patients with hormone-receptor-positive or slowly proliferating tumors. In particular, the absence of ER was associated with the most unfavorable prognosis (3 out of 4 patients relapsing within 4 years from diagnosis), whereas a low proliferation identified tumors with an indolent outcome (only 1 out of 5 patients relapsing at 4 years).

In addition to these biologic variables, whose clinical role has been definitely assessed in tumors from younger patients subjected to different treatment modalities including local-regional [5-7], adjuvant chemical [8] and hormonal [9] treatments, in this subset of patients the clinical predictivity of P53 expression was also investigated. P53 expression, which proved to be one of the most promising prognostic markers in younger patients [10-13], showed an even more remarkable prognostic role in elderly patients. In fact, the risk of relapse was four times higher for tumors highly expressing P53 (90%) than for those with low protein levels (24%). As already observed for tumors from younger patients, the integration of pathologic and biologic variables significantly improved the predictive resolution for the low risk whereas it marginally contributed to the identification of the high risk patients. In fact, singly, good-prognosis markers identified patients with a 20-30%

relapse rate at 4 years. In association, they provided more accurate prognostic information, with the better resolution observed for the association of low ^{3}H-dT LI and less than 3 positive nodes, which was able to identify a subgroup of patients with a 5% relapse rate. Conversely, the single most powerful indicators of a poor prognosis were ER- and P53 overexpression, which identified 77% and 90% of relapsing tumors, respectively; the other markers did not give any additive prognostic information.

In conclusion, these findings are generally similar to those obtained in younger patients [9]. It should be noted that the data were obtained on patients subjected to endocrine treatment, which is known to provide the highest benefit for tumors with hormone receptors and a slow proliferation [14, 15]. However, a separate analysis on the subset of ER+ tumors, conventionally considered hormone-responsive, showed that again the best and worse prognoses were identified by low ^{3}H-dT LI in association with a low number of positive nodes and by the overexpression of P53. Such evidence raised the question whether cell proliferation and P53 could be actually considered specifically responsible for benefit or failure of hormonal therapy in addition to their strong prognostic significance.

All these data have been derived from retrospective analyses and need to be prospectively confirmed. However, particularly for elderly patients, for whom the cost-benefit of treatments should be carefully assessed, it would seem reliable to use biologic findings as a complement to clinico-pathologic features in a 'risk-factor profile system' for treatment planning.

References

1. McGuire WL, Clark GM. N Engl J Med 1992; 326:1756-1761
2. Valentinis B, Silvestrini R, Daidone MG, Coradini D, Galante E, Cerrotta AM, Abolafio G, Arboit L. Breast Cancer Res Treat 1991; 20:19-24
3. Silvestrini R, Daidone MG. In: Senn HJ, Gelber RD, Goldhirsch A, Thurlimann B (eds) Recent Results in Cancer Research 127. Berlin-Heidelberg: Springer-Verlag, 1993; 71-76
4. McGuire WL. J Natl Cancer Inst 1991; 83:153-154
5. Silvestrini R, Daidone MG, Valagussa P, Di Fronzo G, Mezzanotte G, Bonadonna G. Eur. J. Cancer Clin Oncol 1989; 25:1165-1171
6. Meyer JS, Province M. Breast Cancer Res Treat 1988; 12:191-204
7. Tubiana M, Pejovic MH, Koscielny S, Int J Cancer 1989; 44:17-22
8. Silvestrini R, Daidone MG, Valagussa P, Di Fronzo G, Mezzanotte G, Mariani L, Bonadonna G. J Clin Oncol 1990; 1321-1326
9. Silvestrini R, Daidone MG, Mastore M, Di Fronzo G, Coradini D, Boracchi P, Squicciarini P, Salvadori B, Veronesi U. J Clin Oncol 1993; 11:1150-1155
10. Thor AD, Moore DH II, Edgerton SM, Kawasaki ES, Reihsaus E, Lynch HT, Marcus N, Schwarzt L, Chen LC, Mayall BH, Smith HS. J Natl Cancer Inst 1992; 84:845-855
11. Isola J, Visakorpi T, Holli K, Kallionemi OP. J Natl Cancer Inst 1992; 84:1109-1114
12. Allred DC, Clark GM, Elledge R, Fuqua SAW, Brown RW, Chamness GC, Osborne CK, McGuire WL. J Natl Cancer Inst 1993; 85:200-206

13. Silvestrini, R, Benini E, Daidone MG, Veneroni S, Boracchi P, Cappelletti V, Di Fronzo G, Veronesi U. J Natl Cancer Inst 1993; 85:965-970
14. Meyer JS, Lee JY. Cancer Res 1980; 40:1890-1896
15. Paradiso A, Lorusso V, Tommasi S, Schittulli F, Maiello E, Del Lena M. Breast Cancer Res Treat 1988; 11:31-36

Mastology - Breast Diseases
A.S.S. Figueira Fo et al., editors.

Breast cancer in elderly patients : EORTC protocols and new therapeutic prospects

I.S. Fentiman, F. Mignolet and T. Sahmoud
ICRF Clinical Oncology Unit and EORTC Data Centre

ABSTRACT

Breast cancer in women aged over 70 years is a substantial problem and until recently no randomised trials have been conducted. The EORTC breast cancer cooperative group has run 2 parallel trials.

10850	modified radical mastectomy
	tumour excision and tamoxifen (20mg)
10851	modified radical mastectomy
	tamoxifen alone (20mg)

After a median follow-up of 4 years, in 10850 the relapse free survival of both groups was the same, but breast relapse was more common in the excision and tamoxifen group whereas distant relapse occurred more frequently in the mastectomy group. Overall survival was the same for both groups. In 10851 there was significant increase in local relapse, overall relapse, and an increase in mortality in those treated with tamoxifen alone.

Introduction

There is now increased awareness of the problem of breast cancer in the elderly and heightened interest in new therapeutic approachs for such patients. In Britain approximately 1 in 3 patients with breast cancer is aged 70 years or more. As public health improves and smoking decreases so the proportion of elderly women with breast cancer will increase further.

Older women do not have intrinsically less aggressive disease. Although more of them will have lobular, mucoid and papillary carcinoma compared with younger women, there are still substantial numbers with grade III breast carcinoma and up to 50% of these women will have axillary nodal metastases at the time of presentation [1]. This is unlikely to change until health policy is altered to allow a call/recall system for all women age 50 years or more, rather than 50-64 which is the age group presently offered screening mammography in Britain. As a possible alternative routine clinical examination may be of value in this age group because of the increased easy of detection of small cancers within the fatty-replaced breast tissue.

Background

In 1984 when the EORTC breast cancer cooperative group were considering setting up a trial of therapeutic options for elderly women with operable breast cancer there were no data available from prospective randomised trials since women aged 65 or 70 had been excluded from these. The main reason for this was a belief that the morbidity in older women would lead to contamination of trial of excess of non-cancer deaths. Additionally, many felt the treatment options were unimportant because of patients would die of other diseases before their cancer relapsed and became problematic.

There have been several reports of uncontrolled studies in which women with operable breast cancer were given tamoxifen alone and the preliminary results were encouraging [2,3,4]. The use of adjuvant tamoxifen in this group was not routine. The trial carried out by the Danish Breast Cancer Cooperative had suggested no benefit from adjuvant tamoxifen in older women [5]. There was agreement among the surgeons of the group that the standard treatment should be a modified radical mastectomy and not a total mastectomy, since this had been shown to achieve better local control [6].

The main debate arose concerning what should be the test arm of the trial. Some surgeons wished to try to keep many elderly patients out of hospital as possible and wished to make an outpatient diagnosis using fine needle aspiration cytology or core needle biopsy and then give tamoxifen in the hope of shrinking and possibly eliminating the carcinoma. Other surgeons wanted to rid the patient of the lump of which they were complaining then use tamoxifen in an adjuvant role to try to prvent local relapse. Because of the irreconcilable nature of these feelings it was decided to run two parallel trials with individual centres committed to participating in only one of them.

Study design

		Tumour-excision + tamoxifen
Trial 10850	R	
		Modified radical mastectomy
		Tamoxifen alone
Trial 10851	R	
		Modified radical mastectomy

To be eligible for either trial the patients had to be aged 70 years or more with operable breast cancer (T_1, T_2, T_3, N_o, N_1, M_o). They had to be physically and psychologically fit for either procedure and gave informed consent according to local ethical committee recommendations. None had any previous breast cancer nor any other malignancy.

In 10850, patients were treated by either a modified radical mastectomy or by tumour excision. Although the aim was to achieve gross clearance of the carcinoma there was no stipulation for histologically confirmed tumour free margins. Post-operatively patients were given tamoxifen 20 mg daily with the aiming of continuing this on a permanent basis or until relapse of disease. It was assumed that the majority of the relapses would occur within the breast so that a subsequent salvage mastectomy would be possible. Thus in a way the study was a comparison of immediate versus possibly delayed mastectomy. Women randomised to modified radical mastectomy were not given any adjuvant tamoxifen.

In 10851, the diagnosis of cancer was made by FNAC or Trucut biopsy after which they were randomised to receive tamoxifen at the same dosage of 20 mg or modified radical mastectomy. Local progression was deemed to have occurred in this group when there was an increase in size of the primary tumour or axillary nodal metastases by more than 50%. As in the other study it was hoped that those progressing or relapsing would mostly be salvagable by mastectomy.

Results

A total of 236 women entered trial 10850 of whom 116 were treated by tumour excision and 120 by modified radical mastectomy. Mean follow-up was 4 years. Results are given in Table 1. Relapse free survival was similar in both groups although local relapse,

Table 1.

Results of EORTC Trial 10850 at 5 years

	Tumour excision and tamoxifen	Modified radical mastectomy
n	116	120
Relapse-free survival	65%	65%
Local relapse-free survival	72%	85%
Distant relapse-free survival	95%	70%
Overall survival	65%	65%

Table 2.

Results of EORTC Trial 10851 at 5 years

	Tamoxifen alone	Modified radical mastectomy
n	84	86
Relapse-free survival	15%	60%
Local relapse-free survival	20%	90%
Distant relapse-free survival	75%	85%
Overall survival	55%	80%

predominantly in the breast, occurred more frequently in the tumour excision and tamoxifen group. Distant relapse occurred with significantly increased frequency in the mastectomy group but the overall survival of the two groups was similar.

There were 170 patients entered in 10851 of whom 84 received tamoxifen and 86 were treated by modified radical mastectomy. Median follow-up was 4 years. Results are given in Table 2 which shows a significantly increase local progression rate and overall relapse rate in the tamoxifen treated group. There was no significant difference in the distant relapse rate but there was a significantly increasd mortality in the tamoxifen only group.

Thus tamoxifen alone constitutes inadequate primary treatment for otherwise fit elderly women. Although tumour excision and tamoxifen gave similar relapse and overall survival rates to those with modified radical mastectomy it is likely that modified radical mastectomy and tamoxifen would have been better than tumour excision and tamoxifen. This has been confirmed in the Cancer Research Campaign trial which compared "optimal surgery" and tamoxifen with tamoxifen alone [7]. There were more relapses and more deaths in the tamoxifen only group.

Future prospects

One of the byproducts of the EORTC trials was increased awareness by participating surgeons of the needs of elderly women. Thus although mastectomy is very effective in achieving local control the altered body image is repugnant to many older women who therefore reject aggressive surgery. It is going to be necessary to develop alternative approaches. One possibility will be to perform a histologically confirmed complete local excision and axillary clearance and then use tamoxifen in an adjuvant role. Such an approach could be tested in a prospective trial examining whether tamoxifen is necessary under these circumstances.

An alternative is to use current breast conservation techniques, tumour excision, axillary clearance and external radiotherapy. One drawback of this is the protracted course of radiotherapy. A pilot study at Guy's Hospital examined tumour excision, axillary clearance and brachytherapy alone (iridium implant giving 55Gy) [8]. A more recent study has used intermittent caesium implants (45Gy) in 4 fractions over 4 days using a microselectron. This might provide a viable approach for older patients with the ability to deliver all surgical and radiotherapy treatment within a 5-day hospital stay.

Finally, age alone should not be used as an exclusion criterium for trials of treatment for breast cancer. It is important that older women receive adequate primary and adjuvant therapy in order that there lives are not prematurely shortened by relapse after inadequate treatment.

REFERENCES

1. Schaefer, G., Rosen, P.P., Lesser, M.L. et al. Path. Annu. (1984) 19:195-199.
2. Bradbeer, J.W., Kingdon, J. Clin. Oncol. (1983) 9:31-34.
3. Aktar, S.S., Allan, S.G., Rodger, A. et al. Eur J Surg Oncol (1991) 17:30-35.
4. Horobin, J.M., Preece, P.E., Dewar, J.A. et al. Br. J. Surg. (1991) 78:213-217.
5. Mouridsen, H.T., Andersen, A.P., Brucker, H. et al. NCI Monogr. (1986) 1:115-118.
6. Fentiman, I.S. Detection and Treatment of Early Breast Cancer (1990) Dunitz.
7. Bates, T., Riley, D.L., Houghton, J. et al. Surg. Res. Soc. (1992).
8. Fentiman, I.S., Poole, C., Tong D. et al. Eur. J. Cancer (1991) 27:447-450.

Mastology - Breast Diseases
A.S.S. Figueira Fo et al., editors.

Inflammatory carcinoma of the breast

Erazo A, Cervantes G, Torrecillas L. * Onología Médica, Centro Hospitalario 20 de Noviembre, ISSSTE México.

ABSTRACT: Inflammatory carcinoma of the breast, coming up abruptly, of rapid course and most of the time lethal. At the exploration the mammary gland is edematose, presenting redness and increase of local heat , and palpable axillary nodes. Differential di agnostic will be made with bacterial infections, dermatitis, leukemic infiltration, lymphomas, sarcomas, and rarely tuberculosis.

Histological type are the same common to the breast which might be from ductal infiltrative to medullar, but in most cases they are indefferenciated.

Even when inflammatory breast cancer is a very rare entity, it would be interesting to have the highest number of series determining hormonal receptors.

Background. Inflammatory breast cancer constitutes the most aggressive form of locally advanced breast cancer. The first description of this entity was made in 1814 by Bell (1), in 1889 Bryant (2) describes the presence of subdermal lymphatic nodes. In 1924 Lee BJ, Tennenbaum NE (3) named it as "Inflammatory breast carcinoma", while formerly was named as: Carcinomatose mastitis, acute indurated cancer, lactancy cancer, carcinomastoide, encephaloid cancer, and breast lymphocytoma. This variation is characterised for coming up abruptly, dermic infiltration, of rapid course and most of the times lethal.

Clinical features. It is characterised by a general increase of the mammary gland, and tumoral mass is not generally detected, it comes with symptoms which Haagensen (4) qualified as classical criteria for the diagnosis of inflammatory breast cancer.

HAAGENSEN	89 cases
Erithema	30%
Local heat increase	10-36%
Edema, orange skin	13.5-67%
Pain	50-75%
Axillary metastases	60%
Leucocytosis	10%

Mammary gland at touch is edematose, presenting redness, sometimes having a dotted aspect, we also find the presence of a fibrous band surrounding the affected skin, the gland may be hot, presenting orange skin and the presence of palpable axillary nodes.

Incidence. It is considered that it constitutes 1 - 4% of breast tumours, and a third part of patients are premenopausic. In countries as Tunisia a 55% of all breast tumours is reported. The average age is 52 years.

The reported incidence by the NCI from 1975-1981 (5) reflects that out of 60,479 breast cancer cases the 5.1% were diagnosed as inflammatory, performing a clinicopathological diagnostic in 153 cases, and in 2,937 the diagnostic was only clinical.

Pathology. Histological types are the same common to breast cancer, which might be from ductal infiltrative to medullar, but in most cases they are indifferenciated.

This stage is subjected to a lot of controversy with respect to the diagnostic whether it should be clinical or clinicopathological. As from 1974 Ellis & Teitebaum (6) suggested that the finding of dermic infiltration was indispensable to diagnose an inflammatory carcinoma, since its absence was associated to a good prognosis.

Years later Lucas and Perez Mesa (7), while carrying out a retrospective trial and only after an accurate analysis of 58 cases, they reach the conclusion that patients with clinical signs of inflammatory cancer were associated to an unfavourable, independently of pathological findings.

Radiological findings. The mastology may show an increase in the skin thickness, most of the times a tumoral mass may not be observed, only the presence of calcification may be seen.

Differential diagnostic. Bacterial infections, dermatitis, leukemic infiltration, lymphomas, sarcomas, and rarely tuberculosis.

In order to establish the diagnosis it is recommended to: perform an excisional biopsy, though this could be made by punction, biopsy must include skin in all its thickness, to diagnose dermic infiltration, routinely radiological studies such as chest x-rays, mastography, metastatic bone series, bone scan, ct scan, to determine disease extension, as well as laboratory assays with the purpose of evaluating medullar, renal, and hepatic function.

Hormonal receptors. Currently some clinical reports are available for information of hormonal receptors. Most of the previous series could not establish hormonal receptor status, because diagnosis was performed in aspiration biopsy samples.

La Rue and colleagues (8) reported the following data in 59 cases submitted to incicional biopsy.

La Rue and colleaugues.	59 cases
RE + RP +	28%
RE - RP +	5%
RE + RP -	19%
RE - RP -	48%

Even when inflammatory breast cancer is a very rare entity, it would be interesting to have the highest number of series determining hormonal receptors, with the purpose of generating more experience with this biological neoplasia so aggressive.

References:

1. Bell C: A system of operative surgery, vol.2, p.136. Hartford, Hale & Hosmer, 1816.
2. Bryant T: Diseases of the breast, vol. 4, pp 35-322, New York, Woods Medical and Surgical monographs, 1889.
3. Lee BJ, Tannenbawm NE: Inflammatory carcinoma of the breast: A report of twenty-eight cases from the breast clinic of the Memorial Hospital. Surg. Gynecol. Obstet 39:580-595, 1924.
4. Haagensen CD: Disease of the breast, 2nd. ed., pp 576--584, Philadelphia, WB SAunders, 1971.
5. Harres J, Hellman S, Henderson E: Breast disease, 2nd ed., p 775. JB Lippincot #5, 1991.
6. Ellis DL, Teitelbaum SL: Inflammatory carcinoma of the breast: A pathologic definition, Cancer 33: 1045-1047, 1974.
7. Lucas FV, Perez-Mesa C: Inflammatory carcinoma of the breast. Cancer 41: 1595-1605, 1978.
8. La Rue JC, May-Levin F, et al: Oestrogen and progesterone cytosolic receptors in clinically inflammatory tumours of the human breast. Br. J. Cancer 44: 911-916, 1981.

Mastology - Breast Diseases
A.S.S. Figueira Fo et al., editors.

Bilateral breast cancer

C.I. Paula*

*Oncologic Surgeon, Mastologist of the Connective Tissue Department Araujo Jorge Hospital of Goias Anticancer Association.
Director of Teaching and Research Institute.

Address for correspondence: Dr. Carlos I. Paula
Rua 239, n 52, Setor Universitário
74605-070 Goiânia/GO
Brazil

Definition: Bilateral Breast Cancer is a separate primary cancer in each breast.

The occurrence of bilateral breast cancer is reported to be between 5% and 15%. The incidence of cancer in the second breast is approximately 1% per year after treatment of the initial breast cancer, (Robbin and Berg). They estimate the risk as five times that of a patient who did not have a first breast cancer.

Bilateral Breast Cancer can be synchronous or metachronous. Synchronous bilateral breast cancer is primary cancer detected at the same time, in both breasts. Metachronous cancer is a second primary cancer detected in the opposite breast at any time after the first cancer is diagnosed. The majority are metachronous. When the interval between metachronous tumors is long, the first cancer has to have a favorable prognosis and the patient must be relatively young when it is diagnosed.

When cancer is detected in the second breast, the question is if it is a primary or metastatic tumor.

The criteria for the diagnosis of a second primary breast cancer was established by Chaudary, Millis and associates:

1. The demonstration of in situ change in the contralateral tumor is considered absolute proof that the contralateral lesion is a primary tumor.
2. The tumor in the second breast is considered to be a new primary if it is histologically different from the cancer in the first breast.
3. The carcinoma in the second breast is considered to be a new primary if its degree of histologic differentiation is distinctly greater than that of the lesion in the first breast.
4. In the absence of definitive histologic difference, a contralateral carcinoma is considered to be compatible with an independent lesion provided there is no evidence of local, regional, or distant metastases from the cancer in the ipsilateral breast.

A woman who has had breast cancer has a fivefold increase in risk for a second breast cancer.

Aditional risk factors:
1. multifocal cancer
2. lobular carcinoma in situ
3. original cancer at an early age
4. long survival
5. ductal carcinoma in situ
6. family history

The most frequent antecedent of cancer in one breast is the history of having had cancer in the opposite breast (Foote and Stewart).

The incidence of synchronons bilateral cancer is aproximately 1% a 2% and that of metachronous cancer 1% a 6%.

Mamography has increased the number of synchronous cancer.

The incidence of invasive cancer detected by random biopsy of the opposite breast is not high enough to justify routine adoption of this procedure.

The remainder breast must by followed by physical examination and annual mammography.

The treatment of the secondary primary breast cancer should be that appropriate for the stage of the disease.

The prognosis is quite favorable and is dependent on the stage of both the first and the second cancers.

Patients with breast cancer, registered at our Department between 1973 and 1993 were reviewed. The age distribution and the menstrual status is showed in the table 1 and 2. Of the 632 patients, 22 (3.5%) had bilateral cancer (table 3). Eight tumors were synchronous (36.4%) and fourteen metachronous (63,6%).

Table 1
Breast cancer: age distribution

21 – 30	21 (3.3%)
31 – 40	124 (19.6%)
41 – 50	190 (30.1%)
51 – 60	141 (22.3%)
> 60	156 (24.7%)
TOTAL	632

The paraffin blocks contained at the archive will be reviewed for histologic type and invasion and will be matter of future analisys.

Table 2
Breast Cancer: Menstrual Status

Premenopause	413 (65.3%)
Postmenopause	219 (34.7%)

Table 3
Breast Cancer

Bilateral Cancer	22 (3.5%)
Unilateral	610 (96.5%)

Table 4
Bilateral Breast Cancer

Synchronous	8 (36.4%)
Metachronons	14 (63.6%)

Table 5
Bilateral Breast Cancer: Menstrual Status

Synchronous	7 (31.8%)
Metachronous	15 (68.2%)

References

1. Chaudary MA, Millis RR, Hoskins EDL, et al. Bilateral primary breast cancer: A prospective study of disease incidence. Br J Surg 71:711-14, 1984.
2. Donovan AJ. Bilateral breast cancer: Surgical clínics of North America 70(5): 1141-49, 1990.
3. Sterns EE, Fletcher WA. Bilateral cancer of the breast: A review of clinical, citologic and immunohistologic characteristics. Surgery 617-622 october, 1991.

Mastology - Breast Diseases
A.S.S. Figueira Fo et al., editors.

Breast cancer in elderly patients: an overview

Aurelio Picciocchi, M.D., Riccardo Masetti, M.D., Daniela Terribile, M.D., Armando Antinori, M.D., Alessandro Marra, M.D., Miriam Valentini, M.D.

Department of General Surgery I, Catholic University of Rome, Largo A. Gemelli 8, 00168 Rome, Italy

Summary

Approximately 40% of all breast cancers occur in patients 70 years of age or older.

Several studies have indicated that, because of the fear of concomitant medical disease and the presumed short life expectancy, elderly women are less likely to receive optimal standard therapy for their disease. Other assumptions that have favoured the use of lesser treatments are that breast cancer in the elderly may present in a more advance stage and may be a more indolent disease. Evidence to support these assumptions remains however controversial. Treatment with curative intent, similar to that adopted in younger patients, is warranted.

Text

Breast cancer remains the most common malignancy and the leading cause of cancer death in women of all ages. Approximately 40% of breast cancer patients are 70 years of age or older (1). The risk of developing breast cancer increases with advancing age. Data from the Surveillance, Epidemiology and End Results (SEER) Program of the National Cancer Institute show that the yearly incidence rate of breast cancer is as high as 435 per 100,000 in women 80 to 84 years of age as compared to 212 per 100.000 in women aged 50 to 54 years (2). As life expectancy continues to increase, the percentage of elderly women with breast cancer will also increase.

The usual forms of therapy for carcinoma of the breast have been frequently modified in elderly patients. Several studies have confirmed that elderly cancer patients are less likely to receive standard treatment than younger patients by the supposition that the former have a limited life expectancy, are too frail to tolerate curative treatment, have more locally advanced disease at initial presentation, and have less aggressive tumors.

Evidence to support these issues remains however controversial and will be addressed separately in this review.

1) Life expectancy of elderly patients does not seem to be so limited to contraindicate curative treatments. Several epidemiological studies have estimated that

at the age of 70 a women has a life expectancy of more than 15 years; at the age of 80, she is expected to live an additional seven years (2-4). It follows that many elderly patients will live long enough to recur locally if they are undertreated. Delay of appropriate surgery will only enlarge the risks of surgical treatment once it will have become unavoidable (5).

2) The assumption that elderly patients are too frail for curative treatment has withheld many surgeons from performing standard surgical procedures. However, Turnbull et al (6), in an analysis of 4,050 operations demonstrated that the operative mortality was similar in patients older than 70 years to that of all ages (4.8% vs 3.4%). Elderly patients in good health can tolerate expeditious mastectomy with an operative risk similar to that of younger patients. Hunt et al. (7) showed that the average mortality rate in elderly patients undergoing mastectomy is less than 1%. A similar finding was reported by Amsterdam et al. (8). In our series of 182 patients aged 70 years or older treated by mastectomy, there were no operative mortalities and the rate of morbidity (8.4%) was acceptable, mainly related to short-term wound complications (9).

Surgeons' reluctance to perform standard curative procedures is also based on the assumption that in elderly patients concurrent health problems may override the life-threatening risks from breast cancer. Satariano et al (10) reported that the comorbid conditions in elderly women with breast cancer are similar to those of women in the general population. Cardiovascular disease, arthritis and hypertension were the main health problems for women of this age both with and without breast cancer.

Moreover, only a small number of the elderly patients that do present with severe concomitant diseases will not be adequate candidates for standard treatment if properly managed (2,4,10-12).

3) Controversial data have been reported also about the stage of breast cancer at initial presentation in the elderly. Yancik et al. (2) using data from the SEER program, indicated a greater likelyhood for older women to present with more advanced disease than younger women. Satariano et al. (10) compared incidence rates of localized, regional and remote breast cancer in women of the Detroit metropolitan area by age at diagnosis. They found that elderly women had an increased risk for being diagnosed with more advanced forms of breast cancer. Other studies however have failed to demonstrate any significant relationship between the age of the patient and the stage of breast cancer. Clinical staging prior to therapy did not differ among age groups in the study of Chu et al. (13) on 1680 female breast cancer patients treated in 17 community hospitals. Singletary et al (14) in a review of 184 women older than 69 years treated for breast cancer at the University of Texas M.D. Anderson Cancer Center and Mueller et al. (15), in a review of 3,558 patients, reported no stage differences between age groups.

4) Whether it is diagnosed or not in a more advanced stage, breast cancer in the elderly does not present more unfavourable prognostic factors associated with early relapse or short survival.

Several studies have indicated that the rate of estrogen and progesterone-receptor positive tumors increases directly with age: in elderly patients it ranges from 76% to 81% of cases (9-11).

Owens et al. (16), reporting data from a series of 10,009 patients, indicated that elderly women are more likely to have diploid tumors and tumors with lower proliferative rates as measured by the percentage of cells in the S-phase of the cell cycle.

Thus, elderly patients with breast cancer often present two important factors that are associated with good prognosis and this finding is consistent with the hypothesis of a less malignant, slow-growing disease. However, relatively dismal clinical outcomes have been reported in some large series (2,17-18). Possible explanations for this apparent inconsistency might include incomplete staging of the disease and/or suboptimal treatment.

Based on the controversial assumptions discussed above, many surgeons have performed less intensive treatments for breast cancer in elderly patients.
Samet et al. (19) analyzed the appropriateness of treatment in 4388 elderly women with breast cancer in the New Mexico Tumor Registry. They found that the percentage of women who received curative treatment dramatically dropped after age 75. The SEER data (2) confirm this finding, indicating that elderly women tend to receive less extensive surgery. Because of this less extensive surgery, a higher proportion of elderly patients are not properly staged as compared to other age groups (11% vs less than 6%).

Older women are likely to receive less chemotherapy than younger women for all stages of disease (20). They are also less likely to receive radiotherapy after conservative treatment of their breast cancer. Kantorowitz et al. (21) in a retrospective analysis comparing 77 elderly patients treated with segmental mastectomy alone to 50 patients who also receive postoperative radiotherapy revealed a significal reduction in loco-regional recurrences in the latter groups (34% vs 4%). They concluded that radiotherapy may be more beneficial in the elderly than among younger women.

A recent study by Veronesi et al (22) has reached different conclusions. The Authors randomised 579 patients with breast cancer less than 2.5 cm in maximum pathologic diameter to receive either quadrantectomy followed by radiotherapy or quadrantectomy without radiotherapy. All patients underwent axillary dissection. The rate of local recurrence in patients older than 55 years who did not receive postsurgical radiotherapy was 3.8%. They concluded that quadrantectomy without radiotherapy may be considered an adequate treatment in older women.

Several studies have recently reported the use of tamoxifen alone without surgery for operable breast cancer in elderly patients. Horobin et al. (23), reporting 113 elderly patients with breast cancer treated with tamoxifen alone, showed a local recurrence rate of 62%. Robertson et al. (24) randomized 135 patients over the age of 70 to receive either tamoxifen or wedge resection. They found no difference in survival, but a significantly higher number of patients in the tamoxifen group (43% vs 24%) developed a local recurrence and ultimately required mastectomy.

A comparison between various surgical treatments followed by adjuvant tamoxifen versus tamoxifen only was reported by Bates et al (25). A statistically significant higher local recurrence rate at three years was reported in the patients treated by tamoxifen only. These patients then required additional surgery.

In conclusion, many issues about breast cancer in the elderly remain controversial. There is an urgent need for prospective randomized trials to compare the efficacy of different treatment strategies in these patients. Some have been initiated and their preliminary results are anxiously awaited.

At present, critical analysis of the data from the uncontrolled studies examined above suggest that the choice of therapies should be based on physiological rather than chronological age. Treatment for elderly patients with breast cancer should be neither more nor less aggressive than treatment for younger women as elderly patients in good health not only can tolerate curative treatment but can benefit from their application (26-27).

Appropriate surgery allows the best chance for definitive cure with the lowest risk of local recurrence and should thus have a major role in the therapeutic strategy for breast cancer patients regardless of age. Limited surgery plus tamoxifen may be considered an acceptable alternative for treatment of selected patients with significant medical problems. Treatments that do not include at least excisional biopsy, such as tamoxifen alone, do not offer the same long-term chance of cure and disease-free survival. Thus, they should only be justified when high-grade comorbid conditions contraindicate appropriate surgical treatment.

References

1. Silverberg E, Lubera J. CA 1988; 38:2-19.
2. Yancik R, Ries LG, Yates JW. Cancer 1989; 63:976-81.
3. Robins ER, Lee D. Am J Surg 1985; 149:606-9.
4. Dixon JM. BMJ 1992; 304:996-7.
5. Foudraine NA, Verhoef LCG, Burghouts TM. Eur J Cancer 1992; 28A:900-3.
6. Turnbull AD, Gundy E, et al. Clin Bull 1978; 8:139-42.
7. Hunt KE, Fry DE, Bland KI. Am J Surg 1980; 140:339-42.
8. Amsterdam E, Birkenfeld S, et al. J Surg Oncol 1987; 35:180-3.
9. Masetti R, Terribile D, Picciocchi A. Proceedings EUSOMA Consensus Conference, Venice March 1994, p. 113.
10. Satariano WA. J Gerontol 1992; 47:24-31.
11. Greenfield S, Bianco DM, et al. JAMA 1987; 257:2766-70.
12. Fentiman IS, Tirelli U, et al. Lancet 1990; 335:1020-2.
13. Chu J, Diehr P, et al. J Gerontol 1987, 42: 185-90
14. Singletary SE, Shallenberger R, Guinee VF. Ann Surg 1993; 218:667-71.
15. Mueller CB, Ames F, Anderson GD. Surgery 1978; 83:123-32.
16. Owens MA, Beardslee S, et al. Proc Am Assoc Cancer Res 1990; 31:184.
17. Host H, Lund E. Cancer 1986;57: 2217-21.
18. Adami Ho, Malker B, et al. Cancer 1985; 56: 898-902.
19. Samet J, Hunt WC, et al. JAMA 1986; 255: 3385-90.
20. Taylor Sg, Gelman RS, et al. Ann Intern Med 1986; 104: 455-61
21. Kantorowitz DA, Poulter CA. Int J Radiat Oncol Biol Phys 1988; 15: 263-70
22. Veronesi U, Luini A, et al. N Engl J Med 1993; 328:1587-91.
23. Horobin JM, Preece PE, et al. Br J Surg 1991; 78:213-7.
24. Robertson JF, Ellis I, et al. Eur J Cancer 1992; 28:908-10
25. Bates T, Riley DL, et al. Br J Surg 1991; 78:591-4.
26. Clark GM. J Gerontol 1992; 47:19-23.
27. Gazetas P, Estabrook A, et al. Ann Surg 1992; 216:22-6.

Mastology - Breast Diseases
A.S.S. Figueira Fo et al., editors.

Breast cancer and pregnancy. Prognostic factors.

Gerardo Hernandez- Muñoz
Unidad de Mastologia Centro Clinico de Maternidad Leopoldo Aguerrevere
Address for reprints: P.O. Box 66962, Caracas

Abstract

An ample review of the literature is made observing that through time and experience, the prognosis and outcome of patients who are pregnant with a concomitant breast cancer is getting better. Factors that modify the response of the breast tissue are discussed as well as those that depend on diagnostic method.
Since the earliest reports, more than a century ago the prognosis for patients with breast cancer during pregnancy, has gradually improved. Kilgore and Bloodgood reported a 17% 5 year survival rate [1]. Haagensen and Stout reported no survivors [2] and White's collective series, (1953), showed only an 8,6% overall 5 year survival rate. Harrington at the Mayo Clinic is credited with starting to revive optimism on finding a 61%5 year survival rate among those women without axillary metastases [4].
However, studies in the past 30 years have demonstrated convincingly that the poor results are attributable to delay in diagnosis and reluctance to treat patients aggressively during pregnancy rather than to a detrimental effect of pregnancy or lactation itself.

Factors pregnancy dependent

- Age
- Hormone alterations
- Difficulties in diagnosis
- Physician's error
- Patient's fault
- Hostage resistance
- Age of pregnancy
- Abortion

The prognosis of younger women with breast cancer is controversial. There have been several significant reports indicating a more favorable outcome of the disease [5]. Consistent evidence that patients under the age of 35 have the worst prognosis of all age groups [6].

The highest local recurrence observed in patients under 40 years of age, (21 %) reflects the greater prevalence of certain morphologic characteristics compared with older patients: mayor lymphocytic stromal reaction (36% vs. 20%), histologic grade III (42% vs. 28%) and very extensive DCIS (2 1% vs. 6%) [7].
Nugent and O'Connel, clearly show that pregnant or lactating women. under the age of 40 who are identified early with negative axillary lymph nodes, have an expected outcome similar to that of non pregnant women. When 5 year survival rates were compared in these groups, both by stage and overall, no difference was noted [8].

It is reasonably clear that abortion for early stage breast cancer has no proven therapeutic value and is, therefore, not a necessary component of treatment. The considerations that went into decision for ''therapeutic'' abortion or not and the circumstances, such as stage of the cancer and age of pregnancy, that surround it, are not always evident, but the information that is available fails to support its efficacy, [Table 1]

TABLE 1

ABORTION FOR OPERABLE BREAST CANCER WITH PREGNANCY

	Five year survival	
Author	Abortion	Delivered
Hochman-Scheiber[9]	4/6	4/10
Helman-Bennett[10]	4/7	3/3
Peete et al[11]	2/7	3/6
Rissanen [12]	3/4	8/10
King et al [13]	9/21	22/37
Total	22/45(49%)	40/66(61%)

Factors tumor dependent:

- Size
- Axillary status
- Histological type
- Histological grade
- Clinical stage
- Inflammatory carcinoma
- Hormone receptors
- Catepsin D
- Flow Cytometry
- Oncogenic amplification

Delay in diagnosis appears to be the primary and perhaps the only reason for the generally worse prognosis overall for all patients with breast cancer during pregnancy or lactation.

As a consequence of these delays, virtually all articles on patients with breast cancer during pregnancy report a more advanced stage that in non pregnant series.

Steroid hormone receptors may be difficult to demonstrate in breast cancer during pregnancy unless special methods are used. Pregnancy may depress levels of estrogen and progesterone receptors detectable in breast cancer cytosol fractions, resulting in false negative studies because high levels of estrogen circulating in pregnant patients cause receptor translocation into the nucleus and occupy all the cytoplasmatic receptors leaving more available for assay.

Factors dependent of diagnostic method:

- Mammography
- Ultrasound
- Fine needle aspiration
- Biopsy

Pregnancy makes diagnosis of breast cancer more difficult. The enlargement of the breast during pregnancy and lactation tends to obscure parenchymal masse. The effectiveness of mammography is also compromised by the full development and function of mammary parenchyma. Breast ultrasonography should be adequate and safe. Aspiration with fine needle and its disappearance readily serves to differentiate a cyst or galactocele from a solid tumor.

Even more so than in the non gestational state, biopsy of the breast of a pregnant or lactating women calls for careful hemostasis because of increased vascularity; an incisional biopsy can be an excellent alternative.

Effect of subsequent pregnancies on breast cancer prognosis.

Even the early literature suggested that about 7% of women who are fertile after mastectomy, have one or more pregnancies and 70% of these pregnancies were to be expected within the first 5 years. From the meager amount of literature on the topic, it has been generally observed that breast cancer patients who subsequently became pregnant, survive very well, often better than patients with no subsequent pregnancy [14,15,16].

References

1. Kilgore A R , Bloodgood J C: Tumors and tumor -like lesions of the breast in association with pregnancy. Arch Surg, 1929; 18:2279-2098.
2. Haagensen C D, Stout A P: Carcinoma of the breast. Criteria of operability. Ann Surg, 1943; 118:859-870.
3. White T T :Carcinoma of the breast and pregnancy. Ann Surg, 1954; 139"9-18.
4. S W. Carcinoma of the breast. Results of surgical treatment when the carcinoma occurred in course of pregnancy or lactation and when pregnancy occurred subsequent to operation. Ann Surg. 1937;106:690=700.

5. Bennet J C et al. Diagnosis of breast cancer in young women. Aust N Z J Surg. 1991;61:284.
6. Stoll B A. Selection of young women with high risk breast cancer for adjuvant systemic therapy. Clinical Oncol. 1992;4:48.
7. Kurtz J M et al. Why are local recurrences after breast conservative therapy more frequent in younger patients? J Clinical Oncol. 1990;8:591.
8. Nugent P et al. Breast cancer and pregnancy. Arch Surg. 1985;120:1221-1224.
9. Hochman A et al. Pregnancy and cancer of the breast. Obstet Gynecol. 1953;2:268-276.
10. Helman P et al. Breast cancer and pregnancy. S Afr Med J.1963; 37:1236=1239.
11. Peete P M. Carcinoma of the breast in pregnancy. NC Med J 1966;25:514.
12. Rissanen P M. Carcinoma of the breast during pregnancy and lactation. Br J Cancer. 1968;22:663-668.
13. King R M et al. Carcinoma of the breast associated with pregnancy. Surg Gynecol Obstet 1985;160:228-232.
14. Donegan W L . Pregnancy and breast cancer. Obstet Gynecol. 1977;50:244-251.
15. Petrek J A et al. Prognosis of pregnancy associated breast cancer. Cancer. 1991; 67:869-872.
16. G. Cancer de mama y embarazo. En Avances en Mastologia (Ed) Gerardo Hernandez-Mu<\q>oz. Editorial Universitaria. Caracas, 1992 pp. 259-267.

Mastology - Breast Diseases
A.S.S. Figueira Fo et al., editors.

BREAST CANCER DURING PREGNANCY (BCDP): HISTORY AND EPIDEMIOLOGY

Dr. Francisco Sandoval Guerrero

Servicio de Tumores Mamarios
Unidad de Oncologías
Hospital General de México, S.S.

Abstract. The association of breast cancer and pregnancy or lactation is a rare event that represents a difficult management problem. A few of the historical reports that influence the concept of the disease are presented. The principal epidemiological reports that deal with frequency and risk factors are analyzed.

INTRODUCTION

Breast cancer is the most frequent malignant neoplasm in women in many geographic zones and is responsible for a high mortality. An increase in the incidence and a tendency for presentation at an earlier age has been observed. It represents the most frequent malignancy associated with pregnancy and lactation. BCDP implies emotional and ethical aspects that have a difficult management. Because it is a rare event, it is difficult to acquire a vast experience in it's management, which leads to erroneous information in many instances.

HISTORY

In 1880, Samuel Gross described that BCDP carried a bad prognosis due to the fact it presented a rapid growth. It was considered inoperable. In 1886, Halsted performed a radical mastectomy on a woman who was breast feeding her child, and 30 years later, she remained in good health. Kilgore describes a survival of 70 % at 5 years in lactating women with negative nodes and 11.5 % when nodes were positive [1].

Based on these results, this author recommended that BCDP should be treated in the same way as in the non-pregnant woman. This philosophy remained a truism until 1937 when Harrington reported the bad results obtained when pregnant women were treated with radical mastectomies: all 24 patients in the study had died shortly after the study was begun (all patients were node positive) [2].

In 1943, Haagensen and Stout [3] reported their bad experience in BCDP. Of the 20 patients that were reported, 19 were node positive. These reports brought on a negative attitude towards BCDP claiming this was an incurable disease. Haagensen went so far as to contraindicate radical surgery in this case. At a later date, when he had acquired more experience, he observed that several patients had been cured with radical surgery, which prompted him to change his view in 1949 [4].

Several series have been published since then such as Peters' in 1968 [5], as well as Holleb and Farrow's in 1964 [6], in which the bad results that are presented are demonstrated to be a consequence of a delay in diagnosis and the unwillingness to treat these patients aggressively, and not due to an intrinsic effect of the pregnancy or lactation on the neoplasm.

EPIDEMIOLOGY

Under 20 % of breast cancers develop during the woman's fertility years, which explains the rareness of BCDP: pregnancies occur most frequently from ages 20 to 33, and carcinomas between ages 40 and 55. Nevertheless, today's woman's tendency to postpone childbearing will surely favor an increase in the incidence of BCDP [7]. Table 1 shows the different percentages according to several authors.

In Table 2, it is possible to identify the incidence of this disease relative to the number of pregnancies.

Table 1. *FREQUENCY OF BCDP.*

Source	Breast Cancer (#)	Pregnancies (#)	Frequency (%)
White	45, 881	1296	2.9
Peters	7, 163	271	3.8
Da Silva Neto	6, 206	103	1.6
Rabinovich	2, 470	41	1.6
Hernández	783	20	2.5
Romero Jaime	1, 707	23	1.3

Table 2. *INCIDENCE OF BCDP.*

Source	Pregnancies (#)	BCDP (#)	Incidence
White	300, 860	93	3/10, 000
Fin	62, 562	10	1/6, 256
Torres	416, 000	91	1/5, 000
Hernández	363, 384	12	1/30, 307

Table 3. *BCDP IN WOMEN UNDER 35 YEARS.*

Source	Cases	Frequency (%)
Treves-Holleb	108 / 579	18.6
Montgomery	79 / 650	10.7
Rosemond - Maier	79 / 649	12.1
Hernández	8 / 47	17.0

In women under 35 years of age, BCDP increases significantly.

The majority of authors report a mean age of presentation of 34 years. Risk factors associated with the disease are early menarche (33 %), familial breast cancer (20 %), delayed parity (10 %), history of abortions (33 %), and short menstrual cycles.

REFERENCES

1. Kilgore AR. Tumors and tumor like lesions of breast in association with pregnancy and lactation: The treatment of tumors of the breast during pregnancy and lactation. Arch Surg 1929; 18: 2079 - 2084.

2. Nugent P, Connell TX. Breast cancer and pregnancy. Arch Surg 1985; 120: 1221 - 1224.

3. Haagensen CD, Stout AP. Carcinoma of the breast: Criteria of operability. Ann Surg 1943; 118: 859 - 864.

4. Haagensen CD. The treatment and results in cancer of the breast at the Presbyterian Hospital. Am J Roentgenol 1949; 62: 328 - 333.

5. Peters V. The effect of pregnancy in breast cancer. In Prognostic factors in the breast. Forrest APM, Kunkler PB eds. London: ES Livingstone, 1968; 65 - 80.

6. Holleb A I, Farrow J H. The relation of carcinoma of the breast and pregnancy in 283 patients. Surg Gynec Obst. 1962; 115: 65 - 71.

7. Hoover HC. Breast cancer during pregnancy and lactation. Surg Clin North Am 1990; 70: 1151 - 1163.

8. Hernández Muñoz G. *Cancer de mama y embarazo.* In *Mastología..* Hernández Muñoz G ed. Caracas: S. A. I. O., 1984; 91 - 99.

Mastology - Breast Diseases
A.S.S. Figueira Fo et al., editors.

BREAST CANCER DURING PREGNANCY (BCDP) : DIAGNOSIS AND STAGING.

Dr. Ernesto Sánchez Forgach

Unidad de Oncología
Hospital General de México, S.S.

Abstract. Diagnosis of BCDP is often delayed because of changes ocurring in breast tissue which make physical examination difficult. The value of mammography is controversial. Fine needle aspiration is a recommended technique for diagnosis. When biopsies are performed and anesthetic agents are to be used, physiologic alterations brought on by pregnancy have to be considered. The risk - benefit ratio of performing staging procedures is discussed

DIAGNOSIS

During pregnancy, breast tissue undergoes hormonally induced changes which make diagnosis of breast cancer difficult. Moreover, the physical exam of the pregnant patient concentrates almost exclusively to the pregnancy itself. In a study by Meden et al, all the patients with BCDP first noticed the tumor by self-examination [1].

The delay in diagnosis which frequently accompanies BCDP can be attributed to a physician's oversight or reluctance to perform a biopsy during pregnancy [2]. These factors contribute to determine a delay in diagnosis which is the only reason for the generally worse prognosis in these patients [3].

The value of mammography during pregnancy remains controversial. There is an increased density of the breast which tends to obscure the radiological signs of

malignancy. Nevertheless, the radiation exposure to the fetus is less than 100 millirads. While mammography during pregnancy is not the optimal study, it may reveal the presence of occult foci [4].
Other studies which have proven valuable in the detection of neoplasms include ultrasound, and more recently, Magnetic Resonance Imaging.

A mass in a pregnant woman's breast should never be regarded as a change brought on by the pregnancy itself. Although most will prove to be benign, there are certain signs which should alert the physician: a large, irregular mass, skin retraction or fixation, skin thickening, and palpable axillary nodes. If none of these features are present, the mass should be closely followed during a period of up to four weeks. If growth ensues, or if it becomes suspicious, a prompt evaluation is warranted.

A fine needle aspiration (FNA) of the mass is recommended to distinguish between cystic or solid lesions. Although the specificity of FNA is 95% [5], sensibility is rated at 66% [6] mainly due to sampling error or cytopathologic diagnostic limitations. This means that a negative aspiration not necessarily means that a malignancy is not present. Nevertheless, even if a difference in clinical presentation and in cytological findings may be present, FNA in the pregnant patient is as useful as in the non-pregnant woman for therapeutic considerations. If a positive diagnosis is obtained, staging should take place. Otherwise, an excisional or incisional (if a large mass is present) biopsy should take place. In any case, there is a similar diagnostic rate in both populations (22 % in pregnant - 19 % in non-pregnant women) [8].

ANESTHESIA

Biopsies can be performed under local or general anesthesia; when precautionary measures that take into consideration physiologic alterations are in place, the risk is not higher than in the non-pregnant population (Table 1).

The use of anesthetic agents has not been proven to be teratogenic to the fetus. In any case, an experienced anesthesiologist is required.

STAGING

Once a diagnosis of BCDP is obtained, an adequate staging is of the utmost importance to reach a correct therapeutic decision. Tumor and axillary characteristics can be assessed by performing a thorough clinical examination. Since most of the studies in the staging evaluation of a pregnant patient involve radiation exposure, careful consideration as to the risk/benefit of performing them should take place. Some authors consider that in the presence of a T2 tumor and a negative physical exam,
the patient should undergo surgical treatment. Otherwise, a metastatic workup is warranted [13].

The majority of procedures carry the risk of radiation exposure to the fetus, which can be minimized with safety measures such as lead protectors in fetal development areas. In any case, vital information which could alter the management of the patient should not be sacrificed. Hall has determined the radiation risk to the fetus relevant to the development stage (Table 2) [14].

Studies which carry no risk to the fetus include serologic examinations, hepatic ultrasound, and nuclear magnetic resonance of the central nervous system as well as of suspicious bony lesions. Other studies which should be restricted to cases in which a positive result could alter management include chest films and bone scans which are indicated when dealing with a Stage III disease, an elevated lactic dehydrogenase, or in bone pain. In any case, exposure to radiation should be minimized [15].

Table 1. *PHYSIOLOGIC ALTERATIONS DURING PREGNANCY*

1) Cardiac Alterations:	
	- Increased blood volume (35 %)
	- Increased heart rate (10 - 15 beats per minute)
	- Increased cardiac output (30 - 50 %)
	- Decrease in vascular resistance
2) Hematologic Alterations:	
	- Increased platelets (50 %)
	- Increased fibrinogen
	- Hypercoagulability (risk of thromboembolism)
3) Other Alterations:	
	- Respiratory (diaphragmatic compresion)
	- Circulatory (great vessel compression)
	- Gastric (prolonged emptying time)

Modified from Wallack M K, Wolf J A, and Bedwineck J. Gestational carcinoma of the female breast. Curr Prob Cancer. 1983: 7; 1 - 58.

Table 2. *RADIATION RISK TO THE EMBRYO AND FETUS*

Development Phase	Dose	Consequence
Preimplantation (day 0 - 10)	< 10 rad	Death
Organogenesis (day 11 - 56)	> 10 rad (>100 rad = 100 % alterations)	Congenital malformations (microcephaly)
Fetal Growth (after day 57)	Dose is proportional to gestational phase	Postnatal neoplasia

REFERENCES

1. Meden H, Marx D, Rath W, Tsikuras P, Kuhi W, Schauer A. [Breast carcinoma in pregnancy. Clinical, histological and immunohistochemical findings]. Zentralbl Chir. 1992; 117: 216 - 9.

2. Petrek JA. Pregnancy - associated breast cancer. Semin Surg Oncol. 1991; 7: 306 - 10.

3. Hoover HC. Breast cancer during pregnancy and lactation. Surg Clin North Am 1990; 70: 1151 - 1163.

4. Barnavon Y and Wallack MK. Management of the pregnant patient with carcinoma of the breast. Surg Gyn Obst 1990; 171: 347 - 352.

5. Toma S, Nicola G, and Bruzzi P. Single fine needle aspiration in the diagnostic evaluation of breast lumps. Breast 1985; 11: 25 - 29.

6. KlineTS, Josh LP and Neal HS. Fine needle aspiration in the diagnostic evaluation of the breast: diagnosis and pitfalls - a review of 3545 cases. Cancer 1979; 44: 1458 - 1464.

7. Gupta RK, Mc Hutchinson AG, Dowle CS, and Simpson JS. Fine - needle aspiration cytodiagnosis of breast masses in pregnant and lactating women and its impact on management. Diagn Cytopathol 1993; 9: 156 - 9.

8. Byrd BF, Bayer DS, Robertson JC. Treatment of breast tumors associated with pregnancy and lactation. Ann Surg 1962; 155: 940 - 943.

9. Pedereson H and Fisnter M. Anesthetic risk in pregnant surgical patient. Anesthesiology 1979; 51: 439 - 451.

10. Lloyd TS. The safety of surgical operations during pregnancy. South Med J 1965; 58: 179 - 183.

11. Wallack MK, Wolf JA, and Bedwineck, J. Gestational carcinoma of the female breast. Curr Prob Cancer 1983; 7: 1 - 58.

12. Brodsky JB, Cohem EN, Brown BW, et al. Surgery during pregnancy and fetal outcome. Am J Obstet Gynecol 1980; 128: 1165 - 1168.

13. Baker RR. Preoperative assessment of the patient with breast cancer. Surg Clin North Am. 1984; 64: 1039 - 1049.

14. Hall EJ . Effects on the embryo and the fetus. In Hall E J (ed.): Radiobiology for the Radiologist. Hagerstown, Harper & Row, 1973, p. 231.

15. Baker J, Amjad A, Groch MW, et al. Bone scanning in pregnant patients iwht breast carcinoma. Clin. Nucl. Med. 1987; 12: 519 - 524.

Mastology - Breast Diseases
A.S.S. Figueira Fo et al., editors.

Breast Cancer During Pregnancy (BCDP) National Experience and Follow-up

Dr. José Antonio Serrano Migallón

Chief Breast Surgery Department
Oncology Unit
Hospital General de México, S.S.

Abstract. A multicenter study reveals that BCDP accounts for 1.3 % of all breast cancers. Mean age at presentation is 34.8 years, and is frequently associated with an early menarche, delayed parity as well as with familial breast cancer. Most present at advanced stages (75 %). Surgery and chemotherapy are the main forms of treatment. Clinical presentation and prognosis are the same as for the non-pregnant population. Congenital malformations present infrequently.

A retrospective study of 51 patients with BCDP was performed by 3 oncology institutions in our country: *Hospital General de México, S.S., Instituto Mexicano del Seguro Social,* and the *Instituto Nacional de Cancerología.*. Frequency was 1.3% of all breast cancers.

The study included: age, risk factors for breast carcinoma, gyneco-obstetric history, gestational age, time span from diagnosis to treatment, clinical presentation, tumor size, diagnostic procedures performed, clinical stage, treatment, pregnancy outcome, as well as follow-up of the newborn. Patient status was also considered.

AGE

Age ranged from 21 to 44 years, with a mean of 34.8. The mode was 32

Table 1. *AGE AT DIAGNOSIS OF BCDP*

Age	# Patients	Frequency (%)
20 - 24	4	7.8
25 - 29	12	23.5
30 - 34	14	27.5
35 - 39	12	23.5
40 - 44	9	17.7
Total	51	100.0

Table 2. *RISK FACTORS FOR BCDP*

Factor	Patients (#)	Percentage (%)
Early menarche	11	21.5
Familial breast cancer	6	11.7
Delayed parity	7	13.7
No risk factors	27	53.1
Total	51	100.0

RISK FACTORS

Early menarche, late parity, and familial breast carcinoma constitute the most important risk factors. Nevertheless, over half of the patients did not present any risk factors

GYNECO-OBSTETRIC HISTORY

An elevated number of gestations and abortions is noted

GESTATIONAL AGE

Most cases presented during the third trimester (21 cases - 41.2 %); during the second trimester 20 cases (39.2 %) were seen. Finally, the least number of cases were diagnosed during the first trimester (8 cases - 15.7 %). Two presented during lactation.

TIME SPAN FROM DIAGNOSIS TO TREATMENT

A long period of time between detection and medical treatment initiation is usually the rule, with over a third of patients seeking attention after 3 months, and in one case, after 18 months. The mean time span from diagnosis to treatment was 5.8 months.

CLINICAL PRESENTATION

Eighty-eight percent of tumors was detected by patient self-examination. A tumor was present in 90 %, followed by axillary nodes, ulceration, skin retraction, and edema.

The right breast was involved in 58.9 %, the left breast in 37 %, and bilaterally in 2 cases. Tumor size varied from 2 to 15 cm with a mean of 7.6 cm. All patients had histopathologic confirmation of diagnosis, either by excisional, incisional, or by fine needle aspiration. A mammogram was performed in 80 % of patients.

CLINICAL STAGE

Advanced stages present most frequently: 75 % of patients presented with Stage III and Stage IV disease (Table 4).

Table 3. *GYNECO - OBSTETRIC HISTORY*

Factor	Presentation	Mean
Menarche	10 - 15 years	12.3 years
Menstrual cycle	26 - 30 days	28.4 days
Sexual activity initiation	16 - 34 years	23.0 years
Gestation	1 - 9	3.5
Parity	0 - 9	3.1
Abortion	0 - 2	3.1
Age at first delivery	17 - 35 years	24.3 years

Table 4. *CLINICAL STAGE*

Stage	Patients (#)	Percentage
I	5	5.7
II		
II A	5	9.4
II B	5	9.4
III		
III A	14	26.5
III B	11	20.7
IV	15	28.3
Overall	51	100.0

Table 5. *TREATMENT FOR BCDP*

Procedure	Patients (#)	Percentage (%)
QUART	9	16.9
QUART + CT	6	11.4
Tumorectomy + CT + RT + HT	5	9.4
Biopsy + CT + RT	2	3.8
MRM	4	7.5
MRM + CT	6	11.3
MRM + RT + CT	6	11.3
CT	15	28.4
Total	53	100.0

(QUART = quadrantectomy, axillary disection, and radiotherapy. CT = chemotherapy RT = radiotherapy. HT = hormonetherapy. MRM = modified radical mastectomy.)

TREATMENT

Pregnancy resolution was as follows: 30 deliveries, 18 cesarean sections, 2 therapeutic curettages. One patient remains pregnant at 28 weeks. There were 5 premature births, one twin delivery, 3 presented slow intrauterine growth, one newborn presented a club foot, one case of oligohidramnios was diagnosed in a patient that received one cycle of CAF chemotherapy at week 20 of gestation. Two newborn patients died within 72 hours of delivery. The rest of the offspring have evolved satisfactorily (Table 5).

EVOLUTION

Stage I: one patient presented with hepatic metastasis.

Stage II: one patient developed pulmonary metastasis

Stage III A: two patients presented hepatic metastasis which were diagnosed during Cesarean section and one died with systemic disease.

Stage III B: three patients were lost to follow-up (all were alive with disease), two died with systemic disease and one developed supraclavicular metastasis.

Stage IV: three patients died with systemic disease.

Of the remaining patients, 12 are lost to follow-up and 24 patients have no evidence of disease.

REFERENCES

1. Chacón, H M. [Breast cancer and pregnancy. Thesis.] Mexico: Clinical Investigation Department of the *Hospital General de México, S.S.*, 1993.

2. Romero R. Hernandez F, Nava M C. [Breast cancer and pregnancy]. Revista Mexicana de Mastología. 1991; 1: 7 - 17.

3. Lugo M., Ramírez M T, Rosales S, et al. [Breast cancer and pregnancy]. Revista del Instituto Nacional de Cancerología. 1990; 1: 972 - 975.

Mastology - Breast Diseases
A.S.S. Figueira Fo et al., editors.

Breast Cancer During Pregnancy (BCDP): Surgical Treatment.

Dr. Carlos Sanchez Basurto

Department of Surgery
Hospital de Mexico.

Abstract. The surgical treatment of patients with BCDP with a curative purpose is indicated in early stage disease (I and II), as in cases where pregnancy is not present. A modified radical mastectomy is the treatment of choice since radiation therapy is not necessary and should be avoided during pregnancy, specially during the first half. In case conservative surgery is preferred, radiotherapy should be postponed until after delivery. If axillary metastasis are not found, chemotherapy is not necessary. Otherwise, it should be administered in the later stages of pregnancy or after delivery. When treatment is installed in the second half, survival diminishes.

The frequency of breast cancer in young patients in our environment is higher than in other places if one takes into account that at least one out of every four cases of breast cancer occurs in women 45 years of age or younger. In a series performed in the *Hospital de Oncologia, Centro Médico Nacional, IMSS* in Mexico City, the global percentage of patients with BCDP was considerably higher than that reported by other authors (6.6 %) (Table 1) [1].

For Haagensen [2], breast neoplasms developed so rarely during pregnancy or lactation that a single surgeon could rarely get to treat more than a handful of these patients, and his observations tend to be more anecdotal than sustained in statistical evidence.

Survival in a patient with breast cancer is determined by certain conditions:

those inherent to the patient, timing of diagnosis, tumor characteristics, and the treatment performed. The association of breast cancer with pregnancy posses the greatest conflict that can occur within breast neoplasias and is surely one of the worst therapeutic ordeals. Diagnosis is generally delayed because of circumstances related to the pregnancy itself and treatment frequently represents one of the toughest decisions for the physician. Everyone agrees that in the case of BCDP or during lactation, survival is dependent on stage as well as how soon therapy is installed.

Dealing with a group of young patients, it is logical to think that the benefits of conservative surgery should reach them directly. Nevertheless, the obligatory radiotherapy complement obliges us to avoid the procedure in most instances because of the potential damage to the fetus. This is why, in cases diagnosed during the first half of the pregnancy, radiotherapy should be postponed intentionally, which surely reflects on prognosis.

Therapeutic decisions should then be taken according to the stage of pregnancy as well as that of the tumor, with the preference for treatments that do not produce fetal abnormalities or death. Surgery, mainly mastectomy and axillary dissection, is the mainstay treatment and is the standard measure for operable cases during the first half, unless characteristics in a certain case do not represent a risk for conservative surgery.

When the histopathologic specimen of a mastectomy reports a negative axillary dissection, surgery should be the only treatment. Otherwise, if positive nodes are reported, adjuvant treatment is mandatory, as is neoadjuvant therapy in locally advanced or metastatic disease.

Table 1. *Frequency Of Breast Cancer During Pregnancy*

Source	Frequency (%)	Year
Kissanen (Finland)	0.4	1963
Deuit (U.S.A.)	0.4	1963
Robinson (England)	0.7	1965
White (U.S.A.)	2.0	1956
Peters (U.S.A.)	2.5	1990
McDonald (Sweden)	3.0	1967
Benett (U.S.A.)	4.0	1963
Sánchez Basurto (Mexico)	6.6	1970

Table 2. *Pregnancy Following Beast Cancer*

Source	5 Year Survival (%)
Holleb	52
Peters	72
Brown	75
Cooper	75
Rissanen	75
Darlent	79

In the case of breast cancer during lactation, the treatment should be as if this condition were absent. Lactation will be suppressed prior to therapy.

The efficacy of radical treatment depends on the moment at which it is performed related to pregnancy or puerperium. Patients treated during the second half of pregnancy have a worse overall survival than those treated earlier [4].

Pregnancy after a controlled carcinoma of the breast does not worsen the prognosis since survival at 5 years is similar and occasionally higher to non-pregnant patients, although other factors might be involved (Table 2). Table 2

Most authors [3, 5] recommend a time lapse of 2 years before pregnancy in Stage I and II disease when the axilla was negative, and 5 years when positive nodes were present.

Prognosis is not altered by pregnancy interruption [6] Peters and Meakins [1] believe that there is no reason to terminate a subsequent pregnancy unless the patient has clinical evidence or recurrence or metastatic disease. Even in this case, many prefer to go through with the pregnancy specially since prognosis is so dismal.

Prognosis is related to stage at diagnosis. It is also related to stage of pregnancy, with a better survival when diagnosis is made during the first stages.

Prophylactic castration has no moral or medical justification in young patients and the only argument for its performance might be to prevent future pregnancies or to block the oestrogenic stimulus to the tumor [3].

REFERENCES

1. Peters MW, Meakin JW. The influence of pregnancy carcinoma of the breast. Prog Clin Cancer 1965; 1: 471-506.

2. Haagnesen CD. Diseases of the breast. Philadelphia: Saunders, 1956.

3. Barnavon Y, Wallack M K. Management of the pregnant patient with carcinoma of the breast. Surg Gynec Obst. 1990; 171: 347 - 352.

4. Hoover, HC. Breast cancer during pregnancy and lactation. Surg Clin North Am 1990; 70: 1151 - 1163.

5. Rissenan P M. Carcinoma of the breast during pregnancy and lactation. Br J Cancer 1963; 168: 22 - 26.

6. Holleb A I, Farrow J H. The relation of carcinoma of the breast and pregnancy in 283 patients. Surg Gynec Obst. 1962; 115: 65 - 71.

III. 8. Radiotherapy

Mastology - Breast Diseases
A.S.S. Figueira Fo et al., editors.

RADIOTHERAPY OF BREAST CANCER

Philip Angelakis MD, DMRT, FRCR
*Assistant Professor in Radiation Oncology. "HYGEIA" Hospital, Athens, Greece

Abstract: As alternate to mastectomy women suffering from early breast carcinoma can choose breast preserving small surgery and radiotherapy. Minor surgery involves lumpectomy or quadrantectomy and lymphadenectomy with separate incisions. Minor surgery to be safe and also aesthetically sound requires more skill and competence than simple mastectomy and should be undertaken with this in mind. The same holds for postoperative radiotherapy. Aesthetics must have high priority otherwise there is always mastectomy followed by reconstruction. Radiation oncologists must take every step to secure high quality radiotherapy. Small daily or twice daily fractions, moderate total doses, simulation and use of high energy, compensated beams at 100cm FSD are indispensable . Localised ductal carcinoma in situ can also be treated with lumpectomy and radiotherapy.

A. Minor surgery and radical radiotherapy in the treatment of early breast Carcinoma.

Conservative treatment of breast carcinoma with no mastectomy is now an established method of treatment [1–5]. Women in general are aware that carcinoma of breast is not synonymous to mastectomy and seek treatment which will not destroy their somatic integrity. In Fisher's [2] clinical trial in USA and Veronesi's in Milan approach their twentieth year since they were initiated. B. Fisher has shown that ongectomy and radiotherapy has equal result with simple mastectomy and Veronesi has shown that quadrantectomy lymphadenectomy and radiotherapy are equal to radical mastectomy in regard to survival, local control or contralateral breast new carcinoma formation . This is very important as breast preserving treatments are applied to young women.

Indications for minor surgery and radiotherapy in breast carcinoma.

Due to increasing use of low dose mastography with advanced techniques breast carcinomas are being discovered at an earlier stage than in the past.
Size of newly diagnosed breast carcinomas is getting smaller and smaller and more patients today have no metastases to axillary lymph nodes .
All stages O, I and II breast carcinoma cases are eligible for minor surgery and

radiotherapy. After fine needle aspiration positive biopsy a woman has the right to be given the time (1) to decide for her self the kind of treatment she prefers. Mastectomy may be preferred if there are two or more carcinomas in the same breast, the woman is pregnant or there are extensive microcalcifications on mastography distant from the primary tumour.

Probable contraindications are large tumours in small breasts, large pendulous breasts, tumours at the periphery of the breast because of proximity to the skin and chest wall, serious pulmonary disease, serious cardiac disease for left side breast carcinomas, collagen vascular disease or severe uncontrolled diabetes.

Local recurrence after minor surgery and radiotherapy has been connected with extensive ductal carcinoma in situ DCIS and young age. Harris et al [6] have reported 38% local recurrence rate in women younger than 35 years of age and extensive DCIS in and around the breast carcinoma. It is very important to secure clear margins during ongectomy.

Fisher [2] in his multinstitutional trial has shown the value of postoperative radiotherapy. Ongectomy was applied to women with breast carcinoma up to 4 cm´s in size. In lymph node negative cases local recurrence was 12% when radiotherapy was applied and was raised to 37% when radiotherapy was not applied. In lymph node positive cases radiotherapy reduced local recurrence to 6% while it was up to 43% when radiotherapy was not applied. The value of radiotherapy is even more obvious if one takes into consideration that cases with positive nodes were also given chemotherapy which by itself did not protect from local recurrence in 43% of the women so treated.

B. Methods of treatment

Ongectomy involves the excision of the carcinoma together with at least one cm of normal tissue around [5]. Harris et al [6] proceed to second and third excision until the specimen is clear of DCIS . The incision should be directly over the tumour if possible or if not the tumour bed should be marked with clips to allow the radiation therapist to deliver a boost if it is required. Lymphadenectomy is done with separate incision for aesthetic reasons [5].

After stitches have been removed and healing has been completed postoperative radiotherapy follows. The entire breast must be treated uniformly. After lymphadenectomy of the axilla, radiotherapy may not be needed [5]. If the nodes are positive chemotherapy is also given.

The whole breast is treated with tangential parallel and opposed beams from linear accelerators (4-6 MeV) or ^{60}Co teletherapy machines at 100 cm S.S.D or F.S.D. The beams are modified by wedge filter for more homogeneous dose. Simulator or CT scanner are needed for treatment planning. Half beam may be used when independent jaw movements are available.
Daily dose of 180 or 200 cGy are given. We also use twice daily 150 cGy treatments with six hours interfraction time for better aesthetic results.
As time passes breast tumours are getting smaller and smaller and the question has been raised as to whether postoperative radiotherapy is always needed. Veronesi et al [7] reported recently on a clinical trial comparing quadrantectomy with or without postoperative radiotherapy. He recommends radiotherapy after partial surgery for small breast carcinomas at least in women less than 55 years of age. He adds that in the case of lumpectomy if not supplemented by radiotherapy, leads to local recurrence in 50% of patients and cannot be justified without it.
Some radiotherapists give a boost dose to tumour bed, if the tumour is larger than 2 cm, margins are involved or there is no clear statement in the histology report, if the tumour is grade III or there is indication for lymphatic involvement. Boost to tumour bed can be given with a photon beam, electron beam or iridium wire implant. We use a small beam 220° arc rotation to boost radiation dose to tumour bed.

C. Cosmetic results

The aesthetic result of breast preserving treatment is very important, otherwise mastectomy is an alternative. All measures must be taken to satisfy the patients need to come out with a more intact body image and a perception of well being. There is no justification of bad cosmesis. The aesthetic result depends on the size of the breast, the size of the tumour, the position of the tumour in the breast, the surgical technique, the radiotherapeutic technique and the adjuvant chemotherapy.
Large surgical incision performed to remove the primary tumour in continuation with the incision to remove the axillary lymph nodes, large haematomas, wound infection can adversely affect the aesthetic result. In some patients with tumours at the periphery of the breast it may be difficult to obtain adequate margins because of proximity to the skin and chest wall. Subareolar tumours present a problem of obtaining adequate margins without sacrifice of the nipple areolar complex. However this sacrifice may be acceptable to some patients.

D. The integration of postoperative radiotherapy and adjuvant chemotherapy.

Adjuvant postoperative chemotherapy is recommended in early breast carcinoma cases if 1-3 lymph nodes in the axilla are positive for metastases or the primary tumour exhibiting characters of high risk for micrometastatic disease as ER negative, aneuploid , diploid with high S phase fraction, T greater than 2 cm, poor nuclear grade, poorly differentiated tumour, high levels of catepsin D, overexpression of the HER-2neu oncogene and loss of the p53 tumor suppressor gene [9]. On the other hand scepticism is expressed every so often in the medical periodical press [10] as to the effectiveness of adjuvant chemotherapy. The addition of adjuvant chemotherapy to postoperative radiotherapy in early breast carcinoma cases may aggravate the aesthetic result of breast conserving treatment specially when given concurrently [11] . If chemotherapy is to be given, it is essential that it be started as soon after surgery as possible while the systematic tumour burden is minimal. On the other hand, prompt initiation of radiotherapy may be important in reducing the tumour burden prior to chemotherapy to prevent the emergence of drug resistance. A large increase in the rate of local recurrence [2] will also negate the purpose of breast conserving treatment. At this point of time the question of sequencing adjuvant chemotherapy and postoperative radiotherapy in this situation is unresolved. Harris and Recht [12] are conducting a prospective randomised trial to test more formally the effect of sequencing of RT and chemotherapy on outcome. However until the results of this study are available clinicians must make therapeutic decisions based upon published retrospective data. Buchholz et al [13] reported that a delay in the initiation of radiation for a period of six months or greater from diagnosis resulted in a higher local failure rate. Furthermore, this was associated with an increased rate of distant metastases and a decreased overall survival rate.

E. Intraductal breast carcinoma

Recently B. Fisher et al [14] reported on a clinical trial where 818 women with ductal carcinoma in situ were randomly assigned to undergo lumpectomy or lumpectomy followed by breast irradiation (5000 cGy). Sufficient tissue was removed that the margins of the ressected specimens were histologicaly tumour free. The mean duration of follow up was 43 months. Five year event free survival was better in the irradiated women (84,4 percent vs. 73,8 percent) for the women treated by lumpectomy alone. Of 391 of the lumpectomy alone cases 32 developed non invasive and 32 invasive carcinomas (16,4 percent) in the ipsilateral breast. Of the 399 women treated with lumpectomy and breast irradiation ipsilateral carcinoma developed in 28 (7.0 percent) (Non invasive in 20 and invasive in 8). Fisher et al [14] concluded that breast irradiation after lumpectomy is more appropriate than lumpectomy alone for women with localised ductal carcinoma in situ, and considers the five year results to be firm and more appropriate for therapeutic decision making than retrospective anecdotal information.

BIBLIOGRAPHY

1. The American cancer society: Workshop on Management of Limited Breast Cancer 1990 ; Cancer, V. 65, No. 9

2. Fisher B, Redmond C, Poisson R, et al . N Engl J Med 1989; 320: 822-892

3. Veronesi U, Luini A, Del Vecchio M, Greco M, Gallmberti V, Merson M, Sacchini V, Saccozzi R, Savio T, Zucali R, Zurrida S, and Sasvadori B. The N Engl J Medic 1993;328: 1587-1591

4. Sarrazin D, Le MG, Arriagada R, et al: Radiother Oncol 1989; 14: 111-184.

5. National Institutes of Health: June 18-21, 1990. National Institute of Health Publication, USA 1990.

6. Harris RJ, Recht A, Connolly J, Cady B, Come S, Henderson C, Koufman C, Love S, Schmitt S, Osteen R: Cancer 1990; 66: 1427-1438.

7. Veronesi U. N Engl J Med 1993; 329: 1578-1579.

8. Angelakis P, Vrouvas J, Kolitsi G, Kolitsi Z, Kappas C. Radiotherapy 1992; 185(P) : 172.

9. McGuire WL, Clark GM. The N Engl J Med 1992; 326: 1756-1761.

10. Mueller CB. Am J Clin Oncol 1994; 17 (1): 86-92.

11. Abner AL, Recht A, Visini FA, Silver B, Hayes D. Come S, Harris JR: Int J Radiation Oncology Biol Phys 1991; 21: 331-338.

12. Harris RJ, Recht A. Int J Radiation Oncology Biol Phys 1993; 26: 183-184.

13. Buchholz TA, Austin-Seymour MM, MOE RE, Ellis GK, Livingstone RB, Pelton JG, Griffin TW. Int J Radiation Oncology Biol Phys 1993; 26: 23-35.

14. Fisher B, Constantino J, Redmond C, Fisher E, Margolese R, Dimitrov N, Wolmark N, Wickerham DL, Deutsch M, Ore L, Mamounas E, Poller W, Kavanah M. The N Engl J Med 1993; 328: 1581-1586.

Mastology - Breast Diseases
A.S.S. Figueira Fo et al., editors.

Radiation Therapy in Breast Cancer Patients with Negative Axilla.

Dr. Antonio Sola Valverde. Servicio de Radioterapia. Instituto Dr.Caupolican Pardo C. Santiago de Chile.

Abstract

Radiation therapy in breast cancer patients with negative axillary nodes has been subject of discussion. Due to the good prognosis of these patients and the low, but real, risk of complications, some oncologists routinarily do not indicate post operative radiotherapy unless it could be indicated. Careful patient selection and adequate techniques avoiding unnecessary irradiation of normal tissues, heart and lung can provide not only a better quality of life, with less local failures, but improved survival.

Radiotherapy in Breast Cancer.

Since 1894, when Halsted published his technique of radical mastectomy, including axillar lymph nodes removal, surgery has been the main treatment for breast tumors with radiation therapy playing an increasing role in the management of breast cancer. In the early thirties, a conservative approach was already reported (1), and in the 60s and 70s, irradiation allowed treatment of selected cancer patients without mastectomy (2,3,4,5), with good cosmesis (6) and improved quality of life (7). In last years, conservative treatment, nowadays the standard treatment for early stages, has been used even in locally advanced disease after adequate response to neoadjuvant chemotherapy.

Toxicity of Radiotherapy.

One of the major concern subjects in radiotherapy is related to its potential risk of long term damage of normal tissues, (8,9,10) with special regard to lung (11) and myocardial injury (12). High doses of radiation delivered on the heart are responsible for enhanced risk of dying due to cardiac failure ten or more years after the date of exposure. Data from european authors provide evidence on this respect. (13,14) Analysis of techniques used in those patients lead us to conclude that radiotherapy techniques were inadequate. In all series analyzed, serious handicaps are evident, mainly due to the use of kilovoltage irradiation, or attempts made to include internal mammary chain in extensive tangential fields (15), giving high total doses and doses per fraction in large heart volumes. Such techniques are no longer used. (14)

Indications for Radiotherapy:

There are five major indications for giving radiotherapy to invasive breast cancer patients with histological negative axilla:

1. Inadequate axillary specimen for diagnosis. Patients with less than 6 lymph nodes dissected have a 10% higher chance of residual disease in axilla. (16) In this condition, surgery must be considered inadequate, and irradiation is indicated over regional lymphatics. In cases of adequate axillary dissection, no advantages of radiotherapy exist, (17) but higher risk of lymphoedema of the arm (18).

2. Central and inner quadrants and multifocal invasive disease. Patients with medial or centrally located tumor are at risk of developing internal mammary chain recurrence in spite of negative axilla. Irradiation of parasternal lymphatics results in no recurrences at this level, and may improve the survival rates in this group of patients (19,20). Radiotherapy can be given through a direct open field on the 3 interspaces avoiding cardiac muscle irradiation in left-sided breast tumors, or including lymphatic chain in tangential fields.
3. Conservation Surgery. In limited surgery, radiotherapy provides good local control (21), not reached yet by any chemosurgical or hormonal protocol without irradiation. No cure of cancer can be obtained without local control, so radiation therapy must not be considered as an adjuvant in breast conservative procedures even in noninvasive cancer (22), but as an essential part of primary treatment of cancer. Furthermore, evidence is available, adequate irradiation in selected cases provides better survival curves, suggesting that local and regional control can prevent dissemination. Treatment of breast is given through opposed tangential wedged fields, 45-50 Gy/5 weeks, followed by a boost in the scar in patients with histologic findings related to high risk of local recurrence (23) or close surgical margins after tumor excision.
4. Advanced primary tumors. Bulky (T3) or locally advanced (T4) tumors are at high risk of recurrence unless radical surgery is performed. Irradiation of the chest wall may reduce incidence of local failure, improving disease free survival and quality of life.
5. Neoadjuvant chemotherapy. In patients receiving preoperative chemotherapy, both primary and axillary invasion may disappear, making staging difficult. Due to the inadequate tumor control produced by surgery and chemotherapy without irradiation, radiotherapy in tumor bed and peripheral lymphatics is indicated, unless negative axillary nodes are found at diseccion.

Another indication for axillary irradiation is the undissected clinically negative axilla. A good control can be obtained with irradiation alone (5) with low morbidity. Future methods to identify those patients who can benefit with adjuvant systemic therapy may raise non surgical management of axilla. (24)

Conclusions

Radiation Therapy must be used in negative axilla patients too, but only after a carefully selection of patients who will receive its benefits, and techniques to avoid heart and lung irradiation. In such condition, radiotherapy is safe, reliable and its use can produce improved cure rates in breast cancer. Otherwise, long term complications may enmascarate the benefits that Radiation Therapy can provide. (25)

References

1. Keynes G.: Conservative treatment of Cancer of the Breast. British Med Journal 2:643-647, 1937
2. Montague E., Gutierrez A., Barker J., duV. Tapley N., Fletcher G.: Conservation Surgery and irradiation for the treatment of favorable breast cancer. Cancer 43: 1058-1061, 1979.
3. Chu A., Cope O., Russo R., Wang C.C., Schulz M., Wang C.A., Rodkey G..: Treatment of early stage breast cancer by limited surgery and radical irradiation. Int J Radiat Oncol Biol Phys. 6: 25-30, 1980.
4. Veronesi U., Zucali R., del Vecchio M.: Conservative treatment of breast cancer with the QU.A.RT technique. World J. Surg. 9: 676-681, 1985.
5. Baeza M., Solé J., León A., Arraztoa J., Rodriguez R., Claure R., Cornejo S., Cornejo J.:

Conservative treatment of breast cancer. Int J Radiat Oncol Biol Phys. 14: 669-676, 1988.
6. Harris J., Levene M., Svensson G., Hellman S.: Analysis of cosmetic results following primary radiation therapy for stages I and II carcinoma of the breast. Int J Radiat Oncol Biol Phys. 5: 257-261, 1979.
7. Kieber G.M., de Haes J., van de Velde C.: The impact of breast-conserving treatment and mastectomy on the quality of life of early-stage breast cancer patients: a review. J Clin Oncol 9: 1059-1070, 1991.
8. Meyer J.: Thoracic effects of therapeutic irradiation for breast carcinoma. Am J Roentgenol 130: 877-885, 1978
9. Cox J., Byhardt R., Wilson F., Haas J., Komaki R., Olson L.: Complications of radiation therapy and factors in their prevention. World J. Surg. 10: 171-188, 1986.
10. Pierce S., Recht A., Lingos T., Abner A., Vicini F., Silver B., Herzog A., Harris J.: Long-term radiation complications following conservative surgery and radiation therapy in patients with early breast cancer. Int J Radiat Oncol Biol Phys. 22: 915-923, 1992.
11. Lingos T., Recht A., Vicini F., Abner A., Silver B., Harris J.: Radiation Pneumonitis in breast cancer patients treated with conservative surgery and radiation therapy. Int J Radiat Oncol Biol Phys. 21: 355-360, 1991.
12. Corn B., Trock B., Goodman R.: Irradiation-related Ischemic Heart Disease. J Clin Oncol 8: 741-750, 1990.
13. Cuzick J., Stewart H., Peto R., Baum M., Fisher B., Host H., Lythgoe J.P., Ribeiro G., Scheurlen H., Wallgren A.: Overview of randomized trials of postoperative adjuvant radiotherapy in breast cancer. Cancer Treat Rep 71: 15-29, 1987.
14. Cuzick J., Stewart H., Peto R., Fisher B., Kaaae S., Johansen H., Lythgoe J.P., Prescott R.J.: Overview of randomized trials comparing Radical Mastectomy without radiotherapy against simple mastectomy with radiotherapy in breast cancer. Cancer Treat Rep 71: 15-29, 1987.
15. Rutqvist L., Lax I., Fornander T., Johansson H.: Cardiovascular mortality in a randomized trial of adjuvant radiation therapy versus surgery alone in primary breast cancer. Int J Radiat Oncol Biol Phys 22: 887-896, 1992
16. Rose C., Findley P.A., Botnick L., Richter M., Goodman R., Silen W., Harris J., Hellman S.: The role of limited axillary dissection in the treatment of breast cancer by primary irradiation. in Harris' Conservative Management of Breast Cancer. J.B. Lippincott Company. Philadelphia, PA 1983.
17. Dewar J, Sarrazin D, Bemhamou E, Petit JY., Benhamou S., Arriagada R., Fontaine F., Castaigne D., Contesso G.: Management of the axilla in conservatively treated breast cancer: 592 patients treated at Institut Gustave-Roussy. Int J Radiat Oncol Biol Phys 1987 13: 475-481, 1987.
18. Larson D., Weinstein M., Goldberg I., Silver B., Recht A., Cady B., Silen W., Harris J.: Edema of the arm as a function of the extent of axillary surgery in patients with stage I-II carcinoma of the breast treated with primary radiotherapy. Int J Radiat Oncol Biol Phys. 12: 1575-1582, 1986.
19. Fletcher G., Montague E.: Does adecuate irradiation of the internal mammary chain and supraclavicular nodes improve survival rates? Int J Radiat Oncol Biol Phys. 4: 481-492, 1978.
20. Fisher B., Baker M. Margolese R. et al.: Five year results of a randomized clinical trial comparing mastectomy and segmental mastectomy with or without radiation in the treatment of breast cancer. N Eng J Med 321: 665-673, 1985.
21. Pierquin B., Owen, PO., Maylin, C., Otmezquine, Y., Raynal, M., Mueller, W., Hannoun, S.: Radical radiation therapy of breast cancer. Int. J. Rad. Oncol. Biol. Phys. 5: 2185-2192, 1979
22. Solin L., Recht A., Fourquet A., Kurtz J., Kuske R., McNeese M., McCormick B., Cross M., Schultz D., Bornstein B., Spitalier J.M., Vilcoq J., Fowle B., Harris J., Goodman R.: Ten-year results of breast-conserving surgery and definitive irradiation for intraducal carcinoma (Ductal carcinoma in situ) of the breast. Cancer 68: 2337-2344, 1991
23. Osteen R., Connolly J., Recht A., Silver B., Schnitt S., Harris J.: Identification of patients at high risk for local recurrence after conservative surgery and radiation therapy for stage I or II breast cancer. Arch Sur 122: 1248-1252, 1987.
24. Margolese R.G.: Axillary Surgery in Breast Cancer - There still is a Debate. Comments and Critique. Eur J Cancer 29 A:801, 1993.
25. Cuzick J., Stewart H., Rutqvist L., Houghton J., Edwards R., Redmond C., Peto R., Baum M., Fisher B., Host H., Lythgoe J.P., Ribeiro G., Scheurlen H.: Cause-specific mortality in long-term survivors of breast cancer who participated in trials of radiotherapy. J Clin Oncol 12: 447-453, 1994.

III. 9. Prognosis

Mastology - Breast Diseases
A.S.S. Figueira Fo et al., editors.

Genetic alterations in breast cancer: involvement of tumor suppressor genes and oncogenes.

Arnaldo C. Medeiros*(1,3), Maria Aparecida Nagai(2), Ricardo R. Brentani(3).
Departamento de Biologia Molecular/CCEN/LTF/UFPB(1); Departamento de Radiologia/Faculdade de Medicina/USP(2); Instituto Ludwig de Pesquisa sobre o Cancer/São Paulo-Brazil (3).
*To whom correspondence should be addressed at Ludwig Institute for Cancer Research, Rua Prof Antonio Prudente, 109 4º andar, Liberdade, São Paulo, SP, Brazil 01509-010.

Abstract

Several tumor suppressor genes and oncogenes are involved in breast carcinogenesis. These two types of genes are normally involved in the control of the cell cycle. In breast cancer we can find loss of function of several tumor suppressor genes and amplification of oncogenes. Here we describe the possible involvement of overexpression of the c-erbB-2 protooncogene and loss of heterozygosity (LOH) on chromosome 17 in breast cancer and the correlation of these genetic alterations with histopathological features and overall survival. We describe that c-erbB-2 amplification and/or overexpression associated with LOH for loci on chromosome 17 may be indicators of poor prognosis.

Today it is widely accepted that cancer is a genetic disease. This concept implies that during carcinogenesis basic genetic steps occur that change a normal cell into a malignant cell. All these changes are going to accumulate in a clonal manner to contribute to the malignant phenotype.

Breast cancer represents the most common malignancy in women of the western world. The etiology of breast cancer involves very complex factors such as genetic, hormonal and dietary which overlap with the physiological status of the host. Extensive genetic analyses of breast cancer have been done, trying to correlate these genetic alterations with the disease. Most gene alterations found to date have been identified in very advanced carcinomas and little is known about genetic changes in carcinoma *in situ*, the only well-characterized early stage of breast cancer development(1). This implies that at present it is not possible to show a multistep model for breast cancer development. Despite this, much work has been done linking knowledge of the genetic alterations with clinical outcome. The importance of this is that assesment of prognosis may affect treatment of patients with breast cancer. If we know that a patient has a poor prognosis, some form of adjuvant treatment can be provided in addition to the initial treatment at the moment of diagnosis.It is important to select those patients who will benefit from this adjuvant treatment. Besides assessing prognosis, there is another clinical problem where we can also see the importance of the relationship between clinical and basic research. We know that around 30% of treated patients with clinical stage II can relapse and frequently die. Thus it is very important to know the genetic and\or epigenetic factors that contribute for this situation. The type of genetic alteration that have been found in breast cancer include inactivation of tumor suppressor genes, point mutations, chromossomal translocations and oncogene amplification. Studies have been conducted for the analysis of DNA extracted from primary breast carcinomas and normal tissue. These materials are studied using several molecular biological techniques and the results are correlated with the clinical parameters obtained during follow-up time(2).

Inactivation of tumor suppressor genes is a very common genetic mechanism found in breast cancer. These genes normally function as a negative control of the cell cycle and for this reason, they exert the role of controlling cell division, not allowing exagerated cell multiplication. This control is very important in order not to accumulate DNA damage and to prevent transmission of these alterations to the next generations. There are several mechanisms by which these genes can be inactivated, which include deletion of the whole gene, point mutation, and small deletions or rearrangements in the gene. The inactivation can affect one or both alleles. The evidence of several tumor suppressor genes being involved in breast cancer, comes from studies of loss of heterozygosity (LOH), where DNA from normal cells is compared with DNA from tumor cells using polymorphic DNA markers. Loss of heterozygosity has been detected in several chromosomes, often involving loss of several loci in the same tumor, which contribute to the idea of several tumor suppressor genes being involved in the process. Several tumor suppressor genes have been associated with deleted chromosomal regions found in breast cancer. p53 on chromosome 17p (3); Rb on 13(4); DCC on 18(5); and more recently we have described that 29% of patients with primary breast cancer have shown loss of heterozygosity on chromosome 5q21 where tumor suppressor genes called *APC* and *MCC* are located. These allelic losses were analysed for two exons of the *APC* gene and one exon of the *MCC* gene using a LOH-PCR assay(6).

Gene amplification can be a result of an increase in the number of copies of a gene, which can lead to increased production of mRNA and protein expression. This amplification of a specific gene is generated by overreplication which confers a selective advantage for cells that contain an increased copy number of the selectable gene. So far several gene amplifications have been found in breast cancer (7); however the clinical importance of these amplifications needs clearer results. The *neu* oncogene, also known as c-erbB-2, was first identified as a transforming oncogene and has great homology with the epidermal growth factor (EGF) receptor. Liu et al.(8) have found amplification in this protooncogene in 48% of *in situ* carcinomas of the breast. We have analysed alterations of the c-erbB-2 gene in 65 primary breast tumors in order to correlate these genetic alterations with clinicopathological parameters, overall survival and recurrence data. Although no statistically significant correlation was found between c-erbB-2 genetic alterations with prognostic factors in breast cancer, patients in which tumors had shown c-erbB-2 gene amplification (32.3%) and /or overexpression (23.3%) appeared to have a shorter disease-free interval than patients without c-erbB-2 genetic alterations (9). We also have analysed by LOH studies these populations using markers for the short arm of chromosome 17. Allelic loss was 43% at D17S5 and 28% at TP53. Analysis showed significantly shorter disease-free survival in patients whose tumors had LOH for D17S5. To evaluate the possible relevance of LOH at D17S5 and c-erbB-2 amplification as prognostic factors, analysis of these two genetic events in this population showed that patients who had undergone both LOH for D17S5 and c-erbB-2 amplification had a poorer prognosis. This poor prognosis was evaluated as a shorter disease-free interval and an increased risk of recurrence(10). The finding of 29% LOH on chromosome 5q(6), 45% LOH on chromosome 17(10), 32% c-erbB-2 amplification(9) in primary breast cancer contribute to the idea that different subsets of mutations play an important role during tumorigenesis. We also can say that all these genetic alterations may be steps in tumor progression and diversification, and in the acquisition of an autonomous and aggressive behavior. These studies where the genetic events are correlated with clinicopathological parameters have been shown as very attractive specially because if we knew these specific genetic alterations at each stage of the disease we could give an adjuvant treatment besides gaining fuller understanding of the biology of this tumor.

References

1. van de Vijver MJ, Mooi WJ, Wisman P, Peterse JL, Nusse R. Oncogene 1988a,2:175-178.

2. van de Vijver MJ,, Peterse JL, Mooi WJ, Wisman P, Lomans J, Dalesio O, Nusse R. N Engl J Med 1988b,319:1239-1245.

3. Sato T, Tanigami A, Yamakawa K, Akiyama F, Kasumi F, Sakamoto G, Nakamura Y. Cancer Res 1990,50:7184-7189.

4. Lundberg C, Skoog L, Cavenee WK, Nordenskjold M. Proc Natl Acad Sci USA 1987,84:2372-2376.

5. Devilee P, van Vliet M, Kuipers-Dijkshoorn N, Hermans J, Pearson PL, Cornelisse CJ. Oncogene 1991b,6:1705-1711.

6. Medeiros AC, Nagai MA, Neto MM, Brentani RR. Loss of heterozygosity affecting the *APC* and *MCC* genetic loci in patients with primary breast carcinomas. Cancer Epidemiol Biom Prev 1994 in press

7. Kozbor D, Croce CM. Cancer Res 1984,44:438-441.

8. Liu E, Thor A, He M, Barcos M, Ljung B, Benz C. Oncogene 1992,7:1027-1032.

9. Nagai MA, Marques LA, Torloni H, Brentani MM. Oncology 1993,50:412-417.

10. Nagai MA, Pacheco MM, Brentani MM, Marques LA, Brentani RR, Ponder BAJ, Mulligan LM. Allelic loss on distal chromosome 17p is associated wth poor prognosis in a group of Brazilian breast cancer patients. Br J Cancer 1994, in press

Mastology - Breast Diseases
A.S.S. Figueira Fo et al., editors.

The role of p53 tumour suppressor gene in breast cancer

B. Vojtěšek, R. Nenutil and J. Kovařík

Masaryk Memorial Cancer Institute, Zlutý kopec 7, Brno, Czech Republic

Address for correspondence: B. Vojtěšek, Masaryk Memorial Cancer Institute, Zlutý kopec 7, 656 53 Brno, Czech Republic

Abstract

Genetic analyses of breast tumours have identified number of alterations within malignant cell genome. The most prominent abnormalities i.e. mutations and protein overexpression occur in p53 suppressor gene. The present study deals with the analysis of p53 protein level in breast cancer sections using immunohistochemistry. Although the accummulation of p53 protein was observed in 57% of patients no correlation with tumour size and nodal status could be proved. However comparisons of p53 level with tumour grade and proliferation rate showed significant relationship. Our findings indicate that detection of some p53 abnormalities might have meaningful clinical value.

Introduction

It has now been well established that malignant conversion and cancer process itself are associated with a multiple changes within genome that mainly involve genes controlling cell cycle and proliferation. One of the major roles in the maintainance of normal cellular functions has been ascribed to recently discovered regulatory genes known as antioncogenes or tumour suppressor genes [1, 2]. These share the ability of negatively regulating cell growth and they ensure the harmony of physiological cellular processess. Surprisingly various minute molecular alterations in tumour suppressor genes as well as in their protein products occur with spectacular frequency in malignancy. It seems likely that functional impairment of tumour suppressor genes and their proteins may have a conspicuous role in carcinogenesis.

The p53 tumour suppressor gene which is located on chromosome 17p, is the most striking example because its mutation or protein inactivation occur in about one half of all human cancers. In the normal cell p53 protein exerts multifunctional features including the control of cell cycle and differentiation, regulation of DNA synthesis and repair and as recently shown it also affect in negative manner the pathways leading to programmed cell death. The latest data indicate that many if not all of these p53 functions are mediated via its ability to induce transcription of several target genes containing specific p53 DNA binding sequences. Loss of the physiological function of p53 protein as a consequence of gene mutations, post-translational modification or protein neutralization by its specific binding with other cellular or viral proteins, results in the impairment of the integrity of the genome and successively in the cellular dysfunction. While normal p53 acts as a tumour suppressor gene its mutant variants exert efficient oncogenic potential. Mutations in p53 stabilize the protein and this has an important practical consequence in that mutant protein accumulates to levels capable of ready detection by immunohistochemical [3], quantitative ELISA or by immunoblotting techniques [4]. The immunohistochemical results using monoclonal and polyclonal antibodies [5, 6] are often very striking with all the tumour cells staining intensely for p53 against an essentially negative normal cells.

The clinical significance of the assessment of p53 abnormalities is now extensively studied in breast cancer, the malignancy which represents at present one of the major oncological problems, because of the increasing incidence, high mortality rate, long-lasting latency period and unsatisfactory treatment of the disease in advanced stages in particular. Several reports show, that detection of p53 changes in breast cancer tissue may represent new biomarker of tumour aggressiveness. This notion has got further support by clinical studies demonstrating a significant correlation between p53 overexpression and poor prognosis of the patient regardless of the stage of disease [7-10].

Interest in p53 biomarker has recently been augmented by the discoveries of germline mutations in the p53 gene in Li-Fraumeni syndrome [11] and germline p53 accumulation in breast cancer family, with no apparent mutations in p53 gene [12]. Both significant findings may be of value in disclosing breast cancer high risk individuals.

Methods

Seventy one breast cancer patients were included in the study. Tumours were classified according to recent ICD-0 morphologic nomenclature. The Bloom-Richardson scoring was performed to estimate the grading. Standard immunohistochemistry using monoclonal antibody DO-1 for p53 detection and monoclonal reagent PC-10 to determine proliferation activity was employed.

Three stage scoring system was used to evaluate p53 expression i.e. DO-1 negative tumours, DO-1 positivity in less than 50% of malignant cells (Fig. 1) and those exhibiting DO-1 positivity in more than 50% of tumour cells.

Results and Discussion

As a part of long-standing project we present the data showing that slightly over 57% of breast cancer patients manifest accumulation of p53 protein. No relation between DO-1 positivity and tumour size or nodal status could have been noted. As shown on Table 1. the p53 overexpression correlates significantly ($p<0.001$ –

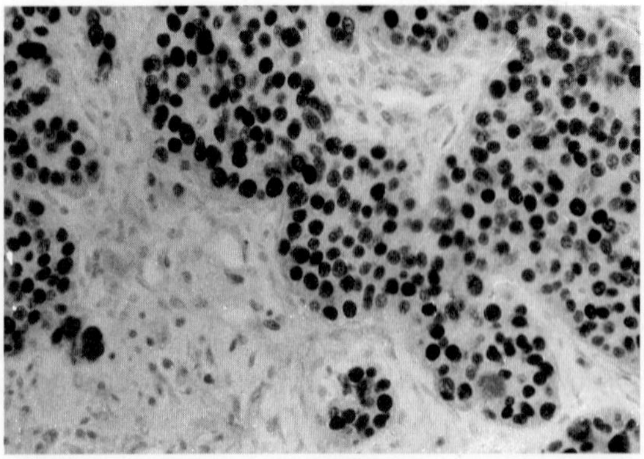

Figure 1. Immunohistochemical staining with anti-p53 monoclonal antibody DO-1 inductal mammary carcinoma grade III using peroxidase conjugated streptavidin biotin technique. Note strong positive staining for p53 protein in majority of tumour cell nuclei (magnification × 250).

Pearson chi-square test) with tumour grade. Over 85% of high grade breast carcinomas contain detectable level of p53 protein. Similar positive correlation was observed between p53 overexpression and rate of proliferation (data not presented). To explain why p53 increased level is lacking to control abnormal proliferation in tumours with high aggressive features two hypothetic mechanisms might be considered. The p53 protein may either be functionally defective per se or the function of wild-type p53 protein overexpressed in some malignant cells is powerless by yet poorly understood defects in the enzyme systems such as cyclin-dependent kinases or some other gene products e.g. WAF 1 [13] which are

Table 1
Relationship between p53 protein expression and tumour grade in 71 breast cancer patients

	Tumour grade			
	I	II	III	Total
p53 negative	16	10	4	30
P53 positive in less than 50% cells	5	13	12	30
P53 positive in more than 50% cells	0	0	11	11
Total	21	23	27	71

known to mediate tumour suppressive effects of p53 protein. From the practical point of view further studies are needed to verify whether p53 overexpression in breast cancer patients could represent an independent and reliable prognostic marker.

Acknowledgments

The authors wish to acknowledge financial support from the Internal Agency of Czech Ministry of Health, grants nos. 1459-3, 1460-3 and 1461-3 and from Grant Agency of Czech Republic 312/93/2329.

References

1. Lane DP, Benchimol S. Genes Dev 1990;4:1-8.
2. Levine AJ, Momand J, Finlay CA. Nature 1991;351:453-456.
3. Cattoretti G, Rilke F, Andreola S, D'Amato L, Delia D. Int J Cancer 1988;41:178-183.
4. Vojtěšek B, Fisher CJ, Barnes DM, Lane DP. Br J Cancer 1993;67:1254-1258.
5. Midgley CA, Fisher CJ, Bártek J, Vojtěšek B, Lane DP, Barnes DM. J Cell Science 1992;101:183-189.
6. Vojtěšek B, Bártek J, Midgley CA, Lane DP. J Immunol Methods 1992;151:237-244.
7. Thor AD, Moore DH, Edgerton SM, Kawasaki ES, Reihsaus E, Lynch HT, Marcus JN, Schwartz L, Chen LC, Mayall BH, Smith HS. J Natl Cancer Inst 1992;84:845-855.
8. Allred DC, Clark GM, Elledge R, Fuqua SA. J Natl Cancer Inst 1993;85:200-206.
9. Thorlacius S, Borreson AL, Eyfjord JE. Cancer Res 1993;53:1637-1641.
10. Iwaya K, Tsuda H, Hiraide H, Tamaki K, Tamakuma S, Fukutomi T, Mukai K, Hirohashi S. Jpn J Cancer Res 1991;82:835-840.
11. Malkin D, Li FP, Strong LC, Fraumeni Jr. JF, Nelson CE, Kim DH, Kassel J, Gryka MA, Bischoff FZ, Tainsky MA, Friend SH. Science 1990;250:1233-1238.
12. Barnes DM, Hanby AM, Gillett CE, Mohammed S, Hodgson S, Bobrov LG, Leigh IM, Purkis T, MacGeoch C, Spurr NK, Bártek J, Vojtěšek B, Picksley SM, Lane DP. Lancet 1992;340:259-263.
13. El-Deiry WS, Tokino T, Velculescu VE, Levy DB, Parsons R, Trent JM, Lin D, Mercer WE, Kinzler KW, Vogelstein B. Cell 1993;75:817-825.

Mastology - Breast Diseases
A.S.S. Figueira Fo et al., editors.

Prognostic value of and antibody response to c-erbB-2 oncoprotein in breast carcinoma patients

Maria I. Colnaghi

Division of Experimental Oncology E, Istituto Nazionale Tumori, 20133 Milan, Italy

Correspondence to: Dr. Maria I. Colnaghi, Division of Experimental Oncology E, Istituto Nazionale Tumori, Via Venezian 1, 20133 Milan, Italy, tel. +39 2 2390565, fax +39 2 2362692

Abstract

A retrospective study was conducted on 1200 histological samples from consecutive breast cancer patients. The indication of a better prognosis for N- patients with tumors overexpressing the c-erbB-2 oncoprotein and showing a lympho-plasma cell infiltration (LPI), suggested a specific action of the immune system of patients in controlling the tumor growth. Indirect immunofluorescence analysis of sera from breast carcinoma patients, whose tumors were characterized for overexpression of the c-erbB-2 oncoprotein and for lympho-plasma cell infiltration, revealed no circulating antibodies specifically directed against the p185 molecule in the 20 samples tested, whereas supernatants of B-cell clones, derived from Epstein-Barr virus-transformed peripheral blood lymphocytes from 10 of these patients contained such antibodies in 6 of the 7 c-erbB-2 and LPI-positive cases.

Monoclonal antibodies employed in histochemistry, in retrospective studies, allowed the identification of markers associated with tumor progression in breast cancer. The c-erbB-2 oncogene, which belongs to the tyrosine kinase oncogene family and codes for a 185 KD glycoprotein, has been suggested to be involved in the pathogenesis of several human tumors [1-4]. In particular, c-erbB-2 gene amplification and overexpression of the gene product have been reported to be associated with poor prognosis of breast carcinoma patients [5].
A retrospective study was conducted on approximately 1200 histological samples from consecutive patients, treated surgically from 1969 to 1971 for breast cancer at the National Cancer Institute of Milan, without any systemic adjuvant therapy and with a 20-year follow-up. The study demonstrated the predictive potential of the c-erbB-2 oncoprotein overexpression in the primary tumor, even in a subgroup of node-negative patients [6], i.e. the population for which the availability of a reliable prognostic factor would be highly useful for better planning of adjuvant therapy. Oncoprotein overexpression was found to be directly related to size, grading and the number of involved lymph nodes, parameters which are associated with a poor prognosis. Surprisingly, c-erbB-2 oncoprotein was found to be more frequently overexpressed in tumors with high lympho-plasma cell infiltration (LPI), which has been reported to be associated with a favourable prognosis as also confirmed by this study [6]. These apparently discordant results, i.e. the association of oncoprotein overexpression with factors related to both unfavourable and favourable prognosis, may be related to the interference of the immunologic status with the predictive potential of the oncogene overexpression. In order to verify this possibility, the association of p185 overexpression with survival was evaluated in relation to the presence of LPI and nodal status. In the lymph node-positive group, patients with c-erbB-2-positive tumors were those with the poorest prognosis, independent of the LPI status. In the negative node group, in

absence of LPI, oncoprotein overexpression had a predictive potential analogous to that found in patients with positive nodes (Figure 1A). On the contrary, in node-negative patients whose tumors showed LPI, the overexpression of the oncogene product was associated with a better prognosis compared to patients with negative tumors (Figure 1B). The indication of a better prognosis for the N^-, LPI-positive and oncoprotein-positive group suggested a specific action of the stimulated immune system of patients in controlling the tumor growth to some extent. Indirect immunofluorescence analysis of sera from breast carcinoma patients, whose tumors were characterized for overexpression of the c-erbB-2 oncoprotein and for LPI, revealed no circulating antibodies specifically directed against the p185 molecule in the 20 samples tested, whereas supernatants of B-cell clones, derived from Epstein-Barr virus-transformed peripheral blood lymphocytes from 10 of these patients contained such antibodies in 6 of the 7 c-erbB-2 and LPI-positive cases. The antibodies contained in two of the positive supernatants immunoprecipitated a 185-kD molecule from oncoprotein-positive cell extracts that was identified as the oncoprotein in sequential immunoprecipitation experiments with anti-p185 oncoprotein monoclonal antibodies. No cells producing antibodies with a similar reactivity were obtained from Epstein-Barr virus-transformed peripheral blood lymphocytes from breast carcinoma patients with c-erbB-2-negative tumors or from healthy donors [7]. These data prove the existence of an antibody response specifically directed against the p185 oncoprotein in breast carcinoma patients that may represent an important effector mechanism in the control of c-erbB-2 overexpressing tumors. The possibility to exploit the oncogene product, not only as a target for passive immunotherapy, but also as a vaccine to further stimulate the patient's immune response against the oncoprotein-positive tumor, opens new areas of investigation regarding epitopes involved in the immune response and the components of the immune system which can be stimulated.

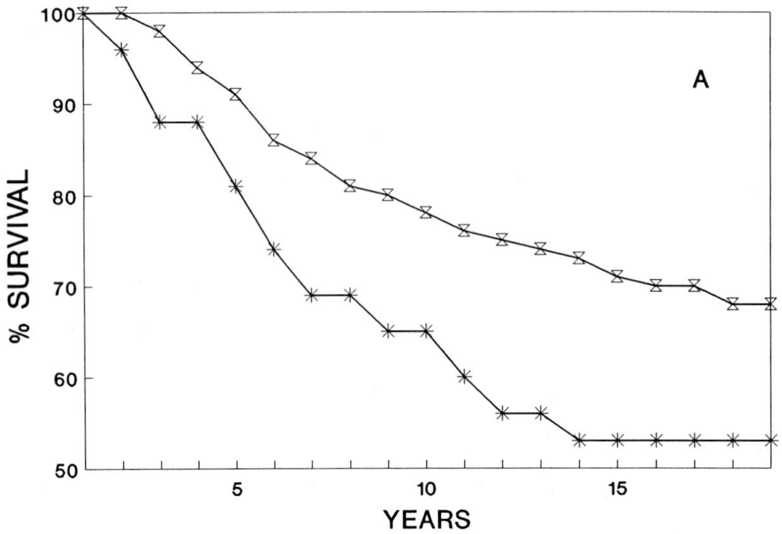

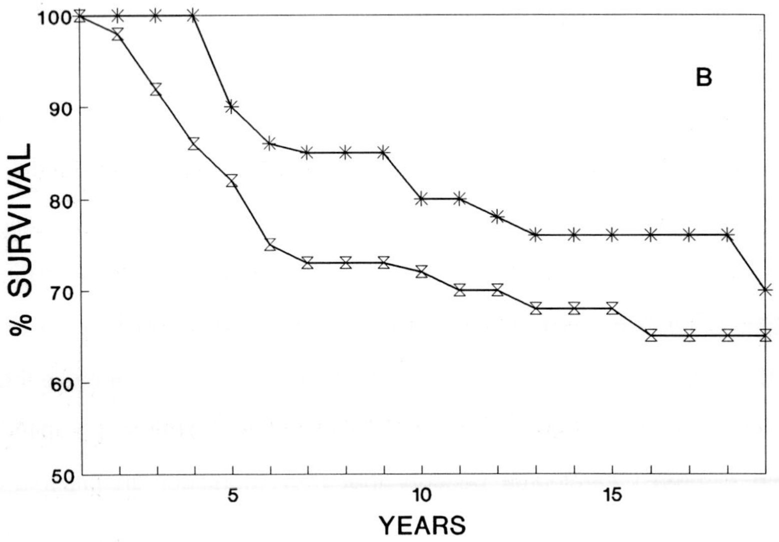

Figure 1A: Overall survival of 373 patients N-LPI- (—✱— Neu+), (—⧖— Neu-).

Figure 1B: Overall survival of 145 patients N-LPI+ (—✱— Neu+), (—⧖— Neu-).

Acknowledgements

This work was partially supported by Associazione Italiana per la Ricerca sul Cancro and by CNR-ACRO

References

1. Berchunck A, Kamel A, Whitaker R, Kerns B, Olt G, Kinney R, Soper JT, Dodge R, Clarke-Pearson DL, Marks P, McKenzie S, Yin S, Bast RC,Jr. Cancer Res 1990;50:4087-4091.

2. Natali PG, Nicotra MR, Bigotti A, Venturo I, Slamon DJ, Fendley BM, Ullrich A. Int J Cancer 1990;45:457-461.

3. Slamon DJ, Godolphin W, Jones LA, Holt JA, Wong SC, Keith DE, Levin WJ, Stuart SG, Udove J, Ullrich A, Press MF. Science 1989;244:707-712.

4. Weiner DB, Nordberg J, Robinson R, Nowell PC, Gazdar A, Greene MI, Williams WV, Cohen JA, Kern JA. Cancer Res 1990;50:421-425.

5. Gullick WJ, Love SB, Wright C, Barnes DM, Gusterson B, Harris AL, Altman DG. Br J Cancer 1991;63:434-438.

6. Rilke F, Colnaghi MI, Cascinelli N, Andreola S, Baldini MT, Bufalino R, Della Porta G, Ménard S, Pierotti MA, Testori A. Int J Cancer 1991;49:44-49.

7. Pupa SM, Ménard S, Andreola S, Colnaghi MI. Cancer Res 1993;53:5864-5866.

Mastology - Breast Diseases
A.S.S. Figueira Fo et al., editors.

THERMOGRAPHY AS PROGNOSTIC PREDICTOR

Dr. Emir Alvarez Gardiol

It is about the condition, the most important this practice registers.
Our thermographic evaluation, surged from the material about contact thermography published by Jacques Tricoire (1) which we learnt to value at the Campinas´ School directed by Professor J.A.Pinotti, and then complimented with the doctrines in infrared thermography sustained by Professors Amalric and Spitalier, from Marseille (France) (2), allowed us to develop in Argentina, since 1978 up to now, a personal and solid experience.

We adopted the classification emerged from the publications of Armando Tejerina (Spain) (3), who describe them as **reactive** and **non reactive thermograms.** When we notice a poor vascularization, regular and relatively symmetric design, low differential gradients of temperature or there is a global hypothermia in both breasts, then we find ourselves in the presence of a non reactive thermogram.

Instead, if we observe a thick and tortuous vascular design, or if it draws a real vascular anarchy, with thermical gradients of more than 3°C, or it establishes a regional hyperthermia, we believe find ourselves in the presence of an hyperreactive thermogram.

Now, if with these conditions, we also have diagnosed a clinical-radiological carcinoma in that breast histologically confirmed, the thermogram, then, has other significance which, in our experience, usually characterise that presentation, resumed in 8 points being the following:

Non reactive thermogram

* Good prognosis. Low cellular kinetics
* Low aggression
* Slow time of tumour duplication
* Great possibility of negative axilla
* Absence of Metastasis
* Increase disease free period
* Prolonged survival
* Optimum for primary conservative surgery

Hyperreactive thermogram

* Bad prognosis. High cellular kinetics
* Great aggression
* Accelerated time of tumour duplication
* Great possibility of positive axilla
* Great possibility of Metastasis
* Short disease free period
* Reduced survival
* Primary surgery is not suggested, placing in front, the systemic therapy

OUR EXPERIENCE

Our work group CEMA (Rosario-Argentina), realized a 10 years follow-up over 496 breast carcinomas, treated between 1978/88, doing a wide excision with axillary dissection of group I and II nodes follow by radiotherapy. If the nodes are positive we used chemotherapy before radiation.
Average age 51 years old.
Averaghe of the follow up, 44 months.

Classification pTNM:

21 in situ	
247 T1 N (-)	75 T1 N (+)
80 T2 N (-)	66 T2 N (+)
1 T3 N (-)	6 T3 N (+)

Resulting 30% with nodes positive and 70% with nodes negative.

We excluded cases with cold tumour (no thermic reaction).

The rest was classified in 2 groups:

203 cases with thermograms of gradients lower than 2.5°C (Low reactives).
241 cases with thermic gradients over 3°C (Hyperreactives).

It was analysed the disease free survival (no recurrences) (DFS), the distant disease free survival (DDFS) and the overall survival (S), resulting statistically significant the three situations.
(presenting three slides).
Differences were more ostensible in node negative patients, after 6 years follow up.
(slide).

CASES

1. J.110, a 48 years old woman with a tumour of 2.5 cm palpable, in upper external situation, the thermogram shows a hot spot over 5°C, of high reactivity.
Not taking into account the thermic gradient, it woul be surgycal.
Procedure: Confirmatory puncture biopsy, chemotherapy, radiotherapy.
Axilla: positive.

2. F. 107, a 47 years old woman, with a tumour of 1.8 cm , of low thermic reactivity (< 2° C). Procedure: Surgery plus Radiotherapy
Axilla: negative.

3. C.709: a 37 years old woman, with palpable tumour, right external situation, 4 cm diameter, high thermic reactivity (>7° C). Fine needle aspiration citology +.
Chemotherapy.
Size reduction at 6 months (no more palpable).
The thermic activity totally disappears.
Surgery plus radiotherapy is suggested.

4. I-850: a fast growing tumour. Duplication in 3 months.
Hypervascularization with high Gradient. Positive Axilla at physical examination.
Procedure: Chemotherapy before Surgery.

5. H. 230: Middle and upper-right tumour, in a 39 years old patient, size of the tumour 2.5 cm, palpable.
Thermic gradient > 5° C.
After a positive FNA citology: Chemotherapy to reduce size. It becomes not palpable, with a concordant thermic reactivity.

COLOUR DOPPLER AND THERMOGRAPHY

The ultrasound technique of Colour Doppler, evidences the anatomic vascularization.
Thermography allows to visualise the local hyperthermia wheter it is blood transported through the blood vessels, as well as the tissue hyperthermia.
Very different principles uphold both methodologies, but they connect their images in a common perception, so it can result anatomical for the Doppler and physiological for the thermography.

Using the "capture of colour" technique, we surch with the transducer over the tumoural formation, at a preset interval (ex: 4- 8 seconds); the final image is freezed and will represent the summation of the space proyection from the high readings of the vessels in the examinated volume.
This gives a good idea of vascularization and even of vascular morphology.
The example we present shows the capture of colour of a carcinoma at the end of 1 second.
The next, at the end of 2 seconds. The last, at the end of 8 seconds.

Then, we show the coloured image of an infiltrant ductal carcinoma, where there are multiple vessels, tortuous and irregulars, following a radial course (see arrows), irrigating the lesion. The thermogram belongs to case I- 850.

Next case shows a 3.5 cm nodule, oval, which we can define suspected as a fiboradenoma, or a phyllodes , or even a medullar carcinoma. The Doppler shows vascular anastomosis, multiple and irregular shunts (arrows).
Histology: Medullar carcinoma.
This images corresponding to the hyperreactive thermograms we described in case H-230.

Cases like the ones we exhibited, show how the Hypervascularization and the Hyperthermia can be put in evidence in a fast and economical way by Tele-thermography. The parameters are coincident with colour Doppler revelations !.

Next we present information which is coincident with ours, from the Mediterranen Academy of Clinical Oncology, founded by Dr Spitalier and Dr Amalric.

Relating to critical analysis of Thermography they say in 1994:

1. It has no value to be used in breast cancer screening.

2. Its diagnostic value is limited, due to the considerable rate in false diagnostic information, wheter they are positive or negative.

3. Great predictive value in benign breast diseases, specially if they are proliferative.

4. Great prognostic value, even in T0 N0, not palpable tumours.

5. Objective identification of fast growing cancers, that need neo-adyuvancy.

6. Useful in monitoring breast conserving surgery, specially recurrence detection in function of initial thermography.

(we put some slides with affirmative statistics from the School of Marseille).

We conclude our presentation with a CRITICAL ANALYSIS of BREAST THERMOGRAPHY which we accept in our GROUP CEMA (Rosario- Argentina).

BREAST THERMOGRAPHY : CRITICAL ANALYSIS

* It should not be use as Diagnostic Methodology.
* As an isolated methodology, should not be use for therapeutical indications.
* Useless in screening programmes.
* Very useful to evaluate aggressivity in breast cancer.
* Specially indicated in T1 and T2 , apparently surgicals, which could require neo adyuvancy.
* Capable of showing the presence of deep focus of Hyperthermia in breat tissue. (even subtelty).
* Fast and easy evidence of hypervascularization in breast areas.
* It has correspondence with an anatomic method: Colour Doppler in breast cancer. Slow and expensive methodology to designs a pattern of breast vascularization.
* It has been overcome as a **prognostic factor** and **risk indicator** by histologycal parameters, progress of inmuno-hystochemical, monoclonal antibodies, hormonal receptors, and the advances in cellular kinetics and molecular biology.

BIBLIOGRAFÍA

1. Tricoire J. La thermographie en plaques. Technique nouvelle d'utilization des cristaux liquides. Presse Med., 1970, 78, 2481-2482.
2. Amalric R., Spitalier J.M., et al. : Dynamic telethermography of 2200 breast cancers. Acta Thermographica, 1978, 3, (1-2)46-52.
3. Armando Tejerina y col.: termografía mamaria: valor predictivo y pronóstico en cáncer de mama. Focus, ISSN-0327-3342. año 3,N° 3, 1992 (16-23).

III. 10. Follow-up

Mastology - Breast Diseases
A.S.S. Figueira Fo et al., editors.

FOLLOW UP IN BREAST-CONSERVING SURGERY

Emir Alvarez Gardiol

The follow up must be organized having in mind the clinical staging at the presentation, the biological behaviour of the disease, the established or to be established therapeutics, and the knowledge we could have about tumor-host relationship.
We use the words **follow up** and **monitorization** , meaning the set up of a vigilance to observe any change it could result useful to control the disease. We are custodying the one who already has the disease, and the mission to prevent it is refered to the possibility of a recurrence or a metastasis..
Target: To guarantee a larger and better survival.
Check up, rhythm and frecuency: being the first two years the most dangerous period to relapse, it will be established a check up for the patient, first monthly, then after two months, after three months and finally after 6 months, a considerable period of time in the follow up of patients bearing carcinomas in early stages.
The follow up must be personalized, relying on the patient and doctor idiosyncrasy, avoiding exagerated dependence but ,without encouraging the prolonged absence to the check up because it could find clinical clinical ostensible recurrences or unexpected systemic colapses. Each appointment serves to actualized the doctor in consideration of the psycho-phyysical events of the check up period.

Importance of each methodology in a conservative treatment:

Physical examination: the anamnesis during a complete physical examination may suggest a systemic metastatic disease. The palpation findings puts aside almost any recurrence.

Mammography: Essential, since it counts with **High Ressolution** and twice important if it has a pre-operatory radiological pattern which constitutes a valuable historycal document. Mammography gives an identification to which we must add the surgical scars (on the skin and in deep tissues), retractions from radiotherapy and the transparences of involution through the time, so that, after a few years, we could have a well defined structural map, capable to predict an eventual recurrence in posterior check ups.

Ultrasound: with high resolution transducers (7.5 and 10 MHz) we can do a creative job with ultrasound. Together with physical examination and mammography completes a remarkable and structural semeiology. The operated and irradiated breast configures a new experience to the clinic, who must interpret the glandular tissue when the oedema is disapearing, the excess of fibrosis is starting and the characteristics of what it will be the definitive sequel of the therapeutic action, is finally settled.
A new semeiology expects us, after 10 years have gone through, realizing a conservative treatment.

Citology with fine needle aspiration (FNA): It is **a challenge for the mastologist** to obtain good and enough material, and also **a challenge for the pathologist** and his experience to interpret it.
Capable to indicate an immediate biopsy or to differ the suspition of local recurrence.
Not to forget that skin recurrences after surgery can simulate benign fibrosis, for a long time, and suddenly they start malignant growing and multiplication. The FNA is not always capable to obtain the proper material for the observation, and offers false negative reports. An excellent method in these days.

Thermography: The pre-therapeutic thermogram serve as a base, when it has been done, to keep a basic panorama of the vascular design, its debit, and also the thermic gradients coming from the tumoral zone.
It should be have in mind the thermographical silence facing small malignant tumours, to which this Round Table refers, the sub-clinics and not palpable ones. In this cases thermography is useless.
In the other hand, it is very useful to evaluate the cutaneous actinic tide consecutive to radiotherapy, allowing to follow its involution until the relatively coolness and subsequently, to observe any area of re-warming, a preanounce of an eventual recurrence.
Chemotherapy follow up: The breast cancer with hiperthermia and positive biopsy demands neo-adyuvancy treatment. The follow up with physical examination, mammography and thermography let us know the extent of the efficacy of the treatment or the persistence of an abnormal hiperthermia, corresponding to poor results.

Metastatic disease

Suspectable in the interview and the physical examination, requests for laboratory and complementary studies.

Thorax: The X-Rays examination could be completed with lineal or computed tomographies, overcoming 20-30% the conventional X-Ray.

Liver: For diagnostic, as well as for therapeutical follow up, the ultra-sound is very useful. In the 10-20% of the difficult to interpretate cases, compliment with CT or MR.

Bones: Bone scintigraphy with technetium 99, very sensible facing initial lesions, anticipatory to radiologycal recognition. Efficiently marks places with multiple metastasis. It is necessary to complete the information of scintigraphy to precise the diagnostic. Guide for diagnostical punctions with CT or MR.

The Laboratory: Alteration in levels of Calcium, leucopenia and plaquetopenia can be orientated to the compromise of the osseous medulla. Alcaline phosphatasa orientate toward the osseous and hepatic systems. It can be completed with the rest of hepatic enzymology.

The tumoural markers are being studied a lot more: the CEA serves to monitorize the clinic evolution.
The CA 15-3 is highly sensible to early detection of recurrence and monitoring of response to treatment.
Others in study: MCA, CA 549, CA M-26, BCA 255.

It has to be remenbered that the management of all these diagnostic methods, proportions an **uncertain clinical benefit** !

References:

1. Alvarez Gardiol, Emir: Mammography, in Focus , ISSN- 0327-3342, pag 36, 1990.

2. Alvarez Gardiol, Emir: et al. Follow up. Monitorizing the patient. : in "Cancer de mama", Editorial El Ateneo, Buenos Aires, 1987, pags323/330.

3. Alvarez Gardiol, Emir: et al. Breast cancer follow up after treatment: in "Dynamic Mastology", Editorial Diaz de Santos, Madrid, chapter 55, 1994, in press.

Mastology - Breast Diseases
A.S.S. Figueira Fo et al., editors.

METHODOLOGY AND PROBLEMS OF THE FOLLOW UP IN CONSERVATIVE TREATMENT .

M.Izquierdo, A.Fernandez-Cid,L.Torre,L.Lopez Marin,R.Fabregas, J.Piera, J.Torralba, B.Navaro,F.Salas,J.Feu,J.Browne,B.Guix,P.Grasses,M.Ribas Mundó, X.Fabregat,A.Modollell,C.Madroñal,C.Baldrich, D.Ribas and J.Penella.

Abstract. The control of an operated and irradiated breast present a great difficulty,as it is necessary to follow a strict protocol which in our Institute is a follows: clinical exploration,mammography,echography and citologycal puncture. The mammography and the clinical exploration have a low sensibility and a low positive predictive value. Echography and citological aspiration improve the results. We think that echography and citology should be incorporated in the follow up protocols of breast cancer conservative treatment.

Introduction

The follow-up of the treated patients with a conservative treatment has a major difficulty, given that you have to control a breast that has been operated and subsequently received radiotherapy.

This means that any recurrence of the breast cancer will be difficult to recognize. If a recurrence is suspected the only method to confirm this diagnosis is to do a biopsy however usually only between 30 an 66% will have a true local recurrence.[1 2 3 4]

Classic diagnosis of local regional recurrence

If we study the efficiency of the different diagnostic methods, we can observe that the clinical exploration yields poor results. Different authors, Solin et al.[2] indicate a diagnosis of only 28% whilst Stomper et al.[3] show a higher rate of 39%.

The rates are low because the surgery and the radiotherapy combined produce a dense fibrosis.

Mammograms are usual method in the locorregional follow-up of these patients and these have proved to be a better method than clinical exploration, although the sensibility diagnosis continues to be low, Solin et al.[2] show a sensibility of 68% and Greenstein et al.[4] 60%.

Where the mammograms have a real difficulty is when the recurrence is situated in the original quadrant.

When the recurrence occurs in other quadrants, the sensibility ratio increases dramatically as much as 80% according to Solin et al[5], whilst Greenstein et al[4] records an increase to 86%.

Furthermore, to date the mammogram provides the best method for the control of the controlateral breast.[6,7,8]

One of the most important mammografic signs which tend to be very difficult to interpret are the microcalcifications in the tumoral bed.

The experience of experts in this field indicates diverse results. Berenberg et al[9] place great importance on microcalcifications an in all the cases they observed with this problem they noted a recurrence.

Other authors such as Dershaw et al.[10] observed that their cases were benign.

It must be noted however that both sets of authors based their results on a very small number of patients.

Identical studies were conducted by Stomper et al.[11] and Solin et al.₂ using a greater number of patientes indicated a ratio of 67% an 58% respectively of recurrences.

Any indication of microcalcification obliges a biopsy.

Approximately 30% of the recurrences present microcalcification and increase radiologic density, in these cases we can establish a secure diagnosis of local recurrence.

New diagnosis of the local recurrence experience of the Institut Universitari Dexeus.

In the Obstetric an Gynaecological Department of Institut Universitari Dexeus we have studied 409 cases of breast cancer treated with a conservative treatment.

The global survival at 9 years is 77,4% free disease survival is 71,4% and locorregional control is 90,7%.

In our follow-up programme we conducted a clinical exploration every 3 months during the first year, and every 6 monoths during the second year and annually thereafter. Mammogram, echography and citological punctures under ecographic control were also conducted annually.

When we studied the diagnostic efficiency we saw the clinical exploration has a sensibility (S) of 37,5% a specification (SP) of 99,7% a positive predictive value (PPV) of 66,6% and negative predictive value(NPV) of 99,1%.

With the mammograms an improvement can be seen as S of 56,2% SP= 99,5% (PPV) 64,2 and NPV of 99,3, although.

The sensibility and the positive predictive value appear low.

The echography has a S=86,6%, SP= 99,2%, VP 76.4% and VPN 99,6%, and citological aspiration has a S= 93,3% SP=99,1%, VPP 77,7% and VPN 99,7%.

The results using this method are an improvement on the results are better the result the mammogram.

In conclusion we think that echography an citology should be incorporated in the follow-up protocols of the breast cancer conservative treatment with the mammogram in order to provide an early diagnosis of any local recurrences.

REFERENCES

1.Spaulding C.A.,Paredes E.S.,Anne P. et al. Detection of recurrence afther breast conservation treatment with radiotherapy. Breast.Dis. 5:75-90. 1992

2.Solin L.J.,Fowble B.L.,Schulz D.J. et al. The detection of local recurrence after definitive irradiation for early stage carcinoma of breast cancer. Cancer. 65:2497-2501. 1990

3.Stomper P.C.,Recht A.,Berenberg A.L. et al. Mammographic detection of recurrent cancer in the irradiated breast. AJR. 148:39-43.1987.

4.Greestein S.,Troupin R.H.,Patterson E.A. et al. Breast cancer recurrence after lumpectomy and irradiation : role of mammography in detection. Radiology. 183:201-206.1992.

5.Solin L.J.,Fowble B.L.,Trpupin R.H. et al. Biopsy results of new calcifications in the postirradiated breast.Cancer. 57:597-602. 1986.

6.Senofsky G.M.,Wanedo H.J.,Wilhelm M.C. et al. Has monitoring of the contralateral breast improved the prognosis in patients treated for primary breast cancer?. Cancer. 57:597-602.1986.

7.Peeters P.H.M.,Verbeek A.L.M.,Hendriks J.H.C.L., et al. The ocurrenceof interval cancers in the Nijmegen screening programme.Br.J.Cancer. 59:929-932.1989.

8.Mellink W.A.M.,Holland R.,Hendriks J.H. et al. The contribution of routine follow up mammography to an early detection of asynchonous contralateral breast cancer. Cancer. 67:1844-1848.1991.

9.Berenberg A.L.,Levene M.B.,Tonnesen G.L., et al. Mammographic evaluation of the postirradiated breast.In Harris J.R.,Hellmans S., Silen W. eds.Conservative management of breast cancer:New surgical and radiotherapeutic techniques. Philadelphia :J.B.Lippincott 265-272. 1983.

10. Dershaw D.D., Shank B., Reisinger S., et al. Mammographic findings after breast cancer treatment with local exicision and definitive irradiation. Radiology. 164:455-461.1987.

11. Stomper P.C., Rech A., Berenberg A.L. et al. Mammographic detection of recurrent cancer in the irradiated breast. A.J.R. 148:39-43. 1987.

Mastology - Breast Diseases
A.S.S. Figueira Fo et al., editors.

Follow-up of breast cancer patients

George N. Peters, M.D.

Baylor-Charles A. Sammons Cancer Center, Baylor University Medical Center, Dallas, Texas

Correspondence: George N. Peters, M.D., 300 Sammons, 3409 Worth Street, Dallas, Texas 75246, USA

After a diagnosis of breast cancer, there is a need for close follow-up by both physicians and patients. The goals for follow-up include 1) early detection of recurrent and new cancers which would allow treatment intervention as indicated, 2) identification of treatment sequelae requiring appropriate interventions, and 3) providing individual practices with the data base necessary to optimize treatment and compare outcomes against national standards. The optimal and most cost-effective means of follow-up and whether early detection of metastasis influences ultimate long-term survival have been matters of debate by clinicians.

Approximately 60% to 80% of breast cancer recurrences are found within the first three years of diagnosis. According to David Schapira, M.D., of the H. Lee Moffitt Cancer Center and Research Institute, Tampa, Florida, 70% of these recurrences are found by patients. Another 16% are found by the physician's physical examination, and mammography detects an additional 2%. The remaining 12% are discovered by bone scan, chest x-ray, and blood chemistry studies. Dr. Schapira and Nicole Urban, Ph.D., of the Fred Hutchinson Cancer Center of Seattle, Washington, therefore advocate that a reasonable approach is to monitor these patients by using minimal intervention. They advocate an annual mammogram plus patient history and physical examination every three months for the first three years and then every four months for years four and five. With minimal follow-up, annual savings would be $1 billion by the year 2000. Extensive intervention would add a complete blood count, blood chemistry studies, and carcinoembryonic antigen testing at each visit, with a chest x-ray and bone scan performed annually. They feel that the most reasonable preventive measure is to educate patients on the signs and symptoms of recurrence. Chest x-rays and liver chemistry tests can detect metastatic disease in 1.2% of asymptomatic patients; bone scans are positive in 0.6% of asymptomatic patients. Dr. Schapira and Dr. Urban maintain that minimal follow-up constitutes standard of care, because with current methods of detection and therapeutic modalities, survival is not significantly improved with more intensive intervention.

In 1992, the American College of Radiology, the American College of Surgeons, the College of American Pathologists, and the Society of Surgical Oncology published standards for breast conservation treatment. Included in these standards of care were those for follow-up care. Important components in follow-up include a patient history and physical examination every three to six months, years one to three. This would vary for patients receiving adjuvant chemotherapy who need more frequent assessment for possible treatment sequelae. In years four to five, examination should be every six months and then annually after the fifth year.

Mammography after mastectomy should be performed on an annual basis. Patients undergoing breast conservation should have postoperative preradiation mammograms to confirm excision of microcalcifications. Mammograms of the involved breast should be done every six months during the first year after excision and radiation. Mammograms of the involved breast (including contralateral mammograms) should be obtained at least annually thereafter.

Although symptomatic patients justifiably are evaluated with other more sophisticated tests such as bone scans, chest x-rays, computed tomography scans, and liver function tests, the efficacy and cost-effectiveness of such studies in routine metastatic screening of asymptomatic patients are undocumented. Under the present guidelines and atmosphere of managed care in the United States, there is a move toward less aggressive surveillance until cost-effectiveness and survival benefits for more aggressive follow-up testing can be ascertained.

References

1. Schapira DV. Presentation at the 15th Annual Breast Cancer Symposium, San Antonio, Texas.
2. Winchester DP, Cox JD. CA-A Cancer Journal for Clinicians 1992;42:134-162.

Mastology - Breast Diseases
A.S.S. Figueira Fo et al., editors.

Therapeutic monitoring of the breast with angiothemography

G. C. Montruccoli, M.D. and D. Montruccoli-Salmi M.D.

Toniolo Hospital, Via Toscana n. 34, 40141 Bologna, Italy.

Summary. Angiothermography records the functional blood flow within the mammary gland, and any modifications due to inflammatory affections or the neoangiogenic phenomena associated with neoplastic or premalignant disease. As well as revealing malignant and premalignant mammary lesions, and providing the clinician with a means to make a constant check-up as to the absence of serious pathology, ATG has a major role in therapeutic monitoring. It provides a means of asessing the effects of the pill or hormone replacement therapy on the activity of the mammary gland, testing the efficacy of treatment with antibiotics of suspected inflammatory affections, and evaluating the effects of preoperative chemotherapy.

Angiothermography (ATG) is a form of contact thermography with liquid crystal plates that differs radically in its interpretative approach from other thermographical methods, to the extent that it could be said to be the modern interpretation of the primitive contact/plate thermography. ATG is based on the concept that the thermographic pattern corresponds to the functional blood flow within the mammary gland: it reveals modifications due to inflammatory infections, or especially to the neoangiogenic phenomena associated with neoplastic or premalignant disease [1,2]. Instead of using the diagnostically confusing classifications characteristic of the older schools of thermography, the interpretation of ATG is based on three main general observations: i) each ATG pattern is unique and is specific to the individual patient ("fingerprint-like"); ii) the form of the individual's pattern is perfectly repetitive in a breast without significant pathology, even after many years; iii) in the case of neoplastic transformation, the pattern always undergoes variations, which are not proportional to the volume of the lesion (so that the signs of even tiny tumours are extremely evident) [1,2].

These characteristics make ATG useful in a range of applications, not least of which the identification small malignancies and premalignant mammary lesions, and the opportunity for a constant, reliable check-up as to the absence of any serious pathology [1-3]. It should be noted that ATG must not be viewed as subordinate or complimentary to X-ray mammography (XRM) and mammary ultrasonography: rather, it needs to be integrated with these techniques with respect to the patient and the clinical state of her breast [1]. For example, in a radiologically dense mammary gland, a point may be identified in which the functional blood flow is for some reason much more significant than in other zones, or even indicative of a pathology. Conversely, the possibility of distinguishing between solid and liquid with ultrasonography or of visualising microcalcifications by XRM may be of similar importance in resolving diagnostic doubts from ATG.

A clear demonstration of how ATG records the functional blood can be had by examining the physiological patterns at puberty and menopause. In the former case, the ATG pattern is particularly intense and diffuse, reflecting the profuse activity of the mammary gland. By contrast, in menopause the pattern "slims" down to the point of almost disappearing in correspondence with the physiological glandular involution. In this context, ATG can be used to monitor the use of the pill to detect any congestion. More importantly, ATG can reveal excessive stimulation of the residual glandular tissue during HRT, with the consequent increased risks of cancer.

ATG also provides a simple and highly reliable way of monitoring treatment with antibiotics of suspected non-puerperal mastitis. In this affection, the ATG pattern in the inflamed area is very similar to inflammatory carcinoma (Figure 1). After one or two weeks of antibiotic therapy, however, the pattern always returns to normal, thereby rapidly excluding any diagnostic suspicion of cancer (Figure 1). It should be noted that with other techniques, a much longer follow up is needed before the same degree of certainty can be reached.

A similar consideration can be made as to the monitoring of antiblastic preoperative chemotherapy. Destruction of a significant percentage of neoplastic cells is always accompanied by a corresponding drop in the blood supply to the tumour. As a result the alterations in the ATG pattern become less and less marked after each successful cycle of therapy. In this way, ATG can provide a reliable visual indication of the success or otherwise of preoperative chemotherapy. In fact, we have found ATG to be a more reliable indicator of tumoral activity than XRM. This is probably due to the fact that whereas ATG registers the tumour's metabolic activity, XRM can only represent the tumour stroma.

In conclusion, some remarks need to be made regarding the rationale of ATG. Much controversy surrounds the prognosis of so-called precancerous lesions such as lobular or ductal hyperplasia with atypia, and even of carcinoma *in situ* [4]. Less controversial, however, is the hypothesis that many years may go by between the onset of carcinogenesis and the possibility of instrumental diagnosis of cancer by XRM, while it has been clearly demonstrated that the onset of breast cancer is always preceded by neoangiogenic phenomena [5]. In this context, ATG is fitted to identify and monitor early cancerous and precancerous lesions at all ages, even in breasts too young for the use of XRM.

Finally, we would like to mention an ongoing study using digitalised enlargements of XRM images that permit visualisation of tiny "neomicrocalcifications" not detectable at conventional photographic enlargement. It has been interesting to note that in many cases of carcinoma *in situ* detected by ATG - and particulaly in lobular ones - no neomicrocalcifications were revealed in correspondence with the lesion. This supports the concept that microcalcifications, when present, are a much later manifestation than neoangiogenesis [1].

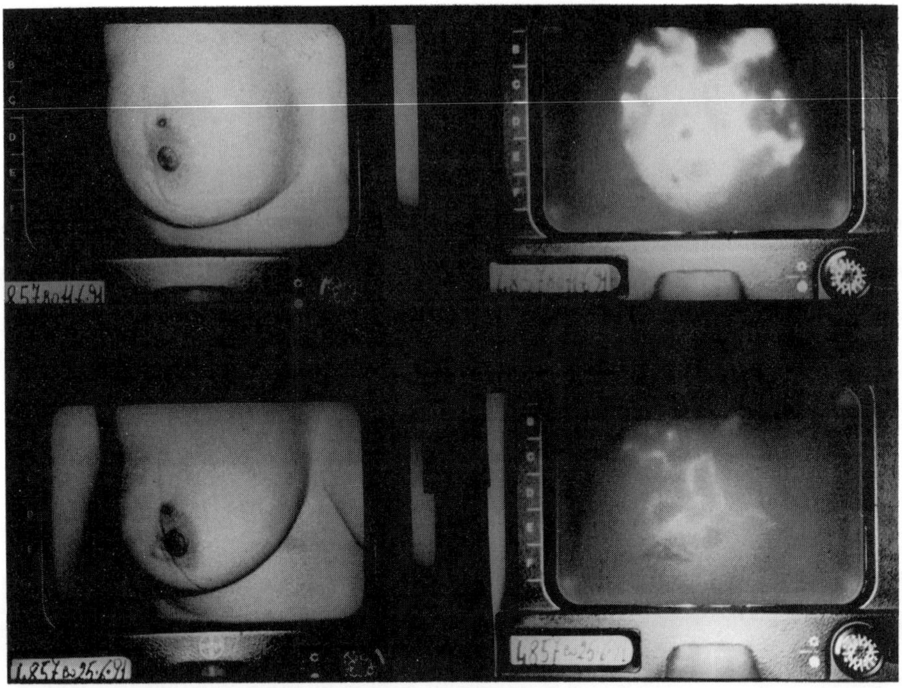

Fig. 1. Case of acute mastitis with antgiothermographic patterns. The higly vascularized intense hot spot (above), angiothermographically similar to cancer, disappeared two weeks later (below) following therapy with antibiotics.

References

1. Montruccoli GC. Diagnosing breast diseases: selecting and integrating diagnostic procedures. In: Women's Health Today, Proceedings of the 14th World Congress of Obstetrics and Gynaecology (in press).
2. Montruccoli GC. The evolution of plate thermography. In: Bonilla Musoles F, Montruccoli GC, Pinotti JA (eds.), Benign Breast Tumors. Valencia: International Federation of Gynecology and Obstetrics, 1994;131-139.
3. Montruccoli GC, Montruccoli DS, D'Errico A, Grigioni WF. Angiothermography in an Integrated Diagnosis for Secondary Prevention of Breast Cancer. In: Lancet Conference - The Challenge of Breast Cancer. London: The Lancet, 1994;49.
4. Fentiman IS. Risk factors for benign breast disease. In: Smallwood JA, Taylor I (eds.) Benign Breast Disease. London: Edward Arnold, 1990;121-141.
5. Folkman J, Watson K, Ingber D. Induction of Angiogenesis During the Transition from Hyperplasia to Neoplasia. Nature 1989;339:58-61.

Mastology - Breast Diseases
A.S.S. Figueira Fo et al., editors.

Breast cancer : Criteria of choice, interest and guidelines of tumor markers in the follow-up

A. Daver, I. Dalifard.
Laboratoire de radioimmunologie, Centre Paul Papin, 2 rue Moll, 49033 Angers cedex.

ABSTRACT: The role of tumor markers is similar to that of other instrumental or laboratory tests. Actually, they are very effective, because they recognize the disease progression in a high percentage of cases. Moreover, in many instance, tumor marker levels increase before any other clinical or instrumental sign of relapse. Aiming to prove a gain in term of survival of an early treatment of recurrences or metastases on the basis of an increase of CA 15-3 and/or CEA without clinical or radiological signs, three random therapeutical assays are in progress. The establishment of a software invention, based on antigen kinetics, like the apparent biological half-life, the doubling-time, and exponential tumor growth in breast cancer follow-up may be the support of the mathematical construction of graphic curve with an accurate definition of the patients' base line and a better therapy adaptation to the clinical evolution of the patient.

During the last ten years, new tumor markers have invaded the biological cancer field, CEA, CA 15-3, CA 549, MCA, TPA/TPS, SP-1, CA M26 and CA M 29 represent the different assays associated with different commercial names and different monoclonal antibodies often recognizing pratically the same epitopes. For the laboratory the choice between the tumor markers will be essentially done now with the ROC curves studies. However, if medical and scientific community are convinced for their usefullness in the follow-up of breast cancer, new parameters like base-line level of each patient, apparent biological half-life, and doubling-time had to be introduced in biological and clinical randomized studies proving their interest in strategical decision. Kinetics evaluation of tumor marker during the follow-up may provide a long lead time with adequate accuracy performances with the goal of the possible treatment of the relapse only on the basis of a biochemical identification.

I THE MUCIN-LIKE GLYCOPROTEINS CA 15-3, CA 549, MCA, CAM 26, CAM 29.
The differential glycosylation of a protein " core " of the polymorphism epithelial mucin (PEM) causes changes in accessibility of different epitopes by monoclonal antibody that may land on in differences in the results of sample evaluation in the same serum. A great part of the PEM is cycled in the cell by an internationalization processing. The extracellular forms and the glycosylated forms linked to the membrane contain more sialylated acids, compared to the precursor molecules and to the internalized and reprocessing glycosylated forms.

1) Monoclonal antibodies specificity

The antibody specificity is directed against the enriched part of metastatic breast cancer cell membranes (DF3) ; cancerous cell lines (BC4 E549, 48, b12, b 15) ; milkfat globules membranes (115 D8, BC4, N 154, M38) (Table I).

2) Characteristics of the different antigens and of their antibodies

The antibodies recognize glycoprotein with 1 or 2 epitopes. The MCA skeleton contains heavy proteins with a lot of lateral chains. The carbohydrate part containing terminal sialylated acids is negatively electric charged. CAM 26 is the only assay with a capture antibody against a sialylated acid epitope which detects more glycosylated forms of alive tumor cells than those secreted by dead cells of necrosis. The epitope of CAM 29 is

Table I : Monoclonal antibody pairs for each antigen (MW = molecular weight)

Antigen	Capture Ab	MW of epitope	Detection Ab	MW of epitope
CA 15-3	115 D8	400 kD	DF3	330 & 450 kD
MCA	b 12	350 kD	b 12	350 kD
CA 549	BC4 E549	400 kD	BC4 N 154	512 kD
CAM 26	M 26		M 38	
CAM 29	M 29		M 38	

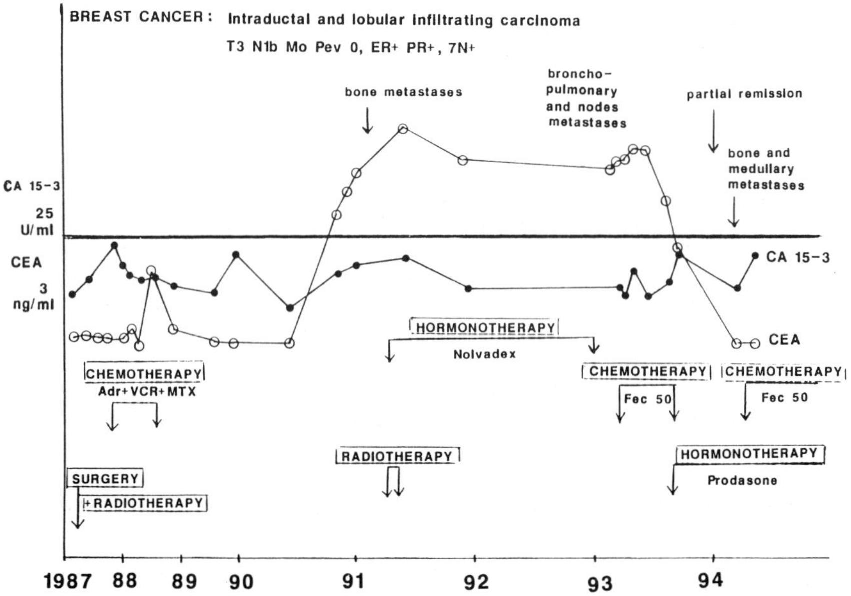

Figure 1
Follow-up of a CEA secreting breast cancer patient.

masked in part by sialylated acid, and is preferentially detected on immaturing internationalized molecules.

3) Normal values of the different assays

The normal values of the different assays differ : CA 15-3 = 25 to 31U/ml ; MCA = 11 U/ml ; CA 549 = 10 to 12 U/ml ; CAM 26 and CAM 29 = 100 and 20 U/ml respectively.

II THE OTHER MARKERS

The other markers, in the breast cancer follow-up, include the well known carcino-embryonic antigen (CEA) as well as the TPS, a new one marker of the cell proliferation.

III CRITERIA OF CHOICE OF THE TUMOR MARKER ASSOCIATION

In the paper of Silver et al. [1], ROC (Relative Operating Characteristic) curves studies allow constructed models for early diagnosis among patients with high risk for breast cancer ; the influence of non malignant pathology on early diagnosis, the discrimination of breast carcinoma from other adenocarcinomas, detection of early recurrence ; and assessment of change in tumor burden. For each model ROC data permitted the unbiased selection of the most appropriate critical values based on the interaction of specificity and sensibility of tumor markers, alone or associated to optimize the clinical and biological information.

IV OUR CHOICE OF THE TUMOR MARKER ASSOCIATION

The two markers selected for the breast cancer follow-up belong from two different origins. We know the origins of mucin-like glycoproteins ; CEA is extracted from liver metastases of colorectal cancer.

For Basuyau et al. [2] the interest of an association of tumor markers in breast cancer may be a cost / efficacy problem ; addition of CEA to CA 15-3 increases sensitivity by 10%, which a loss of specificity. Our suggested recommendations may be :

- CA 15-3 and CEA assays must be done before any treatment ;
- A positive value of one of the two markers involves a follow-up by this marker ;
- The two markers are in the normal zone, carry on the monitoring with CA 15-3 alone ;
- At the time of a clinical evolution without CA 15-3 increase, perform CEA assay or another marker (Figure 1) ;
- For retrospective studies of patients by new markers studies a serum library must be constituted.

V TUMOR MARKER USEFULNESS

1) Role of CA 15-3 in the follow-up

In the therapeutical follow-up, after the initial treatment of :

- Loco-regional cancer (surgery - radiotherapy association) two-third of cases present a normal value at 6 or 12 months even if the initial value is in the normal zone. After surgery a short decrease till normal range is in favour of a good pronostic.
- In straight off metastatic breast cancer, the normalization under chemotherapy treatment is in favour of a good pronostic.

2) Role of CA 15-3 in the recurrences and metastases detection

At the threshold of 35 U/ml, the positive predictive value for recurrences and metastases detection is 97,7%. At the time of metastatic diagnosis, sensitivity is 59% for node involvement , 90% for liver metastases , 76% for bone metastases, 71% for lung metastases, 60% for skin metastases, 21% for brain metastases. One assay performed every 2 months must be the first sign of metastatic evolution in more than 40% of cases. Aiming to prove a gain in term of survival of an early treatment of recurrences on the basis of an increase of CA 15-3 and / or CEA without clinical or radiological signs, three random therapeutical assays are in progress.

• a) Namer [3] (FRANCE) studies the role of the CA 15-3 in the early diagnosis of an evolutionary recovery. The aim of the assay is the detection of an increase of CA 15-3 in the early start of a medical specific treatment and improvement of patients' survival. The recruiting has been made by inclusion at the end of loco-regional treatment of patients with the following criteria : Invasive breast carcinoma without distant metastases ; unknown lymph nodes involvement ; no lymph node involvement with negative hormonal receptors or SBR grade III. The random study divides patients into two groups :

- Group A : Patients have an usual clinical follow-up. They have a specific treatment at the appearance of clinical signs, after paraclinical checking of the diagnosis.
- Group B : CA 15-3 is measured every two or three months during five years. After a first increase superior to 35 U/ml, the assay must be checked again. A specific general treatment after level confirmation must be undertaken.

• b) Jäger et al. [4] (GERMANY) have studied the role of early treated breast cancer metastases. Patients with lymph node involvement, positive hormonal receptors, and monthly CA 15-3 and CEA enter the study. Whose with CA 15-3 and/or CEA above the 97° percentil, have metastases prospective :

- If metastases are detected, patients received standard treatments ;
- If metastases are not detected, a random study is made on 46 patients : The control group included 26 patients with no treatment ; the treated group included 20 patients who received medroxyprogesterone to 1 mg by day. The metastases screening is made every 3 or 4 months. Preliminary results show the median period time between tumor marker increase and metastases detection (1986-1993) is 4 months for the control group patients and above 24 months for treated group patients ; the median survival is respectively 12 and above 36 months.

• c) Hareuveni et al. [5] (ISRAEL) have studied the role of MCA and/or CEA for the early detection of breast cancer metastases. They reported a randomized study on 50 breast cancers with or without lymph node involvement, positive or negative hormonal receptors, with two consecutive assays MCA and/or CEA increase, and without clinical or imagery detection of metastases. Among the 21 patients immediately treated with Tamoxifen, 21 had disease free survival ; among the 29 patients without treatment, 9 had local recurrence or distant metastases, 20 had free disease survival after 15 months of follow-up.

We are waiting about the statistic significance of these results?

VI WHY A SOFTWARE INVENTION?

Introduction of new parameters like the apparent biological half-life and the doubling-time in breast cancer follow-up may provide new informations comparing the different profiles of patients under treatment and must have more confidence in the appreciation of early detection of recurrences and metastases.

Cellular and circulating antigen kinetics, exponential tumor growth may be the support of the mathematical construction of graphic curve with an accurate definition of the patients' base line. In that case, event detection will guided by exponential elevation of the tumor marker, being a best criterion for the selection of the randomized groups than a one cut-off level only. In this same perspective, Gion et al. [6] propose a kinetic use of CA 15-3 in patients which high risks of relapse : The increase of tumor marker should be an early indicator of the relapse. Kiang et al. [7] have also studied four kinetic possible profiles of CEA under chemotherapeutic treatment of breast cancer patients for the early prediction of the therapeutical response. In order to advance in the clinical use of tumor marker in the follow-up of breast cancer patient we need more randomized trials supported by the creation and the adaptation of a software to the biological follow-up which allows :

- A quality control because the patient is his own reference. We probably eliminate in the future the notion of the normal value.
- New definitions of mathematical parameters : like the half-life in the prognostic factors, then in the evaluation of the total survival and of the disease free survival ; and the doubling-time in the therapeutical strategy for individual treatment.
- A better therapy adaptation to the clinical evolution of the patient. A treatment for the early detected matastases. For a same therapeutic protocol, a comparison between the different tumor marker profiles and a better patient stratification.
- The estimation of compared cost-efficacy is also important.

REFERENCES

1 Silver H.K, Archibald B.L, Ragaz J, Coldman A.J. Cancer Res 1991 ; 51 : 1904-1909

2 Basuyau J-P, Brunelle P, Charrot P, Chevallier B, Delapierre F, Graic Y, Julien J-P, Veyret C. Bull Cancer 1993 ; 80 : 213-218.

3 Namer M. Projet de la F.N.C.LC.C.

4 Jäger W, Merkle E, Lang NJ.Tumor Marker Oncol 1991 ; 6 : 56 (abstract).

5 Hareuveni M, Merimsky O, Kovner F, Dotan D, Chaitchik S. Abstract of XXI st Meeting of I.S.O.B.M. Israel 1993 ; 51.

6 Gion M, Fila G, Biasioli R, Vignati G, Mione R, Saracchini S, Rinaldi E, Testa E, Bruscagnin G. Journal Nuclear Med All Sci 1990 ; 34, Suppl 4 : 1-7.

7 Kiang DT, Greenberg LJ, kennedy BJ. Cancer 1990 ; 65 : 193-199.

III. 11. Special aspects

Mastology - Breast Diseases
A.S.S. Figueira Fo et al., editors.

Old Ideas versus New
The History of Breast Cancer Treatment

Melvin J. Silverstein, M.D., Medical Director and Senior Surgical Oncologist,
The Breast Center, 14624 Sherman Way, Van Nuys, California 91405, USA

From Halsted to Rio. In other words, how did we get here from there - from the Johns Hopkins Hospital in the 1890s, to Rio de Janeiro today, a hundred years later; from radical surgery as the only therapy for breast cancer, to the SIS Congress dealing with sophisticated diagnostic tools and multidisciplinary care?

Halsted, faced with locally advanced breast cancer and an unacceptably high local recurrence rate, developed a concept that was both anatomical and mechanical. He felt that breast cancer spread by direct extension, into muscle and skin, and through lymphatics to regional lymph nodes. The nodes, acting as filters, held the cancer cells in check for some unknown time period prior to widespread dissemination. If this were true, it meant that radical surgical intervention in a timely manner could cure cancer.

Halsted initiated his radical operation in New York in 1882. He reported his first 13 cases in *Johns Hopkins Hospital Reports* in 1991. In 1894, he reported 50 cases in the same journal and in 1898, he presented a total of 76 cases to The American Surgical Association. Based upon this tiny group of patients, the use of radical mastectomy became routine. Most physicians throughout the world embraced Halsted's concept, accepting it until the 1970s. "The bigger the cancer, the bigger the operation required to cure it." Many physicians continue to believe it today.

In 1898, Rudolph Matas suggested that breast cancer might spread through the blood stream. His early suggestion that breast cancer might be a systemic disease at the time of diagnosis fell on deaf ears.

In the 1960s, Bernard Fisher, principal investigator of America's National Adjuvant Breast Project (NSABP) proposed a biologic hypothesis. He called it a new paradigm. Fisher felt that invasive breast cancer was a systemic disease at the time it was diagnosed. He set out to prove that variations in local treatment had no impact on survival. This was difficult for most surgeons to accept after almost a century of Halstedian mechanics. Accepting Fisher meant that the surgeon would now play a less important role in the treatment of breast cancer.

In 1973, while on the faculty of the UCLA School of Medicine, I did my last Halsted radical mastectomy. I remember the patient well, having seen her on a number of occasions since the operation. Now an outspoken proponent of breast conservation, she has never forgiven me. She had a 1.5 cm infiltrating ductal carcinoma, a one-stage procedure, a vertical scar, a depression beneath her clavicle, protruding ribs, a skin graft, no significant pre or postoperative counseling, no reconstruction, no informed consent (by today's standards), and no choice. She had the best of what we had to offer in 1973 in the United States. She had the only thing we offered in 1973.

The last 20 years have seen the treatment of breast cancer undergo dramatic changes, the most important of which has been a shift toward breast conservation initially motivated by retrospective data, the Women's Movement, and the media and later supported by prospective randomized trials [1,2]. In 1981, Veronesi and associates [1] were the first to report the results of a prospective randomized study which proved that the survival results of Halsted radical mastectomy could be equaled with a breast conserving procedure called QUART (quadrantectomy, axillary dissection, and radiation therapy).

Today's surgeon must be more than just a technician. Today's surgeon must be familiar with the natural history of breast cancer, the subtle mammographic findings of early breast cancer, the mammographic patterns that suggest different type of breast cancer, the range of diseases that qualify as breast cancer, the techniques for directed breast biopsy, the fact that the "Captain of the Ship" concept is dead and that we take care of breast cancer patients as a team.

Today's *"breast physician"* must be familiar with the heterogeneity of breast cancer, the role of primary chemotherapy, what can and cannot be accomplished by the radiation oncologist for all stages of disease, the meaning of ploidy, S-phase, Her 2-neu (c-erbB-2), P53, the role of high dose chemotherapy with bone marrow transplant or autologous stem cell support, the available prospective randomized studies, the role of the reconstructive surgeon, the methods for detecting recurrence in a radiated breast, and on and on. In addition, todays breast physician should be a patient listener, a psychiatrist, a third or fourth opinion giver, and a willing interpreter of uninterpretable data.

As survival data for infiltrating lesions has accumulated during the last decade, it has been clearly shown that breast conservation therapy with excision of the tumor, axillary node dissection, and radiation therapy is equivalent to mastectomy for properly selected patients. Furthermore, 8-year data from Dr. Bernard Fisher's NSABP protocol B-06 has revealed equivalent survival data when mastectomy is compared with lumpectomy with or without radiation therapy [2].

For many, this has been hard to accept. How is it possible that the results are the same regardless of how the primary cancer is treated? I constantly have discussions with colleagues who think Fisher's systemic disease hypothesis is wrong and that Halsted, Urban , Haagensen, and many others were correct in stating that local treatment is important. Certainly many patients with node positive breast cancer were cured in the era before there was chemotherapy. These patients were cured by surgery, in spite of the fact that they met Fisher's definition of having had systemic disease at the time of diagnosis.

In NSABP B-06, lumpectomy patients who did not receive radiation therapy had a significantly higher risk of local breast recurrence, but there was no increase in mortality, suggesting that local breast recurrence is a "marker" of poor prognosis but not a cause of distant disease [3]. On the other hand, experimental data in laboratory animals clearly shows that metastases can metastasize [4]. If this is true in humans (and why shouldn't it be?) than local invasive recurrences have the potential to cause systemic disease which may not have been present when the primary was originally diagnosed and treated.

If similar data to the NSABP accumulate and become more universally accepted, the diminished role of mastectomy will decrease even further; the need for radiation therapy in every case of breast conservation will also be questioned.

NSABP B-04, a protocol comparing radical mastectomy with total mastectomy (with and without radiation) revealed no survival difference whether or not axillary node dissection was done [5]. With the increasing development of immunohistochemical prognostic factors, axillary dissection may go the way of the radical mastectomy. Ultimately, the surgeons only role, in primary operable breast cancer, may be "lumpectomy" or perhaps even less; radiation therapists will prevent local recurrences, and the true effectors of outcome (survival) could be medical oncologists or immunochemical genetic therapists or whatever they are called in the next century.

Today, the surgical management of breast cancer begins before the biopsy. Clinical evaluation of the patient by physical examination, mammography, and when indicated, fine needle aspiration biopsy helps the surgeon form a prebiopsy opinion regarding the relative risk of malignancy. Stereotactic core biopsy is emerging as an important new minimally invasive tool. It is imperative that the surgeon has thought about breast conservation therapy long before he or she enters the operating room for the initial open breast biopsy.

How suspicious is the lesion that is about to be biopsied? Does this patient want breast conservation therapy if the lesion turns out to be breast cancer? Will she be a good candidate for breast conservation therapy? What can be done to improve her odds? Should she be treated with induction (primary) chemotherapy?

During the last 20 years, Dr. Bernard Fisher has helped to develop a new paradigm for our understanding and treatment of invasive breast cancer. He has done away with the anatomical and mechanical Halstedian cancer model, replacing it with a modern biological model, telling us that invasive cancers are systemic at the time of diagnosis and that local/regional treatments do not impact on survival. Just as many have accepted this, a new problem has arisen: *Mammographically Detected Noninvasive Breast Cancer*, which is certainly not systemic at the time of diagnosis. This is, perhaps, a disease that surgeons can *cure*? In addition, the vast majority of 5 mm (or less) invasive breast cancers are easily cured by the surgeon and without systemic therapy.

When does breast cancer become a systemic disease? Certainly not when the first few cells invade! Perhaps Dickens best summed up our current situation.

"It was the best of times, it was the worst of times, it was the age of wisdom, it was the age of foolishness, it was the epoch of belief, it was the epoch of incredulity, it was the season of Light, it was the season of Darkness, it was the spring of hope, it was the winter of despair, we had everything before us........" [6]

References

1. Veronesi U, Saccozzi R, Del Vecchio M, et al. Comparing radical mastectomy with quadrantectomy, axillary dissection and radiation therapy in patients with small cancers of the breast. N Engl J Med 1981;305:6-11.
2. Fisher B, Redmond C, Poisson R. et al. Eight-year results of a randomized clinical trial comparing total mastectomy and lumpectomy with or without irradiation in the treatment of breast cancer. N Engl J Med 1989;320:822-828
3. Fisher B, Anderson S, Fisher E, et al. Significance of ipsilateral breast tumour recurrence after lumpectomy. Lancer 1991;338:327-331
4. Hart IR and Fidler IJ. Role of organ selectivity in the determination of metastatic patterns of B16 melanoma. Cancer Res 1980;40:2281-2287.
5. Fisher B, Redmond C, Fisher E, et al. Ten-year results of a randomized clinical trial comparing radical mastectomy and total mastectomy with or without radiation. N Engl J Med 1985;312:674-681.
6. Charles Dickens *A Tale of Two Cities* 1859

Mastology - Breast Diseases
A.S.S. Figueira Fo et al., editors.

Diet and breast cancer

Carlos H. Menke, Jorge V. Biazus, José A. Cavalheiro, Eliane G. Rabin

Breast Unit – Hospital de Clínicas de Porto Alegre – Universidade Federal do Rio Grande do Sul – Brazil

Abstract

Experiments with animals, ecologic and analytical epidemiologic studies have shown the relation between diet and BC. We analyze here the most important factors in promoting – or preventing – BC: fat, fibers, vitamins, caffeine, alcohol and smoking. The soundest evidence points to the 'fat-fiber connection' as the main factor responsible for the high incidence rates in Western countries. The association with alcohol seems to exist, but its RR is very low and dose-dependant. Smoking and caffeine have not been proven to have a promoting effect, while the role of vitamins is controversial. Obesity and the kind of diet seems to influence negatively in the prognosis. Intervention trials aim at reducing lipid intake to 15 to 20% of total calories and increasing fiber ingestion to 25 g/day are under way.

This paper updates this discussion including all nutritional factors that may be involved in the promotion – or prevention – of breast cancer (BC). We have included smoking – although it is not a nutrient – because its possible synergism with alcohol (1).

FATS: The so-called 'fat connection' is strengthened by evidence from three different sources: 1)animal experiments – increase of carcinogenesis in rodents after initiation, which suggests a carcinogenesis-promoting effect; 2)ecological studies: they examine the international differences which show high BC rates in countries where diet are rich in fat. In Brazil, interesting regional discrepancies are observed (Table 1). Rio Grande do Sul, the southernmost state in the country

Table 1
Breast cancer incidence in some Brazilian state capitals

(cases/100,000/year)	
Porto Alegre	76.2
So Paulo	65.5
Fortaleza	61.6
Recife	48.2
Belem	40.5
Goiânia	38.8

National Cancer Registry – Ministry of Health, 1990.

and traditionally a place where the consumption of fats and red meat is high, shows rates of incidence similar to those of Uruguay and Argentina and much higher than those of the Northern Region; 3)analytical epidemiology – there are dozens of case-control and cohort studies that show conflicting data. The most widely accepted hypothesis is the hormonal one, which considers the effects of estrogens, which may interfere directly in the ovarian steroid production (2). Another possible explanation is the increase of adiposity in the mammary gland itself, which would make it easier for any promoting substance to be transferred (3).

FIBERS: There is a very important protective role against BC (4,5). They act in three different ways: 1)increasing the weight and humidity of feces and so allow greater estrogen excretion; 2)decreasing the activity of beta-glucorunidase, and intestinal absorption of these hormones; 3) increasing the production of phytoestrogens, which are weak estrogens and compete for the hormonal receptors. Now, we have the 'fat-fiber connection'.

VITAMINS AND OTHER MICRONUTRIENTS: The vitamins listed as protective against BC are A, C, D and E. They generically work as antioxidants and fight free radicals. They are also cell differentiation regulators (Vitamin A). An excellent study (6) showed that low intake of Vitamin A may increase the risk. Vitamin D has been defended by some researchers because BC mortality rate is twice as high in the North of the United States as in the South – higher sun exposure and less acid haze (7). A Canadian study (8) did not demonstrate hypovitaminosis for Vitamin D in 108 BC patients. In experiments with animals and in a few epidemiological studies, selenium metalloid, widely found on the ground, grass and grains, proved to be a protective agent. Hunter et al., however, reached the conclusion that it is not a relevant factor in BC's etiology (9).

CAFFEINE: Caffeine have mutagenic effect producing tumors in rats by raising the levels of adenosine monophosphate in the mammary tissue. In the 80's, it made doctors recommend abstinence from tea, coffee, cola soft-drinks and chocolate, even in cases of fibrocystic changes. It was not confirmed and it has disappeared from literature since 1988 (10).

ALCOHOL: Because of methodological problems, papers available do not allow us to conclude that alcohol increases chances of BC. It has a low RR, less than 2.0 and seems to be consensus that the probable relation of alcohol to BC depends on doses and length of time of use (11).

SMOKING: The literature presents conflicting research results: some show a protective effect due to smoking's antiestrogenic action . Vatten et al. have found an RR of 2.3 in pre-menopause smokers, while Pawlega has not found any relation to BC (12).

INFLUENCE IN PROGNOSIS – DIET INTERVENTION: Several papers have related lipidic diets to worsened prognosis for patients treated for BC (2, 13, 14). There is a clear association between the kind of diet at the time the tumor is discovered and a higher probability of dissemination of the disease (14). Diet intervention may be useful as adjuvant treatment in order to improve survival rates. The intervention trials are under way (15), and almost all of them aim at reducing lipid ingestion down to 15 to 20 % of total calories, while fiber ingestion is raised to 25 g/day. The counter-argument to this strategy is that it is difficult for the population to accept such a drastic change in eating habits when the same results can be obtained through a simple hormone manipulation, such as the prescription of one tamoxifen tablet a day.

DIET COUNSELING IN ROUTINE VISITS: We believe that, together with other measures, the clinician should recommend a special diet to BC high-risk patients (16). These recommendations would be, in general: 1)eat at least 5 servings of vegetables and fruit a day; 2)six servings of bread, cereals and grains; 3)skimmed milk and its by-products, lean meat, chicken without the skin, fish and low-fat processed food; 4)avoid smoking and drinking – not more than one drink a day. In brief, the most prudential dietary advice is: VARIETY AND MODERATION.

References

1. Boyd NF. Nutrition and breast cancer. J NH Cancer Inst 1993; 85: 6-7
2. Schatzkin A, Greenwald P, Byar DP. The dietary fat-breast cancer hypothesis is alive. Jama 1989; 261:3284-3287.
3. Welsch CW. Relation between dietary fat and experimental mammary tumorigenesis: a review and critique. Cancer Res 1992; 52: 2040-2048.
4. Rose DP. Dietary fiber, phytoestrogens and breast cancer. Nutrition 1992; 8: 47-51.
5. Adlercreutz H, Mousavi Y, Hockersted K. Diet and breast cancer. Acta Oncol 1992; 31:175-181.
6. Hunter DJ, Colditz GA, Willet CW. A prospective study of the intake of vitamins C, E and A and the risk of breast cancer. N Engl J Med 1993;329:234-240.
7. Gorhan ED, Garland CF, Garland FC. Acid haze air pollution and breast and colon cancer mortality in 20 Canadian cities. Can J Public Health 1989; 80:96-100.
8. Simard A, Vobecky J, Vobecky JS. Vitamin D deficiency and cancer of the breast: an unprovocative ecological hypothesis. Can J Public Health 1991; 82:300-303.
9. Hunter DJ, et al. A prospective study of selenium status and breast cancer risk. Jama 1990;264:1128-1131.
10. Fentiman IS. Diagnosis and treatment of early breast cancer. Porto Alegre: Artes Médicas, 1993.
11. Plant ML. Alcohol and breast cancer: a review. Int J Addictions 1992; 27: 107-128.
12. Pawlega J. Breast cancer and smoking, vodka drinking and dietary habits. A case-control study. Acta Oncol 1992;31:387-392.
13. Verreault R, Brisson J, Deschenes L. Dietary fat relation to prognostic factor in breast cancer. J Natl Cancer Inst 1988;80:819-825.
14. Holm LE, Nordevang E, Hjalmar E – Treatment failure and dietary habits in women with breast cancer. J Natl Cancer Inst 1993;85:32-36.
15. Nordevang E, Callmer E, Marmur A. Dietary intervention in breast cancer patients. Eur J Clin Nutr 1992;46:387-396.
16. Menke CH, Biazus JV, Cavalheiro JA. Diet and breast cancer. In: Dias EN, Caleffi M, Silva HM, Figueira A. Mastologia atual. Rio de Janeiro, 1994

Mastology - Breast Diseases
A.S.S. Figueira Fo et al., editors.

Multidisciplinary Approach to Breast Cancer: Quality of Life and Treatment

Carlos H. Menke, Jorge V. Biazus, José A. Cavalheiro, Eliane G. Rabim

Breast Unit – Hospital de Clínicas de Porto Alegre – UFRGS – Porto Alegre, RS, Brazil.

Abstract

Breast cancer (BC) demands a multidisciplinary approach due to its high incidence and mortality rates, its unpredictable biological behavior, frequent hormone-dependence, elaborate diagnosis, visibility, and the fact that it causes mutilation and affects the organ that is symbol of femininity. In the beginning, BC was treated only by the surgeon, who was later joined by the pathologist and radiotherapist. The team has grown and today it consists of at least twenty members. We believe that this team should be under the responsibility of one coordinator, the mastologist. The Rehabilitation Program we have conducted since 1982 is presented here. It is divided into seven stages, from diagnosis to terminal phase. In 1993, our group carried out 576 interviews and 65 group sessions; 27 terminal patients and 16 deaths were assisted; 53 mammary prostheses were provided.

Introduction

BC is complex to manage as consequence of the following factors: 1)high incidence and mortality rates; 2)the breast is the organ that symbolizes femininity; 3)it becomes visible after some time; 4)its biological behavior is unpredictable, erratic; 5)many times it presents hormone-dependence; 6)although the breast is an external organ, the diagnosis for breast cancer is not easy; 7) it brings along the fear of mutilation, castration, loss of one's self-image (weight changes, alopecia, arm edema), and a true revolution in family, social and sexual life (1). These factors make BC a multifaceted disease which require wide and varied action. Many times this cannot be provided by one single professional.

DEVELOPMENT OF THE MULTIDISCIPLINARY TEAM: Until the beginning of the 20th Century, BC was treated by surgeons only, and William Halsted and his classic Radical Mastectomy were the best examples of it (2). After the discovery of Roentgen Rays, surgeons shared this field with radiotherapists, so much so that the combination mastectomy plus radiotherapy was the unchallenged therapy for almost half a century. Chemotherapy started in the 60's, and the field then could count on another type of professional, the clinic oncologist (3). Although mammography had been developed much earlier, it was only in the 70's that it became popular. This brought another professional into the team – the radiologist, or better, the mammary 'imageologist', since sonograms also became popular at that time. Along the way, hundreds of pathologists and cytologists turned exclusively to breast pathology. It was at that time, too, that the psycho-social and rehabilitation problems were brought into attention – psychiatrists, psychologists, nurses, physiotherapists, social workers and volunteers all came in. Finally, plastic surgeons joined the team. They brought special importance to reconstructive surgery and helped improve esthetic results of conservative treatment. We mentioned above only those more closely involved in dealing with the disease. However, when recurrence and complications appear, new collaborators may come out: orthopedists (pathological fractures), neurologists (brain metastasis), thoracic surgeons (pleurodesis, resection of chest wall), pain specialists, hematologists and immunologists (salvage chemotherapy and bone marrow transplantation). And we should not forget religious assistants, whenever they are called for.

As we can see, mamy professionals are nowadays involved in the management of BC, and we still have to add those concerned with basic and even clinic research (geneticists, epidemiologists, bio-statisticians, biochemists, and so on). One question inevitably arises: who should be the commander-in-chief in this platoon? Who is responsible for the patient? An overview of Mastology (senology) all over the world shows us that the answers to these questions vary greatly according to Geography. In the Anglo-Saxon countries, mainly the United States, the breast belongs to the general surgeon and not to the gynecologist. In these countries the rule is for the surgeon to operate on the patient and then refer her to the radiotherapist and/or oncologist, who then often becomes responsible for that case (4). There is no such specialization as Mastology there, and the American Society for Breast Specialists is just now coming to existence. Although still in the hands of surgeons and oncologists in Europe, Mastology has been growing in importance there. The Senologic International Society was born in Europe, and the European Mastology Association has been very active. In Latin America and specially in Brazil, the great majority of mastologists come from gynecology. Considered an official specialization by the Brazilian Medical Association and the Federal Medicine Council, Mastology has been developing very fast and is even searched for by the public in general. Therefore, our answer to the question above is that the professional in charge of the BC patient should be the mastologist, who should have some knowledge of all the related areas, and who, in general, gives the final diagnosis and operates on the patient. Anyhow, the doctor-patient relationship in Mastology tends to be very close because of both the psychological morbidity caused by the disease and the frequency of follow-up visits and tests (5).

OUR EXPERIENCE: We present here the organization of our team in the Breast Unit at Hospital de Clínicas de Porto Alegre. It consists of 3 mastologists, 1 nurse specialized in rehabilitation (permanent members), 1 psychiatrist, 3 resident physicians, medical students and trainees (temporary members), and also counts on the invaluable work of the League for the Assistance to Cancer Patients. – LAAPAC, 21 volunteers. Our Unit has existed since 1974, but only from 1982 on was a systematic, multidisciplinary program established to give support to women with BC (6). The team's actions can be divided in several stages, summarized bellow:

Stage # 1 – *Pre-operative*: After the cancer diagnosis is communicated and the therapeutic plan is established by the medical team, the patient is referred to the nurse responsible for the Rehabilitation Program. The nurse listens to her doubts and explains details of the procedures during hospitalization and of the subsequent treatments. A member of the family is interviewed and chosen as spokesperson for the following stages.

Stage # 2 – *During the surgical procedure*: During the surgery special technical care is taken to avoid damage to nerves and to prevent arm edema. At the same time, breast reconstruction is performed, in case it is necessary. Mastectomized patients leave the operating room with an external temporary prosthesis and a bra (7).

Stage # 3 – *Post-operative*: The whole team and a volunteer from LAAPAC visit the patient, when exercises for the homolateral arm and how to take care of the portable drain are taught. Normally in the second day she leaves the hospital (early discharge) and returns on the seventh day (outpatient) for removal of dressing and drain. Sutures are removed between the tenth and the fourteenth days.

Stage # 4 – *Adjuvant therapy*: The result of surgical histo-pathological study is communicated and the adjuvant treatment is discussed. The patient is then referred to radiotherapy and/or chemotherapy, and she is offered the opportunity to participate in the Self-Support Group for Mastectomized Women or in the Chemotherapy Group. She is given incentive to change her temporary prosthesis for a permanent one, made of syllicone and attached to the bra. Readaptation to family and society is encouraged (8).

Stage # 5 – *Follow-up*: The doctors and the nurse see the patient periodically. Attendance to support groups is free. Management of arm edema, if present. The feasibility of late breast reconstruction is considered (9).

Stage # 6 – *Recurrence*: Constant psychological support; pain relief; family involvement (10). If necessary, hospitalization. Religious assistance, whenever requested.

In 1993, 576 interviews with the nurse were made and 65 group meetings took place. The LAAPAC volunteers assisted 130 patients during pre and post-operative stages, 27 terminal patients and 16 deaths. They also supplied 53 prostheses. However, the most important part of this work, carried out for the last 12 years, can not be measured in numbers – it is impossible to calculate how much love and dedication have supported this mission whose only objective has always been better quality of life for the patients.

References

1. Singer PA et al. Sex or survival: trade-offs between quality and quantily of life. J. Clin Oncol 1991; 9: 328-334.
2. Halsted WS. The results of radical operations for cure of cancer of the breast. Ann Surg 1907; 46:1-19.
3. Greenspan EM et al. Response of advanced breast carcinoma to the combination of the antimetabolic methotrexate and the alkylating agent thio-TEPA. Mt Sinai J Med 1963; 33:1-26.
4. Haagensen CD. Diseases of the Breast. Philadelphia: WB Saunders, 1986.
5. Kiebert GM, Welvaart K, Kievit J. Psychological effects of routine follow up on cancer patients after surgery. Eur J Surg 1993; 159:601-607.

6. Menke CH, Rabin EG, Biazus JV. Working pilot plan for a multidisciplinary team in the prevention of breast cancer. Revista do HCPA 1982; 2:75-83.
7. Abidim MR, Durham K, Dooley WC. Use of immediate postoperative mastectomy prostheses. Ann Plastic Surg 1991; 27:387-388.
8. Wingate L et al. Rehabilitation of the mastectomy patient: a randomized, blind, prospective study. Arch Phys Med Rehabil 1989; 21-24.
9. Mc Craw JB et al. Breast reconstruction following mastectomy. In: Bland KI, Copeland EM. The breast: comprehensive managemment of benign and malignant diseases. Philadelphia: WB Saunders, 1991; 656-693.
10. Portenoy RK. Cancer pain management. Sem Oncol 1993; 20:19-35.

IV. Plastic surgery

Mastology - Breast Diseases
A.S.S. Figueira Fo et al., editors.

Reconstruction of the breast: Types and techniques

Antonio S.S. Figueira Fo., Professor of Mastology at the Faculty of Medical Sciences, University of Pernambuco, Head of the Department of Mastology of the IMIP (Institute of Child Health of Pernambuco). President of the Deliberative Council of the Brazilian Society of Mastology. Director of the Breast Institute of Recife. Founder Member and President of the Senologic International Society. **Henrique M. Salvador-Silva**, President of the Scientific Committee of the Brazilian Society of Mastology, Head of the Breast Unit, Materdei Hospital, Belo Horizonte, Brazil. **Ezio Novais-Dias**, Head of the Breast Unit, Department of Gynaecology, São Rafeal Hospital, Salvador Brazil.

Introduction

Women who have undergone a mastectomy experience a psychological state similar to those resulting from the loss of a loved one.

Studies such as that of Goin (1982) show that these reactions are initially of denial (this cannot have happened to me), followed by revolt (why was I chosen), and subsequently despair, in which the women experience a mixture of feelings like sadness, hurt and regret. Finally there comes the reality of daily existence, the certainty of the irreparable loss, with emotional acceptance.

Reconstruction of the breast enhances the quality of life of mastectomized women since, by reducing the physical deformity, it reduces the psychological trauma.

Another important feature of breast reconstruction is, in a sense, the early diagnosis because, on learning of the possibility of having their breast reconstructed, women will see their physician sooner as there is no longer the dread of mutilation (Figueira, 1983).

Historical background

The earliest attempt at breast reconstruction occurred just over a century ago when in 1896 Vincez Czerny in Germany sought to reconstruct the breast of a patient who had undergone a subcutaneous mastectomy, using a lipoma from the lumbar region with satisfactory results (Figueira, 1985).

Tansini, in 1906 in Italy, concerned about the size of the surgical wounds caused by mastectomy, which at that time resected a considerable amount of skin, because, of the locally quite advanced state of the breast tumours, brilliantly employed a myocutaneous flap from the latissimus dorsi to close these wounds. It should be emphasized that Tansini's intention was not to reconstruct the breast but merely to fill the void resulting from the surgical wound.

A number of Tansini's contemporaries also used flaps from the vicinity of the breast. Quinu (1986) performed an abdominal flap transposition to reconstruct the breast wall and Legueu performed rotation of this flap for the same purpose (Davies, 1919).

In 1925, Sauerbruch (Cocke, 1977) used a contralateral breast flap to cover major chest defects caused by radiotherapy, but this results left much to be desired because the mammary gland ended up practically in the middle of the chest. Years later Reinhard (1932) split the contralateral breast down the middle and transferred one half to the mastectomized area, using it to create a neobreast. The remaining half would also give rise to another neobreast. This operation was carried out in various stages and the results were reasonable for that time.

Table 1. Historical background

Year	Author	Contribution
1893	Czerny	Lipoma from the dorsal region for reconstructing breast
1896	Tansini	Rotation of latissimus dorsi flap to breast region
1896	Quinu	Transposition of abdominal flap for reconstruction of breast wall
1899	Legueu	Rotation of abdominal flap to chest wall
1911	Reinard	Abdominal flap
1912	D'Este	Chest flap
1913	Weichert	Transabdominal flap
1924	Kleinschmidt	Abdomino-axillary flap
1925	Sauerbruch	Contralateral breast flap
1932	Reinhard	Bipartition of opposite breast

Adapted from Cocke Jr., W.M., 1977

The bipartition of the opposite breast was popularized in the sixties and seventies by Alexander et al. (1967) and Pontes (1973), with better but, by current standards, unsatisfactory results.

Tables 1 and 2 show some of the contributions made by surgeons over the previous decades to the refinement of breast reconstruction.

In 1974, concerned about many cases of ulcers caused by radiotherapy following mastectomy and about the poor results obtained from the use of free and pedicled skin grafts for covering these ulcers, Olivari 'discovered' the latissimus dorsi myocutaneous flap, using it initially with a similar intent to Tansini, namely to cover extensive chest wounds. Olivari (1976) subsequently went on to use a silicone prosthesis under the flap and in this way achieved very good contours. According to the author himself (1986, 1989), he became aware of Tansini's studies only when Maxwell's paper on them (1978) was published.

Bostwick (May 1978) succeeded in an effective and innovative fashion in systematizing the use of the latissimus dorsi myocutaneous flap in breast reconstruction and in popularizing the technique worldwide. The development represents the start of the era of the third-generation flaps, that is flaps using skin, subcutaneous tissue and muscle. The cosmetic results became excellent.

In 1977, Dreaver (1981, 1986) in Uruguay, described a pioneering technique for breast reconstruction using a vertical ellipsis of skin and adipose tissue coupled to one of the anterior rectus abdominous muscle which, after having its lower vascular pedicle (inferior epigastric artery) ligated, could be transported to the mammary region, without endangering its vascular viability. As the technique was first published in a little-known Uruguayan medical journal his name is seldom remembered as one of the pioneers of breast reconstruction with the myocutaneous flap from the anterior rectus abdominous muscle, but there is no doubt that his studies represent the start of a new era in surgical reconstruction of the breast.

Table 2. Historical background

Year	Author	Contribution
1937	Webster	Thoraco-epigastric pedicled tube
1939	Gilles	Breast reconstruction with pedicled tube
1950	Yannilos	Pedicled tube of contralateral breast
1951	Converse	Jump flap
1953	Whalen	Chest wall reconstruction with bipartition of opposite breast
1953	Bames	Skin fat grafts
1953	Longrace	Skin flaps for breast reconstruction
1963	Zavaleto	Use of greater omentum for breast reconstruction
1963	Cronin	Silicone implant in enlargement mastoplasty
1967	Edgerton	Use of pedicled flap with etherone sponge implant
1971	Snyderman	Silicone implant for breast reconstruction
1974	Furlow	Use of omentum with prosthesis for breast reconstruction
1975	Fujino	Use of microvascular anastomosis in breast reconstruction

Adapted from Cocke Jr., W.M., 1977

Hartramp et al (1982) described a new procedure for breast reconstruction following mastectomy. The technique, which is in fact a refinement of Dreaver's consist of the use of an 'island of skin and fat' attached to the anterior rectus abdominous muscle. They demonstrated clinically that an ellipsis of skin and subcutaneous cellular tissue resected in an abdominal dermolipectomy remains viable if it is attached to just one of the anterior rectus abdominous muscles, even when the vascular pedicle of the inferior epigastric artery is ligated. They also proved that this myocutaneos flap could be transposed to the region and its vascularization would be preserved by the upper epigastric artery.

The major contribution of Hartrampf, the person who has devoted the most effort to this technique, was his demonstration that the flap described in a pioneering fashion by Dreaver could be used in a transverse fashion.

Figueira (1984, 1985), concerned about the stigma caused by elliptic scars following postmastectomy reconstructions, has developed a technique using the incision of a reduction mastoplasty for carrying out the mastectomy and the use of dermomuscular flap from anterior rectus abdominous muscle.

Modern mastology is increasingly concerned to ensure that the woman with breast cancer is mutilated less and less, which is why both breast reconstruction and conservative treatment today form an integral part of the planning of the treatment of this disease. Over the past two decades, with the development of cutaneous expanders, the appearance of more suitable inert materials for reconstruction, and the use of autogenous tissue, together with the refinement of microsurgical techniques for ensuring an adequate blood supply, the cosmetic and functional results of reconstructed breasts have shown a considerable improvement.

In this chapter we shall describe a number of techniques employed for the reconstruction of the breast.

Selection of patients for breast reconstruction using myocutaneous or dermomuscular flaps

In addition to the oncological indications and contraindications for treatment, other factors should be taken into account in the selection of candidates for a breast reconstruction using myocutaneous or dermomuscular flaps from the anterior rectus muscle of the abdomen.

Patients in any more of the following categories should not be submitted to surgery:

1) Patients with little panniculus adiposis below the umbelical scar, which would make it impossible to obtain a suitable flap and would require the implanting of silicone prosthesis.

2) Heavy smokers. The smoking habit should be abandoned at least four months prior to surgery. A higher incidence of necrosis of the pedicled flaps has been observed in chronic smokers as compared to non-smokers.

3) Individuals suffering from chronic diseases (diabetes, rebellious arterial hypertension, peripheral vascular disease, etc.)

4) Obesity. Very obese women possess abundant panniculus adiposus and usually an atrophied anterior rectus muscle of the abdomen, which endangers the viability (blood supply) of the flap.

5) Multiple abdominal scars, especially in patients who have undergone an abdominoplasty and those submitted to cholecystectomy by means of a subcostal (Kocher-type) incision that would damage the upper epigastric artery and its dependent arteries.

6) Emotionally disturbed patients who expect a miracle from the surgery and fail to understand the technical constraints.

Immediate or late

There is some controversy as to when breast reconstruction should be performed, whether immediately after mastectomy or later. The main criticism of performing it immediately is based on the fear that the presence of the prosthesis or flap could interfere with the detection and treatment of local recurrences, which could consequently compromise the patient's survival.

The authors who advocate late reconstruction of the breast stipulate time limits, mostly in random fashion, ranging from six months to five years. It so happens that some patients with malignant EC IIb tumours, candidates, in accordance with the oncological indications described earlier in this book, for an immediate reconstruction, would not survive for five years and would thus live the remaining few years of their lives in a mutilated condition.

Other authors advise late reconstruction of the breast because the patients would thereby experience the mutilation and thus better appreciate the limitations of the surgical techniques. Such a posture is nonsensical, for the patients satisfying the selection criteria mentioned above would not have this problem.

Recent studies show that there are no statistically significant differences in survival in patients who have undergone immediate breast reconstruction as compared to those whose reconstruction was performed some time later (Pinotti et al 1991, Patel et al 1993).

The concern on the part of some surgeons that the size of the operation and the need for a preoperative blood transfusion might lead to an increased aggressiveness of the tumour is without foundation. In a Danish study Eickofoff et all (1991) showed that blood transfusions do not increase recurrence rates after surgery for breast cancer.

The conclusion to be drawn from the literature is that, provided oncological criteria are satisfied, breast reconstruction may be performed immediately after mastectomy without prejudicing the patient's survival.

Preoperative care

An evaluation should be carried out prior to surgery, including a meticulous physical examination, dosage of liver function and tumour markers, ultrasonography of the liver, chest X-ray (PA and profile), bone scan and mammogram. This evaluation is designed to detect any distant metastasis, the presence of which will cause the postponement or cancellation of the reconstruction.

Types and techniques

Implantation of a prosthesis

This is without doubt the simplest of techniques, since it consists of placing a silicone prosthesis under the mastectomy flaps. The major problem with this procedure is the high incidence (ranging from 15 to 70%) of capsular contracture, which invariably results in asymmetry of the breast and consequently a poor cosmetic result in the end. A breast reconstructed with silicone can have various formats, sometimes even similar to a billiard ball, and its consistency can be quite hard.

On some occasions in order to minimize these effects the prosthesis is placed under the greater pectoral muscle. The procedure considerably reduces the incidence of capsules, but on the other hand it may cause suffering to its user, because whenever the pectoral muscles are contracted the prosthesis migrates towards the clavicle or axilla.

Another option is to fashion a muscular pouch by suturing the greater pectoral muscle, detached from its insertion in the rib cage, with the anterior rectus muscle of the abdomen sectioned 10 cm proximally and folded back on itself.

Expanders

Neumann (1957) was the first to recognize the possibility of expanding the soft parts of the human body. He came to this conclusion on the basis of the examples of the African who expanded their lips by inserting wood which produced an enlarged tissue mass. He showed through his studies that the expansion of cutaneous tissues produces a real growth of the latter, and that enlargement is not produced merely by their elasticity.

The main purpose of skin expanders is to increase the amount of tissue in the region of the mastectomy, thereby forming a pouch, so that when the tissue is replaced by the definitive silicone prosthesis there will be a diminution in the incidence of capsular contracture.

The expander, which is a silicone pouch with an antireflux valve, is placed under the greater pectoral muscle after the mastectomy. A quantity of 60-80 ml saline solution is percutaneously injected through this valve every three or four days until a volume of 600 ml is reached. The expander is then emptied, withdrawn and replaced by a silicone prosthesis, the size of which will range from 200 to 400 mm in accordance with the size of the contralateral breast.

Better results have been achieved with expanders than with the simple silicone implant because the greater the amount of skin, the less chance there is of capsular contracture.

Epiploon implant

This technique consists of the exteriorization of the pedicled epiploon through the epigastric orifice and its fixation in the region of the mastectomy, following which it is covered by the skin available in this area. The complexity of this procedure, allied to unsatisfactory cosmetic results, led to its abandonment.

Latissimus dorsi myocutaneous flap

An island of skin, coupled to the latissimus dorsi muscle that is detached from its distal insertion, is totally rotated and positioned in the region of the mastectomy, being supplied by the vascular thoracodorsal pedicle. As this island is very narrow and has little panniculus adiposis the implantation of a silicone prosthesis is always required for shaping the neobreast.

This technique, which had its heyday before the advent of expanders and the myocutaneous flap of the anterior rectus muscle of the abdomen, has fallen into complete desuetude and is nowadays employed only in exceptional cases.

Disadvantages of the technique

1. The patient is in the lateral decubitus position at the start of the operation and is preparatively placed in supination.
2. The portion of skin is very small, larger portions being more easily obtainable by using skin expanders.
3. The need for a silicone implant, which under a small island of skin occasionally causes a capsular contracture.
4. The texture and colour of the dorsal skin are different from those of the anterior chest wall.

Myocutaneous flap of the anterior rectus abdominous muscle

The anatomical basis of the breast reconstruction technique using a myocutaneous flap of the anterior rectus abdominous muscle is the recognition of the axial vascularization of the muscle by the upper and lower epigastric arteries, and the fact that the latter originate perforating branches through the aponeurosis that will supply the entire flap (Daher, 1982).

This technique consists in transposing an ellipsis of skin from the infra-umbelical region, coupled to the anterior rectus muscle of the abdomen, through a sternal tunnel, to the region of the mastectomy. This flap will be supplied by the upper epigastric vascular pedicle. Holmstron (1979) showed that from the umbilicus to the pubis there are three major perforating vessels that are sufficient to maintain this vascularization.

Advantages

1. The operation is performed with the patient in the supine position.
2. There is no need for a silicone prosthesis to be implanted.
3. The amount of skin is immense, making it nearly always possible to mould the neobreast to the size of the contralateral breast.
4. There are no differences in texture or skin colour.

Dermomuscular flap of the anterior rectus abdominal muscle

However satisfactory the results achieved with myocutaneous flaps may be (and excellent results have been obtained), a women will always, owing to the elliptical incisions, whether they be horizontal, vertical or oblique, bear the stigma of having undergone a mastectomy and had her breast reconstructed (Figueira, 1984). This stigma is even worse when the results are unsatisfactory.

To eliminate the scars Figueira (1984, 1985) has adopted a new approach to breast reconstruction using the myocutaneous flap.

The incision of radical or radical modified mastectomy follows the same lines of incision as those of a Pitanguy-type reduction mastectomy (1962, 1964, 1967), respecting the oncological limits and dispensing with the classical elliptical incision.

The technique for rotating the myocutaneous flap is the conventional one. Following its migration to the breast region, the flap is moulded and the excess skin discarded. The tissue remaining from the flap is then decorticated, that is, all the epidermis is removed, leaving only the dermis.

The skin left over from the mastectomy is moulded over the flap, which is now dermomuscular rather than myocutaneous, and which will function as a natural prosthesis.

The final outcome is identical to that of a reduction mastoplasty associated with an abdominoplasty, resulting in the disappearance of the stigma.

Areolomammilar complex

The fashioning of the areolomammilar complex (AMC) may be performed immediately or some time after mastectomy. The AMC of the mastectomized breast may be used as a free graft provided there is no tumour involved (Parry et al. 1977, Pinotti, 1983), which is verified by frozen section of the AMC during the operation.

When it proves impossible to use the AMC, part of the contralateral areola and breast may be employed, or even skin from the inner root of the thigh for the areola and the pulp of the fifth toe for the nipple.

References

1. Alexander JE, Block LI. Breast reconstruction after mastectomy. Plast. Reconstr. Surg. 40:175, 1969.
2. Bostwich JR, Vasconez LO, Juekiewick MJ. Breast reconstruction following radical mastectomy. Plast. Reconst. Surg. 6:862, 1978.
3. Cocke WM. Breast reconstruction following mastectomy for carcinoma. Little, Brown and

Co. Boston, 1977.

4. Daher JC. As reconstruções mamárias com o retalho miocurâneo abdominal. Anais do Simpósio Brasileiro de Abdominoplastia, São Paulo, 144, 1982.
5. Davies, JE. Plastic surgery: Its principles and practice. P. Blakiston Sons and Co. Philadelphia, 1919.
6. Dreaver MJ. Total breast reconstruction. Ann. Plast. Surg. 7:54, 1981/
7. Dreaver MJ. Comunicação pessoal. Recife, 1986.
8. Eickhoff JH, Anderson J, Leyburn C. Preoperative blood transfusion does not promote recurrence and death after mastectomy for breast cancer. Br. J. Surg. 78:1358, 1991.
9. Figueira Fo ASS. Reconstrução mamária. Técnica do retalho miocutâneo do reto anterior do abdômen. Anais so curso de mastologia da XXVII Jornada Brasileira de ginecologia e abstetrícia. Fortaleza, 40, 1983.
10. Figueira Fo ASS. Mastectomia radical seguida de reconstrução imediata com retalho miogorduroso do reto do abdômen (Técnica pessoal). Ango 17 (1):47, 1984.
11. Figueira Fo ASS. Mastectomia radical seguida de reconstrução imediata com retalho dermomuscular do reto anterior do abdômen. Rev. Bras., Cir. 75 (4):313, 1985.
12. Figueira Fo ASS. Mastectomia radical com reconstrução imediata com reto anterior do abdômen (Técnica Pessoal). Anais do XXII congresso Brasileiro de cirurgia plástica. Editora Aplub. Porto Alegre, 544, 1985.
13. Goin MK. Psychological reaction to surgery of the breast. Clin. Plast. Surg. 9(3):347, 1982.
14. Hartrampf CR, Scheflan M, Black PW. Breast reconstruction with a transverse abdominal island flap. Plast. Recons. Surg. 69(2), 216, 1982.
15. Holmstron H. The free abdominoplasty flap and its use in breast reconstruction. In: Ely JF (Ed). Transactions of the Seventh International Congress of Plastic and Reconstructive Surgery. Cartograff. São Paulo, 617, 1979.
16. Maxwell GP, Steuber PH, Hoopes JE. A free latissimus dorsi myocutaneous flap. Plast. Reconst. Surg. 62:462, 1978.
17. Neumann CG. The expansion of an area of skin by progressive distension of a subcutaneous balloon. Plast. Reconst. Surg. 19:124, 1957.
18. Olivari N. The latissimus dorsi flap. Brit. J. Plast. Surg. 29:126, 1976.
19. Olivari N. Comunicação Pessoal. Frankfurt, 1986.
20. Olivari N. The latissimus dorsi flap and breast reconstruction. In: Bohmert H, Leis Jr HP, Jackson IT (Eds). Breast cancer conservative and reconstructive surgery. Georg Thiene Verlag, New York, 252, 1989.
21. Patel RT, Webster DJT, Mansel R, Hughes LE. Is immediate postmastectomy reconstruction safe in the long term? Eur. J. Surg. Onc. 19:372, 1993.
22. Pinott JA, Teixeira LC, Kepke EM, Baroudi R, Matta SM. Mastetomia radical com reconstruçã mamária. Uma nova abordagem, terapêtica. In: Pinotti JA, Teixeira LC, Nisida ACT (Eds). Compêndio de mastologia. Editora Manole, São Paulo, 328, 1993.
23. Pitanguy I. Une nouvelle technique de plastic mammaire. Etude de 245 cas consecutifs et presentation d'une technique personelle. Ann. Chir. Plast. 7:199, 1962.
24. Pitanguy I. Hipertrofias mamárias. Trib. Med. 6:33, 1964.
25. Pitanguy I. Surgical treatment of breast hipertrophy. Brit. J. Plast. Surg. 20:78, 1967
26. Pontes, R. Single stage reconstruction of the missing breast. Br. J. Plast. Surg. 26:377, 1973.
27. Reinhard W. Total mastoneoplasty following amputation or the breast. Deutsche Zeische. F. Chir. 236:309, 1932.
28. Tansini I. Sopra il mio nuovo processo di amputazione dela mamella2. Gaz. Med. Ital. 57:141, 1906.

Mastology - Breast Diseases
A.S.S. Figueira Fo et al., editors.

Breast Reconstruction after Mastectomy by Areolar Approach

João Carlos Sampaio Góes, M.D., Ph.D.

Instituto Brasileiro de Controle do Câncer, Av. Brasil, 549, CEP 01430-000, São Paulo – Brazil

Introduction

The immediate breast reconstruction is a fundamental surgery for the psychological balance of the women submitted to radical surgery treatment of the breast cancer. During the last 15 years is has been progressively accepted by surgeons and required by patients. But the remaining scars from the classic modified radical mastectomy bring the stigma of the applied surgical treatment.

Seeking to get the best aesthetical result as possible we propose the mastectomy by areolar approach with immediate breast reconstruction with a transverse abdominal island flap (TRAM). We use a surgical technique that respects all oncological principles, and also allows us to get results that do not show signs of the previous mastectomy.

Material and Method

We have performed this therapeutic-aesthetic approach for the breast cancer in 34 patients with 4 years of follow-up of the first cases.

We have indicated, in the cases that it is imperative, the total exeresis of the mammary gland and that the external cutaneous lining does not need a large excision in the following clinical situations:

1. intraductal "in situ" or invasive carcinoma
2. comedo carcinoma
3. lobular "in situ"carcinoma
4. ductal multifocal invasive carcinoma with small tumors distant from skin more than 2 cms.

The cutaneous excision is circular and could be done near the areolar or with a bigger margin of excision depending upon the breast volume and upon the oncological necessity.

The glandular dissection should observe the sub-cutaneous level equal to the radical mastectomy, reaching the mammary gland margins and avoiding the extension of the dissection, to keep the positioning of the external cutaneous lining with relation to the thorax.

The inframammary fold must be preserved to allow the ideal positioning of the reconstructed breast, reaching the natural ptosis of the mentioned breast.

The axilar dissection (lymphadenectomy) is performed through the same areolar

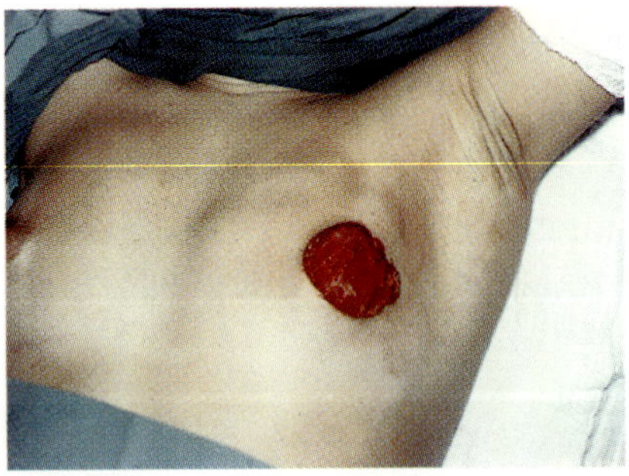

Figure 1a. Radical mastectomy modified by areolar approach, in a 37-year-old patient.

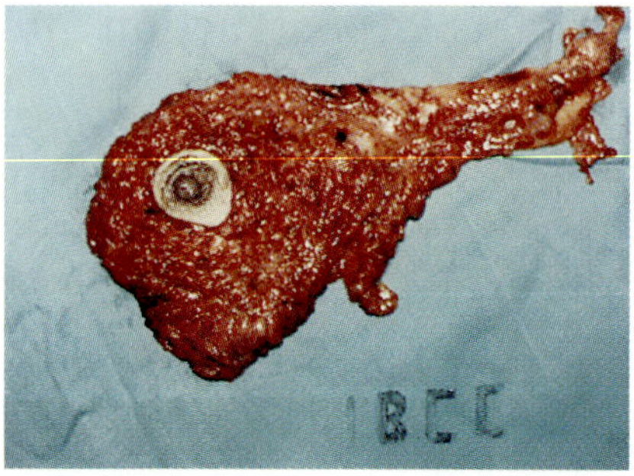

Figure 1b. Surgical specimen removed in monoblock, showing cutaneous periareolar skin and total lymphadenectomy.

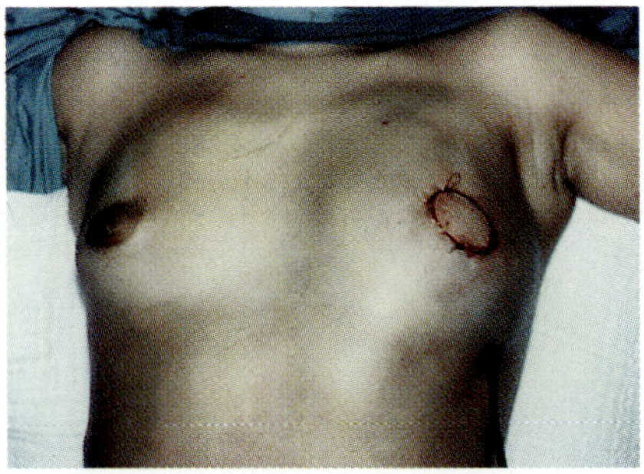

Figure 1c. Immediate reconstruction wth bipedicle TRAM, with circular island skin in substitution of the areola.

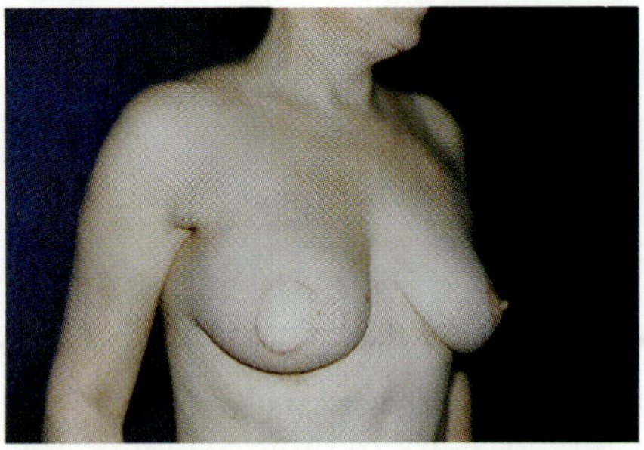

Figure 2a. First surgery of breast reconstruction with bipedicle TRAM after mastectomy by areolar approach.

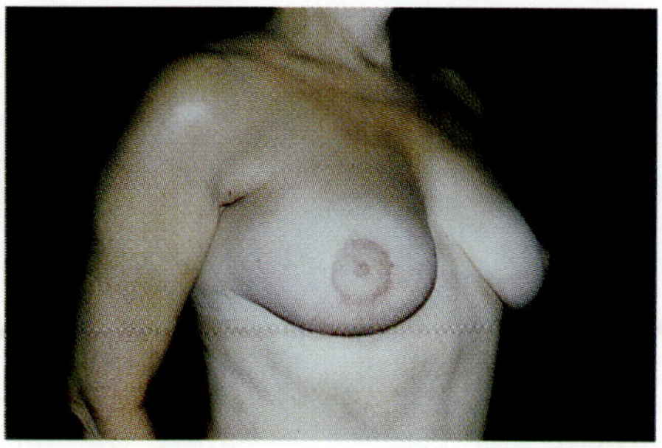

Figure 2b. Second surgery performed neoareoloplasty with skin graft over the mastectomy circular scar. One-year follow-up in a 54-year-old patient.

approach with the help of retractors with local illumination achieving the three levels of the axilar lymphonodus. Within this procedure we avoid axilar scar.

The reconstruction is performed with the rotation of a transverse abdominal bipedicle flap, positioned with the umbelical area on the lower hemisphere to give greater projection in that pole.

The skin flap is totally removed, maintaining only the small circular area with approximately 4 cms diameter to replace the removed areola by the mastectomy.

Cutaneous closing is done by recovering the flap, which exactly fulfils the removed mammary volume, using purse string suture (round block) with mersilene-20 to eliminate tension from cutaneous suture.

During a second surgery we performed the refinements of the shape of the reconstructed breast applying the liposuction and neoareoloplasty with skin graft over the circular area of the skin flap, hidding this way the remaining scar.

Results and Discussion

The obtained results were considered excelent because the reconstructed breast did not present mastectomy scar. Resulting scar is of high-quality and only appears at the areolar area. TRAM flap allows to get a reconstructed, natural, smooth and warm breast and in several cases with certain sensibility. The surgery is definitive allowing further retouches.

The immediate reconstruction brings great aesthetical advantages as it avoids the mastectomy healing process, that causes axilar fibrosis, cutaneous retraction in the surgical area, which considerably minimizes the amount of skin to recover the used flap, and also allows breast shaping with soft and natural limits.

References

1. Benelli, L.: A new periareolar mammaplasty: the “round table” technique. Aesth Plast Surg 14:93-100, 1990.
2. Góes, J.C.S.: Correção imediata da mama após ressecções glandulares amplas. Transactions of the XII Congresso Brasileiro de Cirurgia Plástica, Porto Alegre, 1976.
3. Góes, J.S.Jr.: Diagnóstico radiológico das doenças da mama. São Paulo, Artes Médicas, 1977.
4. Góes, J.C.S.: Patologias da mama. Tumores benignos e malignos. In Melega, Zanini & Psillakis: Cirurgia Plástica Reparadora e Estética. Rio de Janeiro, MEDSI, 1988, p.713.
5. Góes, J.C.S.: Periareolar mammaplasty: double skin technique. Rev Soc Bras Cir Plast 4:55-63,1989.
6. Góes, J.C.S.: Periareolar mammaplasty: double skin technique. Breast Dis 4: 111-127, 1991.
7. Georgiade, N.G.: Aesthetic Breast Surgery. St. Louis, CV Mosby, 1976, p.10.

8. Hartrampf, C.R., Scheflan M. and Black P.: Breast Reconstruction following mastectomy with a transverse abdominal island flap. Anatomical and clinical observations. Plast Reconst Surg 69:216, 1982
9. Hartrampf, C.R. (ed): Breast Reconstruction with living tissue. Norfolk, Hampton Press, 1990.

Mastology - Breast Diseases
A.S.S. Figueira Fo et al., editors.

BREAST CANCER DIAGNOSIS AND TREATMENT AFTER AUGMENTATION MAMMOPLASTY

Melvin J. Silverstein, M.D., Medical Director and Senior Surgical Oncologist,
The Breast Center, 14624 Sherman Way, Van Nuys, California 91405, USA

Abstract: Augmentation mammoplasty reduces the accuracy of mammography and the amount of measurable breast tissue that can be visualized. Augmented women with breast cancer are more likely to present with palpable tumors rather than occult lesions. The survival advantage gained by early mammographic diagnosis is lost in women augmented with silicone-gel-filled implants.

Introduction: In 1986, I was given the opportunity at a meeting of The Los Angeles Plastic Surgical Society to present our data on the mammographic effect of augmentation mammoplasty with silicone-gel-filled implants. The data clearly showed that for most augmented patients, mammography was compromised (an average 28% reduction in measurable area) and if that were true, it meant that breast cancer might not be diagnosed at the earliest possible time. While most plastic surgeons listened with concern, some were clearly angry, and they verbalized it. Others wrapped napkins around their fists to showed how tangential views could be taken that would show the whole "napkin".

In 1987, our group began publishing a series of papers, some dealing with the quality of mammography in the augmented patient, others dealing with the treatment of breast cancer in the augmented patient [1-6]. By 1990, our data and data addressing a variety of other potential implant problems such as silicone leakage, implant rupture, immune disorders, infection, carcinogenicity, etc. began making its way to the media. By early 1992, media coverage of the "silicone problem" was an almost daily event in the United States. By mid 1992, silicone-gel-filled implants had been withdrawn from the market for cosmetic surgery except for tightly controlled clinical trials. The two plastic surgeons at The Breast Center who were doing more than 100 augmentations a year in the late 1980s, did 16 in 1992, all with saline-filled implants.

It has been estimated that more than 1.5 million North American women have undergone augmentation mammoplasty with silicone-gel-filled implants. Numerous studies have now confirmed that silicone-gel-filled implants interfere with mammography in just about all patients. This may be due to compression of breast tissue, capsular contracture, or the implant simply getting in the way of the x-ray beam. The minimum interference is seen in patients with small retropectoral implants and with no capsular contracture [6]. The worst interference is seen in women with larger, subglandular implants and with severe capsular contracture. Since the earliest and most curable breast cancers are nonpalpable (occult) lesions found only by mammography, augmentation mammoplasty, by interfering with mammography, could potentially delay the diagnosis of cancer in many patients when compared with the optimum time of diagnosis for that particular patient.

What I have decided to do here is to bring you up to date on our series of augmented patients who later developed breast cancer and to compare our augmented patients with a number of other reported series of nonaugmented breast cancer patients.

Data: From 1981 through March 1994, 63 women who had previously undergone augmentation mammoplasty, an average of 8.6 years earlier, were treated for breast cancer at The Breast Center. Their average age was 44 years. Fifty-four patients (86%) had unilateral infiltrating carcinomas; nine (14%) had noninvasive (*in situ*) lesions. Fifty-seven of 62 (90%) lesions were palpable. Six (10%) cancers were nonpalpable, discovered mammographically in the absence of physical findings. **Prebiopsy mammography was performed in 51 patients with palpable lesions and failed to reveal an abnormality in 20, a false negative rate of 39%.** Twenty-six patients (41%) were treated with mastectomy, the remaining 37 (59%) with breast preservation. Fifty-four patients underwent axillary node dissection; 27 (50%) had lymph node metastases (if one assumes that the nine undissected patients had negative nodes, the rate of nodal positivity drops to 43%). There have been eight recurrences (13%): one local and seven metastatic. All seven (11%) patients with metastatic disease have died. The 7-year breast cancer-specific probability of survival is 74%. The median follow-up is 70 months. The following table compares five different groups of breast cancer patients.

	BC Augmented	BC Palpable	LA Tumor Registry	NSABP B-06	**BC Screening**
No. Patients	63	1183	5876	1857	**481**
Mean Age	44	53	50	50++	**55**
% *in situ*	15%	8%	7%	4%	**48%**
% Palpable	90%	100%	95%	99%	**0%**
% Positive Nodes	43%	39%	43%	38%	**6%**
7 yr. Survival	74%	77%	75%	76%	**98%**

Discussion: The first four groups: Breast Center augmented, Breast Center palpable, LA Tumor Registry, and NSABP B-06 are all quite similar. Most of the lesions are palpable. *In situ* lesions range from 4-15%, nodal positivity ranges from 37-43%, and the 7-year probability of survival from 74-77%. These lesions represent the typical, average, generally palpable breast cancers found in America today. They are all statistically about the same. The augmented patients in our series do not do any better or any worse than the three other groups with predominantly palpable cancers. And that is the point: most augmented patients with breast cancer present with palpable lesions. But today, the state-of-the-art in breast cancer diagnosis is mammography - a tool that finds nonpalpable lesions.

When we compare the augmented patients or any of the three other groups mentioned above with patients whose cancers were discovered by mammography, there is no comparison. The screen-detected group has lower nodal positivity, more *in situ* lesions, and significantly higher survival rates at every point along the Kaplan-Meier curve. You may say that we are comparing apples and oranges, that it is an unfair comparison, that we have not taken into account the biases cause by self-selection, lead-time, over-diagnosis, and differences in tumor growth time. And you are right, it is an unfair comparison.

But this is 1994! The best tool for early breast cancer diagnosis continues to be mammography. Any elective cosmetic procedure that potentially interferes with mammography must be questioned. Women should be informed of the comparative mammographic and oncologic data, and they should have the right to make the final decision about whether or not they undergo augmentation mammoplasty. It is conceivable that in a given individual, the emotional and psychological benefits of augmentation will far outweigh the potential risks of the procedure. But any woman whose first concern is the earliest possible detection of a breast cancer should not be augmented.

References:

1. Silverstein MJ, Handel N, Steyskal R, et al. Augmentation mammoplasty with silicone-gel-filled implants: Its effect on breast cancer diagnosis and prognosis. Proc. Am. Soc. Clin Oncol. 1987;6:51.
2. Silverstein MJ, Handel N, Steyskal R, et al. Breast cancer in women after augmentation mammoplasty. Arch Surg. 1988; 123:681-685.
3. Silverstein MJ, Handel N, Gamagami p, et al. Mammographic measurements before and after augmentation mammoplasty. Plastic Reconst Surg. 1990;86:1118-1122.
4. Silverstein MJ, Gamagami P, Gierson ED, et al. Breast cancer diagnosis and prognosis in women augmented with silicone-gel-filled implants. Cancer 1990;66:97-101.
5. Silverstein MJ, Handel N, Gamagami P, et al. Breast cancer diagnosis and prognosis in women following augmentation with silicone-gel-filled prostheses. Eur. J. Cancer 1992;28(2/3):635-640.
6. Handel N, Silverstein MJ, Gamagami P, et al. Factors affecting mammographic visualization after augmentation mammoplasty. JAMA 1992:268:1913-1917.

Mastology - Breast Diseases
A.S.S. Figueira Fo et al., editors.

Esthetic Surgery and Breast Conservation

Jorge V. Biazus, Carlos H. Menke. José A. Cavalheiro, Eliane G. Rabin

Breast Unit – Hospital de Clínicas de Porto Alegre – UFRGS – Brazil

Abstract

Breast conservation in the treatment of breast cancer is a world wide discussed question. Since that it was shown that breast conservation had the same or even better prognosis than radical mastectomy, many conservative surgical techniques were created. We were encouraged to develop a new technique using some principles of plastic surgery and the oncologic criteria to treat surgically breast cancer. This procedure is called Oncologic Mammaplasty. It was performed in 96 patients in which standard conservative surgery plus radiotherapy would result in a significant asymmetry. We believe that this surgery will provide a safe treatment of breast cancer with a very good cosmesis and equilibrium of the breast.

Since Veronesi et al (1,2) demonstrated that breast conservation had the same – or even better performance than Halsted mastectomy, a lot of new surgical techniques for breast conservation have been developed to deal with it (2).

Today, breast conservation is the best choice for a surgical approach in the early stages of to this disease. It can be done even to a selected group of patients submitted to primary chemotherapy with a reduction of the tumor size (3).

Many papers came out dealing with the psychological morbidity associated with breast cancer (4,5,6,7,8) showing that breast conservation led to a less negative body-image and best social adjustment.

These previous statements led us to develop a surgical approach that could improve the esthetic results alleviating the psychological distress. We were encouraged to mix basic concepts of plastic surgery and oncologic principles to create a surgical procedure named 'Oncologic Mammaplasty'.

Eligible cases for Oncologic Mammaplasty must fulfill this basic principles:

1. Patient's desire
2. Adequate clinical stage
3. Oncologic safety
4. Individual surgical planning

Once the basic criteria are met, we go through a meticulous pre-operative planning, where some surgical aspects shoud be well defined:

A – The treatment of the disease

1. A wide tumor ressection
2. Complete axillary dissection

B – Esthetic Breast conservative surgery

1. Shape
2. Equilibrium
3. Symmetry

4. Global harmony

This association of esthetic and oncologic therapeutic procedures in breast cancer treatment must respect certain features to reach good results:

1. Patient's age
2. Breast size
3. Breast ptosis
4. Tumor size
5. Tumor site
6. Tumor/Breast ratio
7. Previous scar
8. Glandular structure
   a. fibroglandular predominance
   b. liposubstitution predominance
9. Skin quality – good or poor elasticity

The correct evaluation of this features play an important role in the results of the procedure. Good cosmesis will only be achieved if the surgical planning was able to select the best surgical technique for a specific situation. It means that we have to individualize each case, each treatment.

The tumor size/site and the breast/tumor ratio are the main stands for planning the surgery. Generically, we can state that for tumors located in the upper quadrants we choose one of the inferior pedicules techiniques of breast reconstruction, while for those located in the lower quadrants the superior pedicules are preferable, both followed by a reduction in the contralateral breast.

The periareolar approach can be used whenever feasible, especially in young patients with good skin and fibroglandular predominant tissue.

We consider that the adequate moment to perform the oncologic mammaplasty is during the primary surgical treatment. There are many advantages to doing so:

1. One single hospitalar admission
2. One step surgery/anesthesia
3. Cost reduction
4. Good motivation and immediate secondary gain
5. Better body-image
6. Alleviate immediate psychological morbidity
7. Rapid psychosocial adjustment

Firmly, we believe that oncologic mammaplasty should be discussed with the patients as a good alternative to minimize the tragical effects of breast cancer in the woman's life as a whole (sexual, psychological, professional etc).

This proposal is based on an experience of 96 cases in seven years. The deformity and asymmetry resulting from standard Breast Conservation and Radiotherapy lead us to think in this esthetical way. As far as we are concerned, we believe that breast conservation have to present results as follows:

1. Treatment of breast cancer as itself
2. Good local control
3. Good cosmesis

Breast conservation and immediate reconstruction and an adequate esthetic procedure helps the patients with breast cancer go through it with a better body-image, better psychosocial adjustament and having a better quality of life.

References

1. Veronesi V., Sanozzir R., Del Vecchio M et al. Comparing radical mastectomy with quadrantectomy, axillary dissection, and radiotherapy in pacients with small cancer of the breast. N Engle J. Med 1981, 305:6-11.
2. Veronesi V, Salvadori B., Luini A. et al. Conservative treatment of early breast cancer. Long term]results of 1232 cases treated with quadrantectomy, axillary dissection and radiotherapy. Ann Surg. 1990, 211:250-259.
3. Fischer B, Bauer M., Marsolese R. et al. Five year results of a randomized clinical trial comparning total mastectomy and segmental mastectomy with and without radiation in the treatment of breast cancer. N. Engl. J. Med. 1985, 312:665-673.
4. Sneenw K.C., Aaronson N.K., Yarnold J.R. et al. Cosmetics and functional outcome of breast conserving treatment for early stage breast cancer 2. Relationship with psicosocial function. Radiother Oncol, 1992, nov. 25(3), 160-166.
5. Lee M.S., Love S.B., Mitchell J.B. et al. Mastectomy or conservation for early breast cancer: psychological morbidity. Eur J Cancer 1992, 28 A(8-9), 1340-1344.
6. Hall A., Fallowfield L. Psychological outcome of treatment for early breast cancer: a review. Stress Medicine 1989, vol. 5, 167-175.
7. Fallowfield L. et al. Effects of breast conservation on Psychological morbidity associated with diagnosis and treatment of breast cancer Br Med J 293:1331-1334, nov 22, 1986.
8. Woods, John E. Breast reconstructive:Current state of the Art. Mayo Clin Proc 61:579-585, July 1986.

V. General aspects

Mastology - Breast Diseases
A.S.S. Figueira Fo et al., editors.

Senology as specialty

Lydia Ioannidou-Mouzaka MD, PhD

Assos. Professor at University of Athens, Medical School, President of the Senologic International Society (S.I.S.), 6, Kifissias Avenue, Athens 115 26 - GREECE

Summary

The article is dealing with the difficult and delicate problem of the recognition of the Senology as Independant Specialty. Senology is not a 'luxury' specialty; it is a specialty similar to many others such as cardiology, hematology, nephrology etc. The question of its recognition may be a long lasting attempt, which will require vigour, intelligence, firmness and dialogue between doctors and goverment representatives. The creation of specialised breast centers should be based on the unity of place and on the unity of action. Furthermore, the gathering under the same roof all those who deal with the breast and also securing under the same roof the operation of all up-to-date equipment will help enormously in this attempt.

Introduction

The publication of this article provides a very good opportunity to present in the open our opinion on such a delicate and debatable subject such as the recognition of Senology as an independant specialty, a subject which concerns all those who are involved seriously and responsibly with breast diseases. This subject concerns all of us, and stands in need of an urgent solution.

'Today, the problem is primarily defined by the women themselves. The woman under examination, would like to receive coherent attention together with the appropriate assistance, well adapted to her person. Frequently, she receives a variety of often totally different opinions, because breasts are the subject of examination of gynaecologists, radiologists, surgeons or oncologists. All this, creates an inconsistent situation, since the breast is not only dealt with by senologists, but it is generally dealt with by various specialists all trapped by the influence of their own specialty, who consequently treat the breast from a fixed point of view. So, the radiologist insists on taking more and more images, the surgeon is inclined to se his scalpel more easily, the gynaecologist tends to analyse the breast from a hormonal stand-point. As far as the oncologists are concerned, they are so engrossed in cancer, that they seem to forget that healthy breasts may exist!!'[1]

Why this discrepency?

'The word Senology does not even appear in the dictionaries, despite the fact that the Medical Establishment has for many years acknowledged many other specialties such as cardiology, dermatology, nephrology or hematology'. It appears that the breast is not considered as important as the heart, the skin or the kidneys'. I strongly believe that time has come to follow the exemple of our colleagues in Argentina and Brazil, where the specialty of Senology has been recognized for many years. More precisely, in Brazil, this specialty of Senology was recognized in 1978, and the chair at the University dates as from 1987.

'Senology' as you very well know is a specialty which deals with the breast without underrating any of its aspects either functional or pathological.'It deals with breast feeding, breast imaging, cancer, ultrasounds, the benign disorders, and the socio-psychological aspects of the woman with out separating the breast from her female personality'. Today, it is well known that the woman's psyche influences her breast and even a prolonged psychological stress implicates for breast cancer development[2]. 'Many women, in despair because of a separation, a bereavement, a divorce, or any contestation of their existence, feel a pain in their breasts and apply for an examination with their hands on their chest holding up their breasts'.

The Senologist, despite his scientific qualifications, must know how to listen to the woman and how to allocate the necessary time, appropriate for each case. It is his own obligation to elicit and pinpoint the real reason which drove the woman to visit him, apart from the typical report that 'She is suffering from mastodynia'. Furthermore, the Senologist must be both, sensible and sensitive. Persons who do not possess sensibility should not be doctors and especially should not be senologists.

Senology exist since 1963

'It is very strange that this specialty 'Senology' which was founded in 1963, has no administrative entity. Neither the Ministers of Public Health, nor the medical associations recognise its necessity. Senology does not exist officially. Nevertheless, many doctors not specialized in this field advertise on the entrance to their surgery that they are Senologists, and it is surprising to note that nobody protests and that the Medical Associations do not interfere'. It is obvious that time has come to establish a specialty which will deal exclusively with the Breast: 'The Senology'.

'Happily, doctors are becoming more and more aware of the absurdity of this situation, and they are reclaiming a more solid formation of a breast medicine, open to everybody. Even if they are general practicioners, radiologists, gynaecologists or belong to other fields many of them wish to orient themselves to Senology'.

The school of the senologic international society

So, in line with this request the Board of Directors together with the members of the Standing Committee of the S.I.S, decided in Oporto, in December 1992, to found the International School of Senology of the SIS. After confronting many unfavourable circumstances, and after overcoming many obstacles and difficulties, thanks to the endless efforts of Prof.J.L.Lamarque, Director of this School, and of his collaborators, the school is due to start its operation in May 1995. The field of action of these new specialists is enormous.

'The breast is a difficult and a very complex field. One must be acquainted with the clinical aspects, the breast imaging together with its radiological techniques; must have a formation in oncology, must be receptive to psychological aspects, and finally must have the knowledge to take the responsibility of making the diagnosis and in case that he is not of surgical formation must be able to orient the patient to therapeutical procedures. In this educational field of Senology we have to be very prudent. The formation must not last a few days or a few 80 weeks as it happens now-a-days. Following the theoretical formation, it is advisable to apply an extensive practical training for at least one year in an endeavour to consolidate the knowledge in practice. Failing to accomplish this, we are at the risk of producing an abundance of inefficient senologists, which is a fact that finally will have an adverse effect on all of us.

If the foundation 903-580 and the starting of the operation of the International School of Senology of the S.I.S has lasted 3 years, you can imagine how long may take the procedure of the establishment and the confirmation of Senology as a Specialty. 'This is a long lasting attempt, which requires vigour, intelligence, firmness and dialogue between doctors and goverment representatives'.

All those elements are fundamental qualities that all we senologists possess, and that is why I am sure that at the end our intensive efforts will have a successful result.

'Senology is not a 'luxury' specialty; it is a specialty similar to many others. That is why, the Senologists who have the will to exist must overcome all sorts of obstacles.We must remain cool and brave. In our struggle, the female population take our side, as it knows very well that their breast deserves complete recognition'.

The need of specialised breast centers

If we want to be successful we must make the neccesary preparations and must take the necessary steps.Every single Senologist must realize that the creation of specific reception structures for breast patients will help enormously in this effort. 'Private or public, specialized breast centers must be established, based on the unity of place and on the unity of action. We must try to gather under the same roof all those who deal with the breast and also to secure under the same roof the operation of all up-to-date equipment applying in every single examination the rules of Quality Control. The dispersion creates a very big system error and at the same time it creates a psychological handicap to the already distressed woman. It is completely irrational and unacceptable to conduct the clinical examination in one place, the mammography or the echography in another and the FNA and the biopsy somewhere else perhaps quite distant from the afore mentioned places. Despite the fact that the breast is an organ in the visible part of the body, and easily accessible for any examination, it hides many diagnostic traps to those who may tend to underestimate it and who try to escape from the generally accepted basic principles.

Breast cancer, in the very beginning displays a deceitful and hypocritic character. Diagnostic pitfalls are common and frequently change. The certitude of a correct diagnosis is the result of a number of examinations which complement one another. Every examination is based on a different source of information.'Hence, mammography informs about the variety of densities of the breast. Ultrasonography detects the variations between the consistence of the tissues. Cytology informs about the nature of the cellules'.

In this way, the simultaneous performance of all relative examinations and the synthesis of the data, provide the necessary information from different views, minimize the possibility of errors, individualise a correct diagnosis and personalise the treatment. All examinations are useful, and they complement each other. None of them is the best or the most specialized. Each one has its place but also its own limitations.

Criticism

I think it is worth mentioning that the Science of Medicine or any medical action or method may in the course of time have experienced different confrontations. Every examination passes through various phases: discovery, controversy, approval or rejection, always in accordance with its results and in accordance with the ideas at that time. All the above, apply also to Senology. I remember during the ten years from 1975 to 1985 the enthusiasm with which breast thermography was met. Today it has almost been completely rejected as a non reliable examination. I also remember on my return home from Strasbourg in 1978 how severely I was criticized by colleagues of various specialties for puncturing breast tumors. Today, 16 years later the breast is being punctured by Senologists or by other physicians, not connected with Senology. During the 1970's Mammography met with tremendous opposition, because of the consequences of radiation. Its use was coming to a halt as happened with xerography. On the contrary, today, Mammography is recommended to be effected yearly after the age of 50 and it is utilised even before the age of 50.

Breast Ultrasounds have also reached the same level of success. While at the very beginning ultrasounds were used exclusively to distinguish cystic or solid formations, today their use and acceptance has reached such a high level of success that two years ago the International School for Breast Ultrasound was founded in order to meet this method's requirements.

In every examination there is bound to be a percentage of 'false negative' results to a certain degree. This is the reason why various examinations are required to supplement each other in such a way that the percentage of 'false negative' may be kept to a minimum if not completely eliminated. This is what every woman expects who entrusts herself to us and who presents herself for an examination. That is why, as I mentioned before the principle of the unity of place and of action remains the best guarantee of quality. 'Senology has become a medical, a historical and a human necessity. Let us move on, let us act together as one body, to fight in order to make Senology an official and recognised specialty, independent and powerful in the face of others.

References

1. Gros D. Les Seins aux fleurs rouges. Edition Stock. Paris 1994.
2. Ioannidou-Mouzaka L, Mantonakis J, Toufexi H, Tsiliakos St., Agnantis N.J. Le surmenage psychique prolongé est il un facteur étiologique du cancer mammaire? J.Gynecol. Obstet. Biol. Reprod 1986, 15, 1049-1053.
3. Ioannidou-Mouzaka L. Sénologie. Le Sein 1993, 2(1):2
4. Ioannidou-Mouzaka L. Escuela International de Senologia. Rev. Senologia Y Pathol. Mam. 1993, 6(1):1-2.
5. Ioannidou-Mouzaka L. Senology; yesterday, today, tomorrow. Iatriki, 1993, 64(1): 23-24.
6. Quality Control in Mammography. Ed. Founding members of MANOMED. Montpellier 1994.

[1]The specialty which deals with the breast has been known as SENOLOGY, since 1963, a name which was proposed by the late Charles Marie Gros, who had conceived thirty years ago the necessity to invent a special discipline for breasts, which unfortunately has not yet been officially recognized as a specialty.

[2]Paragraphs under quotation marks are taken from the book 'Les Seins aux fleures rouges' by Dominique Gros.

Mastology - Breast Diseases
A.S.S. Figueira Fo et al., editors.

Hormonal replacement therapy and breast pathology

Douglas J. Marchant, MD. Emeritus Professor of Surgery, Emeritus Professor of Obstetrics and Gynecology, Tufts University School of Medicine, Adjunct Professor of Obstetrics and Gynecology, Brown University School of Medicine, Providence, Rhode Island, Director, Breast Health Center, Women & Infants Hospital, Providence, RI

Address for reprints: Douglas J. Marchant, MD, Director, Breast Health Center, Women & Infants Hospital, 101 Dudley Street, Providence, RI 02905-2499

ABSTRACT

In our current aging society, more than 30 million women have an average post-menopausal life expectancy of 28 years. Coronary artery disease is the leading cause of death in older women, and osteoporosis results in an estimated 1.5 million fractures per year. Various studies have suggested that post-menopausal estrogen replacement therapy could reduce the morbidity and mortality associated with these conditions. The benefits and risks of estrogen replacement therapy are reviewed, and recommendations for management and future research are suggested.

GENERAL CONSIDERATIONS

We live in an aging society. Two-hundred years ago, less than 30% of women lived long enough to reach menopause. Now, 90% of women reach the climacteric. There are approximately 56 million women in the United States who are older than age 35 years, and more than 30 million women have an average post-menopausal life expectancy of 28 years.[1] With the increasing use of adjuvant therapy for breast cancer, many young women experience ovarian failure and symptoms of the menopause.

Coronary artery disease is the leading cause of death in older women, and results in considerable disability in women 65 years of age and older. Osteoporosis causes an estimated 1.5 million fractures per year, and it has been estimated that the number of fractures may double by the end of this century. The annual cost of fractures related to osteoporosis is 7-10 billion dollars per year.[2] Several studies have suggested that post-menopausal hormonal administration including newer low dose continuous estrogen replacement therapy might reduce the morbidity and mortality both from osteoporotic fractures and coronary artery disease, although, not all studies have observed these benefits.[3-6]

MENOPAUSE

Few would deny that the menopause is an estrogen deficient state, it is, however, not a disease, and, every women who lives long enough, will become menopausal. Studies show that post-menopausal women and those who have undergone premature oophorectomy have a higher risk of coronary artery disease than those with intact ovaries.[2] This suggests that menopause has an unfavorable effect on lipid metabolism, which may contribute to an increase in the risk of coronary artery disease.[7] Recent data support the recommendation that hormone replacement therapy may prevent some of these changes.[2] Low density lipoprotein levels appear in men at approximately age 20 years, and in women, at menopause. Studies regarding the efficacy of estrogen replacement therapy suggest that estrogens increase high density lipoprotein levels and decrease low density lipoprotein concentration, thus reducing the risk of coronary artery disease. In some reports, this evidence is strong, consistent and biologically plausible, and the degree of protection seems to be clinically significant and exceeds any known risk.[7] Before recommending, however, that all post-menopausal women receive life-long replacement therapy, a closer look at the data is appropriate.

To date, no large scale trials have been completed in women to address the use of estrogen replacement therapy, and the dose and administration of estrogen are important additional considerations. Sequential and continuous therapy, both increase high density lipoprotein levels. Sequential therapy, however, does not prevent the estrogen induced decrease in low density lipoprotein concentrations, but continuous therapy may. The daily administration of 0.625 mg of conjugated estrogens, and 2.5 mg of medroxyprogesterone acetate may not elicit these actions on lipids. Additional studies are required to identify women most likely to benefit from estrogen replacement therapy and to determine the effects of added progestational agents. A risk analysis including considering the increase in the risk of endometrial cancer (which can be controlled with the addition of progestins) and the possible increase in the incidence of breast cancer is essential.

The data concerning the treatment and prevention of osteoporosis are more difficult to analyze. A critical issue in the measurement of bone loss. There are no inexpensive techniques for assessing bone mass, however, ultrasonographic methods may solve this problem when they become available.[8-12] Some studies have indicated that in women with a low bone density, bone loss can be slowed or prevented by exercise and calcium, or exercise and estrogen and progesterone replacement.[10] At least one report suggests that exercise and estrogen replacement therapy were more effective than exercise and calcium supplementation, but such therapy was associated with more side effects and required increased medical surveillance.[10]

DISCUSSION

There is no question that estrogen replacement therapy improves symptomatology associated with vasomotor disturbances and secondary effects such as insomnia and those attributed to genital atrophy. Vasomotor symptoms affect 75% of post-menopausal women but only 30% seek medical help for these symptoms.[13] It is also true that some menopausal women have psychological symptoms that are not convincingly linked to the endocrine changes of menopause. Vasomotor symptoms usually are relieved during the first few cycles of treatment and the effectiveness of estrogen is indisputable. Some studies have indicated that a progestogen also will relieve vasomotor symptoms or vasomotor disturbances. The vagina and urethra share a common embryologic origin and estrogen deficiency causes atrophy of both. These changes are relieved by the use of estrogen replacement therapy.

Recent studies have evaluated the bleeding patterns of post-menopausal women taking combined or sequential regimens of conjugated estrogens with medroxyprogesterone acetate (MPA). Approximately one half the women who took the continuous combined conjugated estrogens -- MPA regimens -- had amenorrhea. Women who took sequential regimens had good cyclical control with minimal irregular bleeding, and some studies noted that more than one half of women who took conjugated estrogens alone had amenorrhea.[14]

In an effort to minimize progestin exposure, studies have explored cyclic hormone replacement therapy using a quarterly progestin regimen. In one study, quarterly medroxyprogesterone acetate appeared as safe as the monthly schedule and was preferred by most women. This regimen did not increase the risk of endometrial hyperplasia and produced an acceptable menstrual pattern.[15]

Recent studies have indicated that long term thyroid hormone use at thyroxin-equivalent doses was associated with significant osteopenia at the ultra-distal radius, mid-shaft radius, hip and lumbar spine. Estrogen replacement therapy appears to negate thyroid hormone-associated loss of bone density in post-menopausal women. For post-menopausal patients with benign thyroid nodules, goiters and low risk papillary thyroid cancers, a TSH level at or below the normal range represents appropriate control and estrogen replacement therapy should be considered for this group of patients.[16]

CONCLUSIONS

Hormonal replacement therapy does not provide complete relief for the problems of the post-menopausal woman, nor is it the elixir of eternal youth. It is not without risks, and in the usual dosages recommended, it is not tolerated by all women. Instead of attempting to justify estrogen replacement therapy on the basis of available data or the lack of it, more effort should be expended in the area of molecular genetics to identify which patients are at higher risk for breast cancer and endometrial cancer, and which patients are at higher risk for coronary artery disease and osteoporosis.

REFERENCES

1. Edman CD. The climacteric. In: Buchsbaum HJ (editor) The menopause. New York: Springer Verlag, 1983;23-33.
2. Marchant DJ. Estrogen-replacement therapy after breast cancer: risks versus benefits. Cancer Supplement 1993;71:2169-2176.
3. Matthews KA, Meilahn E, Kuller LH, Caggiula AW, Kelsey SF, Wing RR, et al. Menopause and risk factors for coronary heart disease. N Engl J Med 1989;321:641-6.
4. Colditz GA, Willett WC, Stampfer MJ, Rosner B, Speizer FE, Hennekens CH, et al. Menopause and the risk of coronary heart disease in women. N Engl J Med 1987;316:1105-10.
5. Mishell DR, (editor). Interdisciplinary review of estrogen replacement therapy. Am J Obstet Gynecol 1989;161(suppl):1825-64.
6. Utian WH, (editor). Current perspectives in the management of the menopause and postmenopausal patient. Obstet Gynecol 1990;75(suppl):1-81.
7. Stampfer MJ, Colditz GA, Willett WC, Manson JE, Rosner B, Speizer FE, et al. Postmenopausal estrogen therapy and cardiovascular disease. N Engl J Med 1991;325:756-62.
8. Prior JC, Vigna YM, Schechter MT, Burgess AE. Spinal bone loss and ovulatory disturbances. N Engl J Med 1990;323:1221-7.
9. Johnston CC, Slemenda CW, Melton LJ. Clinical use of bone densitometry: current concepts. N Engl J Med 1991;324:1105-9.
10. Prince RL, Smith M, Dick IM, Price RI, Webb PG, Henderson NK, et al. Prevention of postmenopausal osteoporosis. N Engl J Med 1991;325:1189-95.

11. Tilyard MY, Spears GFS, Thomson J. Treatment of postmenopausal osteoporosis with calcitriol or calcium. N Engl J Med 1992;326:357-62.
12. Marslew U, Overgaard K, Riis BJ, Christiansen C. Two new combinations of estrogen and progestogen for prevention of postmenopausal bone loss: long term effects on bone, calcium and lipid metabolism, climacteric symptoms, and bleeding. Obstet Gynecol 1992;79:202-10.
13. Belchetz PE. Hormonal treatment of postmenopausal women -- drug therapy. N Engl J Med 330:1062-1071.
14. Archer DF, Pickar JH, Bottiglioni F. Bleeding patterns in postmenopausal women taking continuous combined or sequential regimens of conjugated estrogens with medroxyprogesterone acetate. Obstet Gynecol 83:686-692.
15. Ettinger B, Selby J, Citron J, et al. Cyclic hormone replacement therapy using quarterly progestin. Obstet Gynecol 83:693-700.
16. Schneider DL, Barrett-Connor EL, Morton DJ. Thyroid hormone use and bone mineral density in elderly women. JAMA 271:1245-1284.

Mastology - Breast Diseases
A.S.S. Figueira Fo et al., editors.

Hormonal Replacement Therapy and Breast Cancer

José Aristodemo PINOTTI - Full Professor - Department of Obstetrics and Gynecology of University of São Paulo School of Medicine.

Filomena Marino CARVALHO, MD - Pathologist of Hospital das Clínicas of University of São Paulo.

Alfredo C.S.D. Barros - Assistent Professor of Gynaecology, University of São Paulo and Full Professor of Gynaecology and Obstetrics, University of Santo Amaro.

I- Introduction

Breast cancer is one of the greatest death causes among occidental women, representing a serious problem in public health today. The steroids role in breast cancer is mainly suggested by the epidemiological data available. During this century, drastic changes have been observed in the reproductive customs, like nulliparity and late childbearing. Associated to these factors, we have an increase of steroids hormone consumption through oral contraceptives and hormonal replacement therapy (HRT). The effects of steroids in the breast, its possible risks and benefits, and finally, the problem of the HRT use in women with treated breast cancer should be discussed.

II- Steroids effects on mammary gland

The proliferative activity of the mammary gland is regulated by a complex mechanism involving the synergic interaction of proteins, steroids and other hormones. The estrogen plays a central role in breast development during puberty, but the total differentiation needs a synergic action of thyroxine, prolactin, growth hormone, insulin and cortisol.

The experimental model of steroids action in Sprague-Dawley rat supports that the mammary gland of these rats is more susceptible to carcinogens when the cellular proliferation is more accentuated, being reduced when the differentiation is completed. The administration of estroprogestative combinations, like the norethynodrel-mestranol, induces the mammary glandular differentiation in the Sprague-Dawley rat, reducing significantly the cancer incidence, either in low dosages, as used for contraception, or in high dosages. On the other hand, the administration of medroxyprogesterone acetate increases cancer incidence when used in high doses, although not altering significantly the risk when the doses are low. These effects are modified according to the animal's age, being more evident in the older animals (16).

The mammary cycle differs substantially from the endometrial one. In the breast, although alterations occur during the menstrual cycle as well as in the different age ranges, the classical proliferation and secretion phases are not recognised. On the contrary, the maximum proliferative activity is observed in the second phasis of the cycle, around the 21st day (15).

III- Effect of the antiestrogens in the mammary tissue

Tamoxifen is a non-steroidal compound which, when given to women producing estrogens, competes with their effects. It possesses weak estrogenic action in hypoestrogenic women, but sufficient to maintain bone density and prevent coronary disease by lowering the circulating cholesterol (9).

The use of tamoxifen in Sprague-Dawley rats shows suppression of the development of tumors induced by DMBA (8,12). It was also demonstrated synergic action with retinoids in chemoprevention of mammary carcinoma (13).

In vitro studies suggest that tamoxifen antiestrogenic action results from direct binding to the estrogen receptor with consequent alterations in the receptor conformation, RNA transcription, and reduction in cell proliferation. Its antiproliferative activity may also be mediated through growth factors. The antiproliferative effect may also be related to the inhibition of protein kinase-C, its binding with calmodulin and its ability of decreasing the insulin-like growth factor-I.

Although tamoxifen was considered safe as to side effects, recently, however, many cases appeared resulting from the association of its use and endometrial cancer and even with other neoplasias, (20,17). Tamoxifen is a safe and reliable medicine for the treatment of breast cancer, but its utilization requires a close monitorization of patients and prompt evaluation of any uterine bleeding or pelvic complaint.

IV- Relation between Hormonal Replacement Therapy (HRT) and breast cancer

The benefits of HRT are undeniable since the relief of vasomotor symptomatology, prevention of osteoporosis and substantial evidence of decreased relative risk of cardiovascular disease have been well established (18). On the other hand, the relationship between HRT and breast cancer risk remains a matter of discussion.

Although there still exist a polemic about the estrogen-based HRT effect on the breast cancer risk, this relation could never be convincingly demonstrated.

Populational studies with constant use of estrogens in postmenopause in general show a relative risk near or a little above 1.0 (10,11,14,4) which may reach 1.5 after 15 to 20 years of use. Nevertheless, this fact is being questioned (2). The increase of risk with length of use is at least partly related to the inclusion of women in premenopause or those who received estradiol. Based on the analysis of more than 50 studies, Gambrell(4) concludes that the estrogen therapy, even of long-term, does not increase the risk of breast cancer.

The HRT based on estrogen-progestogen combinations presented itself as an alternative to the estrogen administration, particularly in women with uterus. The effect of such combinations on breast risk is not yet sufficiently known for the epidemiological data available is small.

In a study comparing the relative risk of breast cancer among users of estrogens and progestagens combinations, estrogens, progestagens and non-users of steroids,Gambrell and col.(5) conclude that the HRT reduces significantly the breast cancer risk and suggest that the addition of progestagens gives additional protection, not obtainable with pure estrogens. On the other hand, Hunt and col(7) in United Kingdom and Ewertz(3) in Denmark did not observe any tendency for risk reduction with the increase of progestagens.

Bergvist and col(1) in Sweden originated a great discussion on the progestagens effect when they published their study on 10 cases where they observed a relative risk of 4.4 (CID 95%, 0.9-24.4) in women using combinations of estrogen and progestagen for a period above 6 years, and based on their results, these authors suggest that the possibility of risk increase with the use of progestagens be verified, though they point out that the number of patients is very small.

The available epidemiological data, although contraditory, suggest a certain protective effect with the addition of progestagens to HRT, but more studies are needed for a better knowledge on the behaviour of the mammary cells under the influence of these and other natural or synthetic steroids. Another important aspect to be verified on the use of progestagen in HRT is its real protective cardiovascular effect, undeniable for estrogens. Some progestin may revert the cardiovascular protective effect of the estrogens. In this connection, the progestagens with the minimal androgenicity should be preferred. (6).

V- HRT in breast cancer patients

Breast and endometrium cancer were always considered as absolute contraindications for HRT. Nevertheless, there is a lot of studies questioning this position. Wile and col(19) studied 25 women with breast cancer and submitted to HRT and did not find any adverse effect. Although the series is small and the follow-up is not sufficiently long (mean 35.2 months), this work calls our attention for the possibility of improving the life quality of the breast cancer patients.

Wren (21), in another study, concluded that there is no clinical evidence that the HRT administered to those patients benefits the recurrence. This author suggests that HRT should be offered to women with a disease-free interval of equal or above 10 years and also for the patients presenting important symptoms resulting from estrogenic defficiency. In the first case, the treatment should be based on estrogen-progestogen combinations with high levels of progestagens, while for the others, a pure progestagenic therapy should be tried, followed by the addition of an estrogen, if possible.

VI- CONCLUSIONS

There are plenty of evidences showing that the HRT brings more benefits than risks, improving markedly the women's life quality and their longevity.

Before deciding on the utilization of steroids, each case should be individually evaluated taking into account cancer risk, clinical conditions and possibility of adequate medical control. In histerectomized patients without risk factors and in good clinical conditions, the option should be for conjugated estrogens. Evidently, the presence of the uterus does not contraindicate the estrogen-HRT, but requires an adequate periodical control of the uterine cavity. The addition of progestagens in low doses may be considered, particularly for women with high risk of endometrial cancer.

In women with breast cancer and in those postmenopausal with increased risk for breast cancer the possibility of hormonal replacement by tamoxifen should be considered, as it maintains the bone density and reduces the blood cholesterol. If a estrogenic or estroprogestative HRT is needed, this should be administered in low dosages and in the shortest possible time.

VII - References

1- Bergvist L, Adami H-O, Persson I, Hoover R, Schairer C: The risk of breast cancer after estrogen and estrogen-progestin replacement. N Engl J Med 321: 293, 1989a.

2- Colditz GA, Stampfer MJ, Willet WC e col: Prospective study of estrogen replacement therapy and risk of breast cancer in postmenopausal women. JAMA 264: 2648, 1990.

3- Ewertz M: Influence of non-contraceptive exogenous and endogenous sex hormones on breast cancer risk in Denmark. Int J Cancer 42: 832, 1988.

4- Gambrell DR, Jr: Estrogen replacement therapy and breast cancer risk. A new look at the data. The female patient 18: 50, 1993.

5- Gambrell RD, Maier RC, Sanders BI: Decreased incidence of breast cancer in postmenopausal estrogen-progestogen users. Obstet Gynecol 62: 435, 1983.

6- Harlap S: The benefits and risks of hormone replacement therapy: an epidemiologic overview. Am J Obstet Gynecol 166: 1986, 1992.

7- Hunt K, Vessey M, McPherson K, Coleman M: Long-term surveillance of mortality and cancer incidence in women receiving hormone replacement therapy. Br J Obstet Gynaecol 94: 620, 1987.

8- Jordan V: Effect of tamoxifen or initiation and growth of DMBA induced rat mammary carcinoma. Eur J Cancer 12:419, 1976.

9- Jordan VC: The strategic use of antiestrogens to control the development and growth of breast cancer. Cancer 70: 977, 1992.

10- Kaufman DW, Miller DR, Rosenberg L, e col: Noncontraceptive estrogen use and risk of breast cancer. JAMA 252: 63, 1984.

11- Key TJA: Hormone replacement therapy and breast cancer risk. Approaches to breast cancer prevention. In Stoll BA (ed): Approaches to breast cancer prevention, Dordrecht, Kluwer Academic Publishers, 1991.

12- Maltoni C, Pinto C, Paladoni G: Project of experimental bioassays on chemoprevention agents performed at the Bologna Institute of Oncology: Report on Tamoxifen control of spontaneous mammarian tumors in Sprague-Dawley rats. Cancer Invest 6: 643, 1988.

13- McCormick D & Moon R: Retinoid-tamoxifen interaction in mammary cancer chemoprevention. Carcinogenesis 7: 193, 1986.

14- Nachtigall MJ, Smilen SW, Nachtigall RD, Nachtigall LE: Incidence of breast cancer in a 22-year study of women receiving estrogen-progestin replacement therapy. Obstet Gynecol 80: 827, 1992.

15- Potten CS, Watson RJ, Williams GT e col: The effect of age and menstrual cycle upon proliferative activity of the normal human breast. Br J Cancer 58: 163, 1988.

16- Russo J & Russo IH: Biological and molecular basis of mammary carcinogenesis. Lab Invest 57: 112, 1987.

17- Seoud M A-F, Johnson J, Weed JC: Gynecologic tumors in tamoxifen-treated women with breast cancer. Obstet Gynecol 82: 165, 1993.

18- Session DR, Kelly AC, Jewelewicz R: Current concepts in estrogen replacement therapy in the menopause. Fertil Steril 59: 277, 1993.

19- Wile AG, Opfell RW, Margileth DA: Hormone replacement therapy in previously treated breast cancer patients. Am J Surg 165: 372, 1993.

20- Wolf DM & Jordan VC: Gynecologic complications associated with long-term adjuvant tamoxifen therapy for breast cancer. Gynecol Oncol 45: 118, 1992.

21- Wren BG: Hormone therapy following breast and uterine cancer. Baillieres Clin Endocrinol Metab 7: 225, 1993.

Mastology - Breast Diseases
A.S.S. Figueira Fo et al., editors.

HORMONE REPLACEMENT THERAPY AFTER BREAST CANCER.

P. Sismondi, N. Biglia, M. Giai, R. Ponzone, L. Sgro, R. Roagna

Department of Gynecological Oncology- University of Turin

SUMMARY

The currently accepted dogma is to avoid the hormone replacement therapy (HRT) for postmenopausal women previously treated for breast cancer. Recently some physicians have suggested to reconsider the use of HRT in patients successfully treated for breast cancer. This position is based not on scientific data but on a review of various "natural experiments"; at present clinical studies on the use of HRT in breast cancer patients are scant and give only preliminary results. Any recommendation concerning the safety of HRT in these patients must consider the conflicting data regarding the effects of estrogen and progesteron on human breast tumor and the possibility that there is an action of these hormones on occult micrometastases. Because freedom from recurrent breast cancer can never be guaranteed, there will be patients with breast cancer in whom a relapse will develop coincident with HRT exposure. The patient should have a clear understanding of this possibility; the final decision must rest within the patient and her treating physician and may be subject to medico-legal interpretation. An alternative to the traditional HRT in these women may be the use of tamoxifen. Tamoxifen has become the endocrine treatment of choise for all stages of breast cancer; moreover, tamoxifen has some estrogen-like effects that could be benificial to maintain bone density and prevent the development of coronary heart disease.

INTRODUCTION

Many reports have confirmed the beneficial effect of hormone replacement therapy (HRT) in the prevention of osteoporosis and cardiovascular diseases and on the quality of life.

Recently some physicians have suggested to reconsider the use of HRT in patients "successfully treated" for breast cancer (BC).[1-7] This position is based not on new scientific data but on a review of various "natural experiments" suggesting the safety of HRT. Other Authors advocate caution in prescribing a traditional HRT for a woman with any significant risk of recurrence.[8] The debate concerns in particular the definition of "successfully treated" tumor. The biology of BC does not permit to assume that local treatment and even the use of adjuvant therapy have cured the BC successfully; it is possible that some patients have minimal but asymptomatic micrometastases that are "at immunologic peace" with the host. In discussing the role of HRT in women treated for BC we must consider the possibility that we are not initiating cancer but that there is an effect of estrogen and possibly progesterone on occult micrometastases. In these patients the benefit obtained by HRT, in term of reduced risk of cardiovascular diseases and fractures, may be vanified by a little increase of cancer-related death, differently from general population, where the mortality for gynecological neoplasia is much lower than the mortality for myocardial infarction and osteoporosis. The annual probability of dying for BC in a woman with a node-negative breast tumor is 3.000/100.000, whereas the overall annual mortality associated with stroke, fractures and cardiovascular diseases is 750/100.000. A woman previously treated for a node-negative BC has a fourfold probability of dying for the tumor than for cardiovascular diseases or for the complications of a fracture. A 50% reduction of the risk of non cancer-related death will be cancelled by a 12.5% increased risk of death for recurrence of the primary tumor. In case of node-positive BC (annual mortality rate 9.000/100.000) a 4% increase of the risk of death for neoplasia could cancel a 50% reduction of the risk of death for other causes. In this review we analyse the epidemiological and clinical evidences regarding the effect of estrogens and progesterone on BC risk; the use of tamoxifen as an alternative to the traditional HRT is also discussed.

EPIDEMIOLOGIC DATA

In the absence of prospective studies some informations may be derived from situations in which patients are exposed to high levels of hormones at time when they might have been harbouring BC cells. Several studies have shown that women with BC during pregnancy have the same prognosis as those who are not pregnant of similar age and stage of disease.[9] Pregnancy after BC treatment does not adversely affect survival; survival rates in women who conceived even within 6 months after BC treatment appear not different from those in a control group.[9] There is a paucity of information about the outcome of patients who may have been exposed inadvertently to oral contraceptives (OC) during the genesis and progression of their tumors. When these women were compared with those with BC of similar age who had never used OC, a trend toward an earlier stage of presentation in users was observed, but no adverse effect on the survival rates for users was noted.[10] Data concerning BC risk and HRT are reassuring; a recent meta-analysis suggests that the use of 0.625 mg/day of conjugated estrogen (CE) does not increase the BC risk; women who received 1.25 mg or more per day of CE had a BC relative risk of 2.0 or less in all studies.[11]

CLINICAL DATA

At present, clinical studies on the use of HRT in BC patients are scant and only preliminary results are available. Stoll treated a group of symptomatic postmenopausal women previously operated for BC and clinically free of recurrence with a combination of CE (0.625/day) and norgestrel (0.15 mg/day) for a period of 3-6 months; after 2 years of follow-up no case of tumor reactivation was observed.[12] Wile reports his experience with 25 women previously treated for BC who subsequently received HRT (CE 0.625-1.25 mg/day with or without progesterone); 17 patients (group I) began HRT less than 24 months after primary breast cancer therapy.[3] The averaged period of observation while receiving HRT was 35.2 months; three patients have had a recurrences during this period, all in group I. The overall survival rate for the entire group was 96%; overall survival of high risk group I, with a mean follow up of 30.4 months was 94%. A case-control study has been conducted on 25 BC patients who began HRT after breast cancer therapy and were disease-free at the initiation of HRT. After an average follow-up of 25.5 months no adverse effect upon cancer outcome could be detected.[7] All the Authors in favour of the use of HRT in BC patients maintain that a number of factors should be considered: 1) size of tumor, nodal and hormonal receptor status; 2) length of time since tumor was first diagnosed; 3) desires and symptoms of patient.[13] There is no doubt that a large proportion of women suffering from BC will be cured of their disease. Depending on the size, type and other prognostic factors the long-term survival varies from 50-95%. The dilemma is just who is cured and who has a metastatic spread? At present there is no way to determine which woman has persistent cancer cells and which has been cleared of the disease. The most likely group of women to achieve this state are those who have a small, non aggressive intraduct BC; they have a 98% chance of surviving 10 or more years with no evidence of recurrences. Several women have no evidence of secondary spread 10 or more years after the primary treatment. Although there can be no guarantee of cure, it can be assumed that the majority of these women will not have a recurrence and can be regarded as "cured". In these cases is probable that HRT will not increase the risk of recurrence.[13] Some women are found to have a BC in premenopausal years and after the initial treatment are allowed to menstruate regularly till they pass

through a normal menopause. If there has been no evidence of secondary spread by the time they achieve menopause, some Authors think that there is no contraindication to the use of HRT after menopause.[1,3,13] On the other hand, it must be considered that a recent meta-analysis of clinical trials on adjuvant therapy has show that ovarian ablation in premenopausal patients with breast cancer determines a significant reduction of the annual risk of death and recurrence, similar to that obtained with adjuvant chemotherapy.[14]
The major problem concerns the women recently treated for BC when the initial prognosis appears to give a good chance of being "cured"; yet, there always remain considerable doubt that an individual woman is free of the disease. The currently accepted dogma is to avoid a therapy regimen which includes a mitogen such as estrogen.

TAMOXIFEN

An alternative to the traditional HRT in these patients may be the use of tamoxifen.[15,16] Tamoxifen has become the endocrine treatment of choice for all stages of BC; the low incidence of side effects and proven survival advantage observed during adjuvant therapy has encouraged the use of long-term treatment.[14] Besides, tamoxifen reduces the incidence of second primary BC and prevents mammary tumorigenesis in animal models; its use has been advocated as chemopreventive agent in health population at high risk of breast cancer.[15] The antitumoral effect of tamoxifen is mediated by its anti-estrogenic action on the breast and by the influence on several growth factors; moreover, the drug has some estrogen-like effects that could be beneficial to maintain bone density and prevent the development of coronary heart disease.[15]

CONCLUSION

Any recommendation concerning the efficacy and safety of HRT in patients treated for BC must consider the conflicting data regarding the effects of estrogen and progesterone on human breast tumors. Based upon the known beneficial effects of HRT and the lack of evidence suggesting harmful effect on BC, some Authors think that there is no reason to deny a regimen with low dose of CE and progestogen to these women, especially in case of small node negative tumors or when a long period of time with no evidence of recurrence is passed from the first diagnosis. On the contrary, other Authors believe that currently it is not recommended that HRT be used routinely for BC patients. Because freedom from recurrence can never be guaranteed, there will be women in whom recurrent disease will develop coincident with renewed hormone exposure. The patient should have a clear understanding of this possibility; the final decision must rests within the patient and her treating physician and may be subject to medicolegal interpretation.[1,8] In this era of extensive medical ligation there is an understandable reluctance to offer estrogen to women with a history of BC. The use of tamoxifen may be a sound alternative for these women, assuring at the same time a survival advantage for all stages of BC and a beneficial effect on menopausal symptoms. All the Authors agree on the need that prospective controlled trials be conducted on this problem.

References

1- DiSaia PJ. Hormone replacement therapy in patients with breast cancer. Cancer 1993;71:1490-1500.

2- Maguire PJ. Estrogen replacement therapy and breast cancer. J Reprod Med 1993;38,3:183-185.

3- Wile AG, Opfell RW, Margileth DA. Hormone replacement therapy in previously treated breast cancer patients. Am J Surg 1993;165:372-3375.

4- Creasman WT. Estrogen replacement therapy: is previously treated cancer a contraindication? Obstet Gynecol 1991;77:308-312.

5- Spicer D, Pike MC, Henderson BE. The question of estrogen replacement therapy in patients with a prior diagnosis of breast cancer. Oncology 1990;4:49-62.

6- Stoll BA. Hormone replacement therapy in women treated for breast cancer. Eur J Cancer Clin Oncol 1989;25,12:1909-1913.

7- Wile AG, Opfell RW, Margileth DA, Anton-Culver H. Hormone replacement therapy does not effect breast cancer outcome. Proc Annu Meet Am Soc Clin Oncol 1991;10:A106.

8- Marchant DJ. Estrogen replacement therapy after breast cancer. Risks versus benefits. Cancer 1993;71:2169-2176.

9- Danforth DN. How subsequent pregnancy affects outcome in women with a prior breast cancer. Oncology 1991;5:23-35.

10-Rosner D, Lane WW. Oral contraceptive use has no adverse effect on prognosis of breast cancer. Cancer 1986;57:591-596.

11- Dupont WD, Page DL. Menopausal estrogen replacement therapy and breast cancer. Arch Int Med 1991;151:67-72.

12- Stoll BA, Parbhoo S. Treatment of menopausal symptoms in breast cancer patients. Lancet 1988;1:1278-1279.

13- Wren BG. Hormone therapy following breast and uterine cancer. Baillière's Clin Endocrinol Metabol 1993;7(1):225-242.

14- Early Breast Cancer Trialist's Collaborative Group: Systemic treatment of early breast cancer by hormonal, cytotoxic or immune therapy. Lancet 1992;339:71-85.

15- Craig Jordan V. The strategic use of antiestrogens to control the development and growth of breast cancer. Cancer 1992;70:977-982.

16- Gelety TJ, Judd HL. Menopause: new indications and management strategies. Curr Opin Obstet Gynecol 1992;4(3):346-353.

Index of authors